The Therapist's Use of Self

W0113786

This book encourages and trains students and practicing marriage and family therapists to bring themselves into the therapy room, offering guidelines and strategies for being more present and personal with their clients.

Mental health professionals are often taught and trained that therapy is serious business, to be cautious and conservative with therapeutic decision-making, and to stick to empirically supported and specific tools in sessions. What gets lost in this positivistic, formulaic, and scientific way of working are therapists' own unique voices, their creativity, flexibility, and the sense of playfulness that make the change process fun and upbeat. *The Therapist's Use of Self* equips therapists with the skills they need to deepen their alliances with clients, to liberate themselves from an over-reliance on models, and to bring their whole selves to the therapeutic encounter. Chapters cover pioneers in the field before exploring ways to bring ideas from outside the therapy room, including from music, art, literature, and film. The book includes a key chapter on teletherapy, and each chapter presents major therapeutic tools and strategies, case examples, the resulting outcomes, and key takeaways.

Students of psychology, social work, nursing, and marriage and family programs, as well as mental health professionals will benefit from this book with a plethora of therapeutic tools, guidelines, and strategies for catalyzing change with even the most challenging couples and families.

Matthew D. Selekman, MSW, LCSW, is a couple and family therapist in private practice and the director of *Partners for Collaborative Solutions*, an international family therapy training and consulting firm in Evanston, Illinois, USA. He is an approved supervisor and clinical fellow with the American Association for Marriage and Family Therapy.

"This book had me at the start; the analysis of the family therapy pioneers was the best I'd ever read. But then Selekman takes it a quantum leap further—capturing the true essence of conceptualizing and doing couple and family therapy, drawing on contemporary research and his own wisdom accrued from extensive experience in the trenches."

Barry L. Duncan, *Psy.D., developer of the Partners for Change Outcome Management System, USA*

"Selekman has done it again. A book for any practitioner, chock-full of wisdom, guidance and encouragement to be more of ourselves as a therapist. After an affectionate review of the old masters of family therapy, Selekman gives us a creative and wide-ranging set of ideas to help us become more courageous as therapists. An aspiring read!"

Guy Diamond, *Professor Emeritus, University of Pennsylvania School of Medicine, USA*

"Matthew Selekman's brilliant new book about the therapist's use of self is exactly the book the field of relational and systemic therapies needs at this time. Wonderfully anchored in and appropriately paying homage to the pioneers of the field, Selekman provides the reader with a much-needed update of how to be most positively engaged and effective in these times. Building on a clear vision of the use of self in therapy that includes a very practical use-of-self toolkit, he offers inventive frameworks for therapeutic decision-making and ways of collaborating with clients to find innovative ways to resolve problems. Filled with poignant clinical examples and the wisdom of a seasoned therapist who has supervised couple and family therapy around the world, this is a book every couple and family therapist and student in the field should read and contemplate."

Jay Lebow, *Ph.D., ABPP, Senior Scholar and Clinical Professor, The Family Institute at Northwestern and Northwestern University, USA*

"As I began reading the first two chapters, my experience was of a travel along a memory lane, remembering the workshops and seminars I had the opportunity to enjoy with those incredible persons. By chapter four I was more on the transition to present time. Then I remember the *time machine exercise* Selekman uses. And of course, the next chapters moved me to the future use of his exercises. (And in there you'll find *the time machine*) Definitely a very good book. From past, to present, to future use."

Ricardo Figueroa Quiroga, *President: Mexican Council for Clinical Hypnosis, Mexico*

The Therapist's Use of Self

Being the Catalyst for Change
in Couple and Family Therapy

Matthew D. Selekman

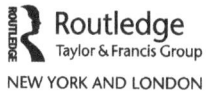
Routledge
Taylor & Francis Group

NEW YORK AND LONDON

Designed cover image: Salvador Dalí (1904–1989), *Apparition of Face and Fruit Dish on a Beach*, 1938, oil on canvas, 45 × 56 5/8 in (114.3 × 143.8 cm), Wadsworth Atheneum, Hartford The Ella Gallup Sumner and Mary Catlin Sumner Collection Fund, 1939.269

Photography credit: Allen Phillips/Wadsworth Atheneum

First published 2024
by Routledge
605 Third Avenue, New York, NY 10158

and by Routledge
4 Park Square, Milton Park, Abingdon, Oxon, OX14 4RN

Routledge is an imprint of the Taylor & Francis Group, an informa business

© 2024 Matthew D. Selekman

The right of Matthew D. Selekman to be identified as author of this work has been asserted in accordance with sections 77 and 78 of the Copyright, Designs and Patents Act 1988.

All rights reserved. No part of this book may be reprinted or reproduced or utilised in any form or by any electronic, mechanical, or other means, now known or hereafter invented, including photocopying and recording, or in any information storage or retrieval system, without permission in writing from the publishers.

Trademark notice: Product or corporate names may be trademarks or registered trademarks, and are used only for identification and explanation without intent to infringe.

Library of Congress Cataloging-in-Publication Data
Names: Selekman, Matthew D., 1957- author.
Title: The therapist's use of self : being the catalyst for change in couple and family therapy / Matthew D. Selekman.
Description: New York, NY : Routledge, 2024. | Includes bibliographical references and index. |
Identifiers: LCCN 2023033708 (print) | LCCN 2023033709 (ebook) | ISBN 9781032369174 (hbk) | ISBN 9781032369167 (pbk) | ISBN 9781003334460 (ebk)
Subjects: LCSH: Family psychotherapy--Methodology. | Couples therapy--Methodology. | Marital psychotherapy--Methodology. | Psychotherapist and patient.
Classification: LCC RC488.5 .S444 2024 (print) | LCC RC488.5 (ebook) | DDC 616.89/1562--dc23/eng/20230921
LC record available at https://lccn.loc.gov/2023033708
LC ebook record available at https://lccn.loc.gov/2023033709

ISBN: 9781032369174 (hbk)
ISBN: 9781032369167 (pbk)
ISBN: 9781003334460 (ebk)

DOI: 10.4324/9781003334460

Typeset in Garamond
by KnowledgeWorks Global Ltd.

To my loving and supportive wife Åsa and Hanna,
my angel and other love

To my wonderful father who has always been
a big source of inspiration and support with
my career pursuits

Contents

About the Author

Matthew D. Selekman, MSW, LCSW is an Approved Supervisor and Clinical Fellow for the American Association of Marriage and Family Therapy, a licensed clinical social worker, and addictions counselor. He also is the Director of *Partners for Collaborative Solutions* (www.partners4change.net), an international family therapy and brief therapy training and consultation practice in Evanston, IL. He is the Clinical Supervisor for 360 Wellness & Coaching in Lake Forest, IL. Matthew received the Walter S. Rosenberry Award in 2006, 2000, and in 1999 from The Children's Hospital in Denver, Colorado for having made significant contributions to the fields of psychiatry and the behavioral sciences. He is the author of eight professional practice-oriented books: *Working with High-Risk Adolescents: A Collaborative Strengths-Based Approach*, *Changing Self-Destructive Habits: Pathways to Solutions with Couples and Families* (with Mark Beyebach), *Collaborative Brief Therapy with Children*, *Gorging, Vomiting, and Self-Injuring: A Brief Therapy Approach* (with Giorgio Nardone), *The Adolescent and Young Adult Self-Harming Treatment Manual: A Collaborative Strengths-Based Brief Therapy Approach*, *Working with Self-Harming Adolescents: A Collaborative Strengths-Based Therapy Approach*, *Pathways to Change: Brief Therapy with Difficult Adolescents* (2nd edition), and *Family Therapy Approaches with Adolescent Substance Abusers* (with Thomas Todd). He has presented workshops on his collaborative strengths-based family therapy approach with children, adolescents, and adults extensively throughout the United States, Canada, Mexico, South America, Europe, Turkey, South Korea, Singapore, Indonesia, Hong Kong, South Africa, Australia, and New Zealand.

Foreword

It is a pleasure and an honor to write the foreword to a book full of stimulating information and suggestions such as this magnificent work by Selekman. The author, starting from his personal evolution as a therapist, refers to some inspiring "giants of psychotherapy," to his specific trainer and to important colleagues with whom he has collaborated.

He succeeds in deciphering the strategic development of family and couple therapy by highlighting different theoretical perspectives and methods of application. All this, reflecting his personal style as a therapist, following the definition of "collaborative strengths-based brief therapy," as he wrote for the *International Dictionary of Psychotherapy* (Routledge, 2019).

Thanks to his prolonged clinical experience, Matthew has elaborated truly effective methods to overcome severe psychopathologies such as: self-harming behaviors; alcohol and drug abuse; and complicated couple and family problems.

In this brilliant text, he addresses the therapist's personal abilities to use his or her personality and special skills to guide clients to achieve their therapeutic goals, overcoming their resistance to change in an original way with *self-disclosure techniques* along with a series of creative stratagems attuned to different clinical situations and to the uniqueness of each human system. I consider this book a "must read" for all people involved in human change processes.

Giorgio Nardone
Centro di Terapia Strategica
Arezzo, Italy
June 3, 2023

Preface

Throughout my career, when I had attended the workshops of well-known couple and family therapists, I had rarely heard them pay homage to their mentors and trainers, what words of wisdom had resonated with them, the signature techniques and strategies they had taught them, and what inspired them the most about them as people. The workshop leaders present their couple and family therapy models like they and their colleagues came up with the core assumptions and major therapeutic techniques and strategies of their approaches in isolation. The bottom line is there is no such thing as an original idea, something or somebodies played a role in the past in shaping and inspiring one's ideas. My inspiration for writing this book was two-fold: one, that it is important that we pay homage to our couple and family therapy mentors and pioneers that came before us and paved the way for us to become competent couple and family therapists; and two, that there are very few texts out there in our field that goes in depth covering the subject of the therapist's use of self, how to become more daring and improvisational in sessions, and expand our therapeutic range by bringing in ideas from outside of our field to spark creative ideas for crafting bold and intriguing questions and for co-designing novel therapeutic experiments with couples and families. The plethora of therapeutic tools and strategies and the creative ways we can use ourselves presented in this book can easily be integrated into any couple and family therapy approach. At this point, I provide a roadmap for what is to come chapter-by-chapter.

In Chapter 1, I pay homage to the following couple and family therapy pioneers: Milton H. Erickson, Michele Weiner-Davis, John Weakland, Harry Goolishian, Michael White, Virginia Satir, and Peggy Papp. I refer to these pioneers as *the co-authors*. Each pioneer's position on the use of self and signature techniques and strategies are covered. This is followed by presenting recent research on therapist effects on treatment outcome and a comparative analysis of the seven pioneers' clinical work.

Chapter 2 pays homage to the clinical wizardry and artistry of Salvador Minuchin, Harry Aponte, and Carl Whitaker. I refer to them as *the directors*, in that they are like theater directors and possessed charismatic leadership in their masterful work with couples and families. Using the same format as the first chapter, I cover their position on the use of self and their signature techniques and strategies. I close out the chapter by comparing and contrasting the pioneers and discuss what couple and family presenting problems and dynamics responds best to their approaches.

Chapter 3 addresses the strengths and weaknesses of relying solely on practice evidenced-based wisdom to guide our therapeutic decision-making. I present important research findings on pattern recognition with a wide range of professionals that have jobs that required quick on their feet intervention responses, such as experienced police officers, firefighters, military servicemen and women, airport control tower workers, and so forth. Additionally, I present the latest research on the characteristics of wise therapists and individuals and how we can use these important findings to inform our clinical practices. To help counter-balance relying too heavily on one's practice evidenced-based wisdom, I present eight mental traps and cognitive biases that can lead us down the wrong paths with our therapeutic decision-making, which could lead to premature client dropouts occurring and worse yet, treatment failure. I discuss how we can identify when each of the mental traps and cognitive biases are in operation and effective steps we take to prevent them from misleading us. Finally, there are two case examples presented, one in which relying on practice evidence-based wisdom was right on target and the other case illustrates how I fell prey to overconfidence and other mental traps and cognitive biases, which resulted in the couple dropping out of treatment.

Chapter 4 presents the therapist's use of self-toolkit. I present eleven different ways therapists can use themselves as the catalysts for change. Case examples are provided after each therapeutic technique or strategy is presented to illustrate them in action.

In Chapter 5, I present what I call *therapeutic brick walls*, that is when we get stuck or the treatment process has come to a standstill. I discuss three sets of contributing factors that lead to therapeutic brick walls occurring, they are: therapist-generated, client-generated, and therapist-client-eco-systemic-generated. I describe each of the contributing factors and rapid and constructive steps therapists can take to ameliorate them and get unstuck.

Chapter 6, covers improvisational methods, idea-generating skill-building exercises, and games we can use with couples and families in a virtual tele-health therapy context. I discuss some of the advantages of doing tele-health couple and family therapy and how constraints bring out the best in us and our clients in terms of co-designing creative and high-quality solutions together.

Chapter 7 discusses resources for enhancing our inventiveness and expanding our therapeutic range and style. What is unique about this chapter is it demonstrates how there are a goldmine of metaphors and creative ideas outside of our brains in the world from such diverse fields as art, architecture, film, theater, literature, philosophy, science and technology, and nature that we can utilize for tapping both our and our clients' inventiveness for crafting intriguing questions and co-designing therapeutic experiments. Finally, I cover idea-generating strategies we can use to come up with high-quality solutions and make creative use of our talents and life passions that we can bring to our clients.

Chapter 8 presents the therapist's use of self-developmental framework, which describes in great detail important developmental tasks that therapists should attempt to master at the beginning, intermediate, advanced, and master levels with their conceptual, perceptual, and executive skill development. Training exercises are provided that are geared to strengthen therapist use of self-skills, expand their therapeutic range, and empower them to be more daring and inventive in their work with couples and families.

Finally, Chapter 9 summarizes the major themes of the book and future directions for research on the therapist's use of self.

Acknowledgements

This book would not have been possible if it were not for the wonderful family therapy supervision, training, and mentoring experiences I had had with Salvador Minuchin, Thomas Todd, Michele Weiner-Davis, John H. Weakland, Harry Goolishian, Harlene Anderson, Jay Haley, Michael White, and John Schwartzman. Thanks to their superb teaching abilities and their wisdom they paved the way for me to become a confident and competent couple and family therapist. Out of this illustrious group of pioneers, I would like to share some of the major therapeutic ideas I learned and achieved mastery with due to the great training, supervision, and mentoring I had received from Minuchin, Weiner-Davis, Todd, Haley, Weakland, Goolishian, Anderson, and White.

Minuchin had taught me how to "dance" with families and have fun in sessions, weave tapestries of metaphors, how to "kick" (challenge) and "stroke" (compliment) couple partners and family members, do enactments, and use oneself as a powerful catalyst for change. I also learned how to be invisible in a session by looking down at my left foot when trying to get family members to directly talk with one another, rather than with you.

Weiner-Davis had taught me the short road to change by seizing clients' self-generated pretreatment changes, past successes, and their strengths and resources to rapidly co-construct solutions with them. Her passion, great sense of humor, and incredible ability to get clients to compliment themselves on their resourcefulness and create a context ripe for change in one session was unmatchable.

Todd, Haley, and Weakland had taught me how to use strategic indirect change strategies with couples and families that are stuck in rigid patterns of interactions and viewing their problem situations in narrow ways. Todd showed me effective ways to use these indirect change strategies with alcohol and substance-abusing couples and families. Three of Weakland and his colleagues' greatest contributions to our field was the importance of finding out from clients in great detail all of their attempted solutions, including what former therapists and treatment program staff had tried with them, so as not to replicate what has not worked; to make sure you have identified the true customer for change in the client system; and inviting clients to determine what the "right problem" to change first is and negotiating it into solvable terms with them.

Goolishian and Anderson drove home with me the importance of honoring and staying close to clients' stories and avoid at all costs, being a narrative editor, particularly with therapy-veteran couples and families who have long stories to tell. Additionally, they taught me how to collaborate with helping professionals from larger systems using respectful curiosity and multi-partiality, that is siding simultaneously with everyone's different views, without privileging your own perspective. This important training has helped me to rapidly foster cooperative partnerships with involved helping professionals from larger systems.

Finally, one of the most important contributions to the family therapy field was White's externalization of the problem strategy. From the training I had received from him, I learned how to use this strategy particularly with couples and families who had been oppressed by their presenting problems for a long time and seemingly had a life of their own. Thanks to the above trainers, supervisors, and mentors I was inspired to create my own unique couple and family therapy approach called *collaborative strengths-based family therapy*, which integrates the best elements of these pioneers' approaches, incorporates mindfulness practices, art therapy methods, expressive writing, drama techniques, and offers practical guidelines for tailor-fitting what we choose to do with our clients based on their goals, theories of change, and unique needs.

Credit List

Re-Authoring Lives: Interviews and Essays, Michael White, pp. 86–87, Copyright © 1995 by Dulwich Centre Publications Pty Ltd. Reproduced by permission of Dulwich Centre Publications Pty Ltd.

The Therapist's Story, Virginia Satir, p. 25, in Michele Baldwin (Ed.), *The Use of Self in Therapy*, 3rd Ed., Copyright © 2013 Routledge. Reproduced by permission of Routledge.

The Therapist's Story, Virginia Satir, p. 26, in Michele Baldwin (Ed.), *The Use of Self in Therapy*, 3rd Ed., Copyright © 2013 Routledge. Reproduced by permission of Routledge.

The Process of Change, Peggy Papp, p. 142, Copyright © 1983, Guilford Press. Reproduced by permission of Guilford Press.

Therapist's Presence, Absence, and Extraordinary Presence, p. 96, in Louis G. Castonguay and Clara E. Hill (Eds.), *How and Why are Some Therapists Better than Others? Understanding Therapist Effects*, Copyright © 2017, American Psychological Association. Reproduced by permission of the American Psychological Association.

Psychotherapy of the Absurd: With a Special Emphasis on the Psychotherapy of Aggression, Carl Whitaker, *Family Process, 14* (1), p. 9, Copyright © 1975, Wiley-Blackwell. Reproduced by permission of Wiley-Blackwell.

Continuing the Experiential Approach of Carl Whitaker: Process, Practice, and Magic, David Keith, p. 3, Copyright © 2015 David Keith. Reproduced by permission of author David Keith.

Reshaping Family Relationships: The Symbolic Therapy of Carl Whitaker, Gary Connell, Tammy Mitten, and William Burberry, pp. 27; 93, Copyright © 1999 by Taylor & Francis Group. Reproduced by permission of Taylor & Francis Group.

Cultural Humility versus Cultural Competence: A Critical Distinction in Defining Physician Training Outcomes in Multicultural Education, Melanie Tervalon and Jann Murray-Garcia, *Journal of Health Care for the Poor and Underserved, 9* (2), p. 120, Copyright © 1998, John Hopkins University Press. Reproduced by permission of John Hopkins University Press.

Gay Affirmative Therapy for the Straight Clinician: The Essential Guide, Joe Kort, pp. 26; 156–157, Copyright © 2008 by W. W. Norton & Co. Reproduced by permission of W. W. Norton & Co.

Toward a Psychology of the Oppressed: Understanding the Invisible Wounds of Trauma, Ken V. Hardy, pp. 134; 144–145, in Monica McGoldrick and Ken V. Hardy (Eds.), *Re-Visioning Family Therapy: Addressing Diversity in Clinical Practice*, 3rd Ed., Copyright © 2019 Guilford Press. Reproduced by permission of Guilford Press.

No-Single Issue Lives: Identity Transitions and Transformations Across the Life Cycle, Elijah C. Nealy, pp. 375; 379–380, in Monica McGoldrick and Ken Hardy (Eds.), *Re-Visioning Family Therapy: Addressing Diversity in Clinical Practice*, 3rd Ed., Copyright © 2019 Guilford Press. Reproduced by permission of Guilford Press.

Wayne Shorter: A Final Interview, Michael Jackson, *Downbeat Magazine, 90* (5), p. 30, Copyright © 2023, Downbeat Magazine. Reproduced by permission of Downbeat Magazine.

Masters of the Use of Self

Couple and Family Therapy Pioneers that Perfected the Craft of Being the Catalysts for Change – Part I

Back in 1986, I brought in a challenging family for Salvador Minuchin to consult with me on during our week-long live supervision family therapy training with him. The presenting problems were the seventeen-year-old son Tim's heavy hallucinogen abuse, failing in school, running away from home, and regularly breaking his father's rules. Roger, the father, believed that his mother's lack of contact with him for seven years after their divorce had contributed to his "emotional and behavioral difficulties" and his adopting as his identity being a modern-day hippie and dressing the part (wearing a fringed leather jacket, jeans with large bell bottoms, and sandals), much to the father's dismay, who was quite conservative with his style of dress and a businessman. Minuchin observed from the beginning of our consultation that Roger would look at him while speaking for Tim and diagnosing him as being "emotionally troubled" and a "drug addict," like trying to be Minuchin's co-therapist. In challenging this pattern of interaction and refusing to serve as Roger's co-therapist, Minuchin changed the subject and shared what was on his mind: "The yuppie and the hippie. Very nice … Wall Street and Abbey Road." The father and son both smiled while listening intently to what Minuchin had to say. He further added while looking at Roger: "You are like Tom Hayden [former social activist] with the 'straight-looking clothes' and he became a politician. But he was a betrayer … he betrayed the cause and started wearing clothes like you with creased pants and dressed straight like you." Tim proclaimed, "I'll never dress like that, man!" Roger added, "I used to have long hair and dress like Tim and liked some of the same music." Minuchin shared, "So you are a betrayer." Minuchin underscored both how similar the father and son were and challenged both Roger's pathological view of his son as being "emotionally troubled" and a "drug addict" and the way his dad spoke for and about his son to others, rather than talking directly to him. Later in the consultation, as a way to challenge the diffuse boundaries in the father-son relationship and challenge Tim as serving as the symptom-bearer in the family, he asked him, "When you get high on acid, do hallucinations of your father appear?" Tim firmly reacted with, "No way, man!" This was the first time I had ever observed Tim really assert himself. Eventually, Roger and Tim started talking directly with one another in the session minus the pathology language, and Minuchin and I became invisible

DOI: 10.4324/9781003334460-1

while they spoke together by looking down and away from them, which forced them to have to look at one another when talking (Minuchin, 1986).

Minuchin's use of metaphors, provocation, and humor are beautiful examples of using oneself as the catalyst for change. Like all of the couple and family therapy pioneers discussed in this and in the second chapter, many therapists familiar with their artful and skillful use of themselves in the therapeutic process would agree that what sparked therapeutic breakthroughs and paved the way for workable realities with the couples and families they worked with was their creative use of themselves, not their therapeutic models. Once the pioneers discovered how best to cooperate and/or be what each couple partner and family member needed from them in their therapeutic relationships through careful observation and responsive listening often determined how best for them to intervene to help the clients to achieve their goals and co-create possibilities together. The couple and family therapy pioneers covered in this and in the second chapter are wide-ranging in terms of the therapeutic operations they employed in a given session to spark therapeutic breakthroughs. However, what they chose to do was purposeful and what they thought would help the clients in the best way possible. With some of the pioneers, they view the clients as the true experts on their problem stories and what their desired outcomes would look like, served as co-collaborators with them, and utilized all that the clients brought to the therapeutic encounter to co-construct solutions. I refer to these masters as *the co-authors*, and are covered in this chapter. While other pioneers were much more directive and assumed a leadership role early in the treatment process believing that the best way to help stuck couples and families entrenched in rigid patterns of interactions, role behaviors, and fixed belief systems was to create a crisis in sessions as a powerful way to liberate them from their difficulties, which could lead to transformation and long-lasting systemic changes. These pioneers believed that couples and families are most amenable to change at the highest point of crisis. I refer to them as *the directors*, whom are showcased in Chapter 2.

In this and in the next chapter, I present ten couple and family therapy pioneers representing ten different couple and family therapy approaches who I and many therapists would consider masters of the use of self, they are: Milton H. Erickson (Ericksonian Psychotherapy), Michele Weiner-Davis (Solution-Focused Brief Therapy), John H. Weakland (MRI Brief Strategic Therapy), Harry Goolishian (Collaborative Language Systems Therapy), Michael White (Narrative Therapy), Virginia Satir (Experiential Family Therapy), Peggy Papp (Experiential & Ackerman Systemic Family Therapy), Salvador Minuchin (Structural Family Therapy), Harry Aponte (Structural Family Therapy) and Carl Whitaker (Symbolic-Experiential Family Therapy). After years of participating in long and short-term intensive trainings with the majority of the pioneers, watching many hours of their training DVDs, and reading the seminal works written by the pioneers themselves or their colleagues and proteges, I decided that they were the masters of the use of self I wanted to pay homage to in this book. The reason why I included Milton H. Erickson among this elite group of couple and family therapy pioneers is that Erickson often is touted as the father of brief and family therapy in terms of his profound influence on most of the above pioneers' use of themselves as the catalysts for change and their therapeutic approaches. Erickson worked a lot with couples and families in his private practice. With each of the pioneers in this and in the next chapter, I cover his or her position on the use of self with their particular therapy approach and his or her signature techniques and strategies used in the therapeutic process when working with couples and families. This will be followed by a comparative analysis of the different ways each of the pioneers used themselves in the therapeutic process and their rationale for doing so.

The Co-authors

As co-authors, the seven pioneers presented in this chapter made careful use of clients' strengths, resources, best hopes, and expertise to empower them to pen the preferred future stories they wished to have. By seizing couples' and families' exceptions or sparkling moments both in and out of sessions, utilizing their past successes, opening up space for the sharing of the unexpressed, and abandoning unproductive problem views, rigid role behaviors, and attempted solutions, these seven pioneers helped liberate them from their problem-saturated dominant stories. The co-authors covered in this chapter are: Milton H. Erickson, Michele Weiner-Davis, John H. Weakland, Harry Goolishian, Michael White, Virginia Satir, and Peggy Papp.

Milton H. Erickson

Erickson approached couples and families and human difficulties in general from a normative perspective and avoided at all costs using what we would call DSM-V labels today and deficiency language. He found the psychotherapy concept of *resistance* to not be a useful way of viewing therapist-client interactions and truly believed that all clients want relief from their oppressive difficulties and it is the therapist's job to carefully observe and look for clues how clients want to cooperate with them. In fact, Erickson believed that within each human being there is a vast reservoir of strengths, resources, resiliencies, past successful blueprints for problem-solving and coping, and self-healing capacities (Short, 2020; Havens, 1996). He also believed that the therapist's expertise is in skillfully utilizing the clients' expertise to empower them to achieve their goals (O'Hanlon, 1987). By doing so, the therapy process is much more efficient and lengths of stay in treatment are greatly reduced. Psychotherapy outcome research has indicated that 40% of what counts for treatment success is the therapist's skillful use of *client extra-therapeutic factors*, that is making maximum use of all that the clients bring to the therapeutic relationship (Duncan, 2019, 2010; Sparks & Duncan, 2010). Erickson was known for having many single-session positive treatment outcomes with a wide range of client presenting problems and the changes that had occurred continued to stick years after the therapies had been completed (O'Hanlon & Hexum, 1990). Critics of brief therapy and the possibility of single-session cures often ask, "How could this be possible?" "Is this just client flight into health?" However, disciples of Erickson believe through the use of his keen sense of observation and superb listening skills; his conveying with a high level confidence to his clients that change *will* happen and it is an only a matter of *when*; his use of humor and absurdity; his carefully tailor fitting what he did therapeutically to the unique needs, best hopes, and characteristics of his clients; and by utilizing to the maximum degree their strengths, resources, interests, life passions, their key words and beliefs, greatly contributed to producing long-lasting changes with them, after one or a few sessions with him. Erickson strongly believed that the therapist's approach should fit the couple or family's unique situation and characteristics, not try and fit them into the box of the therapist's choice and beloved therapy model. He believed that if the therapist can get the clients onboard to experiment with doing things differently, even something small in their couple or family relationships and in other areas of their lives would trigger a cascading effect of further changes. So, for Erickson, it was behavioral change that produces client insight, not the reverse. Finally, Erickson operated from a present and future orientation. He would only tap the couple's or family's pasts to extract successful problem solving and coping strategies to use with their current difficulties. Finally, Erickson believed that the therapist's job is to strive to create a therapeutic climate ripe for change and the client's job is to do the work. We should never be working harder than are clients in the change effort (Havens, 1996).

Position on the Use of Self

Erickson believed that therapeutic flexibility is a must and that the therapist needs to strive to foster cooperative partnerships with his or her clients. Based on the couple partner's or family member's cooperative response patterns verbally and nonverbally would dictate whether or not Erickson would operate in a direct or indirect way in his interactions with them and with determining the best fit of specific therapeutic experiments designed, selected, and offered to them (Haley, 1985a). For example, with a highly concerned wife who comes in for help with her alcohol abusing husband who is ready to do anything to help him, Erickson would first learn about all of her attempted solutions to try and change him and in a more direct way, offer a therapeutic experiment or two to do things differently in her interactions with her husband. If the alcohol abusing husband came alone because he contended that his wife would not stop her incessant "nagging and lecturing" about getting help for his "drinking problem," Erickson would strive to build a strong therapeutic alliance with him so that he was not perceived as a threat to him but an ally. As part of this process, he would most likely compliment the husband on how "sensitive and respectful" he is of his wife's wishes for him to seek help by just showing up for the appointment she had made for him. If it is clear that the husband rationalizes his drinking as "under control," is "not a problem," and he uses it to get relief from "work and marital stress," Erickson would work in a more indirect way with him by restraining him from changing too quickly, since alcohol has been like a good friend and comforter for him. Erickson would then begin to seed helpful ideas in a nonchalant manner like "I wonder if you cut back just a little bit on your drinking if your wife would notice, be encouraged, and 'nag and lecture' less?" This would be followed by a message to take the change process slowly and then seeding another useful thought for the husband to ponder. Once the change process starts to happen, Erickson would often receive a call from the partner or they may end up joining future sessions, which provides confirmation that change is really happening. To help keep the husband on his toes and normalize the inevitability of slips, Erickson would predict that he may experience an alcohol slip down-the-road because slips sometimes go with the territory of change but that he was confident he would quickly get back on track.

Erickson listened for key client words that were used frequently in a session. He would not only be curious to know the meaning of those words but he would use them in his questions and in his rationales for trying out particular therapeutic experiments between sessions. Erickson also would use the client key words in a hypnotic embedded command (Havens, 1996). For example, I once worked with an explosive 8-year-old boy who had severe temper tantrums, destroyed everything in sight, and at times, would hit and kicked his parents when angry and frustrated. In our first session, he used the word "happy" about six times. When asked about what he meant by the word "happy," he said the following: "My parents would stop yelling so much, we would not argue, and we would get along better." At the end of our family meeting, as part of my getting the family fired up for a ritual designed to help tame the Temper (externalized the problem), I shared with the family and then looked at the boy, "It is important that you all work together as a team and not allow that Temper to make you argue and get the best of you, because you like to be "happy." The boy responded to my embedded command with, "Happy."

Another way Erickson used himself with clients that presented with vague explanations of their problems or goals, the couple partners or family members had mutually exclusive explanations about the problem or goals, or to disrupt their excessive use of intellectualizing about their difficulties, was to use his *confusion technique* (Erickson, 1964). When using his confusion technique Erickson would change the subject at hand and talk about something out-of-context, the comments he would share would have two or more possible interpretations, and by doing the above, he would overwhelm the couple partners' or family members' conscious processing abilities (O'Hanlon, 1987). This would often lead to the clients providing more clarity about what they wished to change in solvable terms.

Signature Techniques and Strategies

Erickson often shared personal stories and stories about how other clients conquered their difficulties, anecdotes, analogies, and metaphors which may or may not parallel the clients' difficulties but often would spark epiphanies for them and paved the way for solution-finding. He found that stories, anecdotes, analogies, and metaphors were quite effective at engaging clients' attention, quieting their serious and rational left brains, and tapping their unconscious minds and right brains to picture images and useful themes and accentuate their creative problem-solving capacities (Short, 2020; Havens, 1996; O'Hanlon, 1987). Erickson was a masterful storyteller and his stories were often embedded with wisdom, humor, transcending adversity, and surprising twists that lead to the protagonists finding solutions.

As part of the utilization process, Erickson would make use of elements of the clients' longstanding problems, symptoms, problem-maintaining patterns, and fixed beliefs and not only normalize or reframe these difficulties as ways to cope but as well-intended attempted solutions for trying to resolve life difficulties. It was not uncommon for Erickson to ask a couple what part of their old problem-maintaining interaction they would wish to keep for memory-sake as a reminder of how far they have come or use in a new and more productive way. Another example would be to ask a client with a habit problem like substance abuse, bulimia, or self-injury the following questions: "If weed/bulimia/cutting were to pack its bags today and leave your life for good but you could keep one aspect of it that you liked, what would you wish to keep?" "What would be the disadvantages of your giving up weed/bulimia/cutting?" Since at some point clients' longstanding symptoms or problems have served them well as coping strategies and they are acclimatized to or used to having them present in their lives, a sudden change can be a threat to status quo and raise their anxiety levels, which is the perfect storm for a slip. This is why Erickson believed it is important to predict the possibility of slips occurring, to help keep clients on their toes and doing more of what works, and so if slips should occur, they don't view these events in a disastrous way and as an indicator that they are back to square one (Haley, 1985a).

One of Erickson's most famous techniques was his *crystal ball* technique, which he used in a variety of ways (Erickson, 1954). At times, he would use it to have clients gaze into the past to relive pleasurable and meaningful experiences so he could gain access to what worked for them and could be utilized with their current difficulties. Since the future did not exist for clients yet, it could serve as fertile soil for the compelling and ideal treatment outcome reality they desire to have. Erickson would have them gaze into the imaginary crystal ball and describe in great detail how things will look in the future when their current difficulties are solved and absent. Sometimes Erickson would have clients pick one or two ideal future outcomes and walk him back to the here and now spelling out the steps they took to achieve those positive outcomes. By doing so, he gained access to clients' strengths and resources, building blocks for solution construction, and potential treatment goals. The crystal ball technique had inspired de Shazer's popular *miracle question* goal-setting question (de Shazer, 1985).

Erickson used *pattern intervention* strategies to disrupt entrenched longstanding problem-maintaining patterns that were serving as the problem life support system for the couple or family's difficulties. With pattern intervention strategies, Erickson would do the following: prescribe the symptom or problem/primary problem-maintaining pattern of interaction occur at different times for different durations of time; locations where it would occur; change the order of couple partner and family member involvement; add something novel to the usual context(s) in which the problem/primary problem-maintaining pattern of interaction typically would occur; exaggerate the doing of the symptom/problem/primary problem-maintaining pattern of interaction to an absurd level; and set up a situation where it would be an ordeal to engage in the problematic behavior or pattern of interaction. Erickson would only try the above strategies after building solid alliances with couples and families, where trust had been built, and where a more direct approach was not working (Havens, 1996; O'Hanlon, 1987).

In his work with couples and families, sometimes he would work with individual couple partners and family members where they would separately serve as the agents of change for their couple and family relationships. When he would see the other couple partner or family members a little later in the session, he would pay close attention to where everyone sits. If the seat(s) the other couple partner or family members had been sitting in were those of the wife or the mother or father, Erickson would point that out and have them experiment with perspective-taking. For example, Erickson might ask the acting out son now sitting in his mother's chair to try and imagine from her perspective through her eyes and mind how she views him (the son) and their family situation. By doing so, this can help a family member gain a new perspective on their behavior or situation through the eyes and mind of another member, and possibly lead to him or her being more understanding and empathic with that family member and do something different with his or her behavior to please the other (Haley, 1985a, 1985b).

Michele Weiner-Davis

Michele Weiner-Davis, known as a "pathological optimist," for her ability to rapidly create hope and possibilities with "impossible" couple and family clients that had already been to many therapists that had also labeled them "resistant," "uncooperative," and "noncompliant." Weiner-Davis had joined the core team at the Brief Family Therapy Center in Milwaukee, Wisconsin and along with Steve de Shazer and Wallace Gingerich were the first to do research on client pretreatment change and develop specific questions to quickly gain access to this client goldmine of building blocks for solution construction (Weiner-Davis, de Shazer, & Gingerich, 1987). Not only were Weiner-Davis and I colleagues at one of a handful of youth and family service agencies in the world that used solution-focused brief therapy as the primary treatment framework but I had the luxury of receiving live and videotape supervision and regularly observing her work and serving as a team member using this approach. Since I was running and providing clinical supervision for our adolescent substance abuse program at our agency, Weiner-Davis and I regularly traveled up to the Brief Family Therapy Center to receive supervision-of-supervision with Eve Lipchik, one of the core co-developers of the solution-focused brief therapy approach. Both Steve de Shazer and John H. Weakland from the MRI Brief Therapy Institute in Palo Alto, California, served as our consultants and provided case consultation and live supervision when they visited our agency.

In addition to providing workshops worldwide and serving as a keynote speaker at many major conferences and a guest on talk shows and giving *Ted Talks*, Weiner-Davis is a prolific author and published the following seminal works: *In Search of Solutions: A New Direction in Psychotherapy* (co-authored with Bill O'Hanlon, 1989), *Divorce-Busting: A Revolutionary Program for Staying Together* (1992), *Healing from Infidelity* (2017), and *The Sex-Starved Marriage* (2004). Weiner-Davis has devoted the second half of her illustrious career to specializing in working with troubled couples who have had multiple unsuccessful treatment experiences and whose marriages or intimate relationships were hanging on by a thread. Weiner-Davis's book *Divorce-Busting* was the first highly practical and positive self-help book for the public and therapists alike that drove home the powerful message that a lot of the reasons why couples divorce our solvable problems, such as: poor communications and conflict resolution-skills, money management issues, power and control inequity, lack of sexual intimacy, and even infidelity. This book has helped many couples save their marriages and relationships and led them to seek Weiner-Davis out for consultation and ongoing treatment. In response to the tremendous public demand for her services and therapists wanting to learn her divorce-busting techniques and strategies, she opened Divorce Busting Centers in Woodstock, Illinois and in Boulder, Colorado. Presently, she offers one and two-day intensives to couples and has found this to be quite meaningful work (Weiner-Davis, personal communication, May 25, 2022).

Position on Use of Self

Since Weiner-Davis works a lot with demoralized couples hanging on by a thread with their marriages and high-conflict couples, the therapist has to be highly active, flexible, take charge when necessary, and provide structure in sessions. At the same time, she validates each partner's thoughts and feelings, comes to understand their different perspectives on their couple problem story, and learn about all of their and their past therapists' attempted solutions to resolve their difficulties. Like a super sleuth detective, she listens carefully for couples' past successes and self-generated pretreatment changes worthwhile seizing and utilizing in their presenting problem areas. Weiner-Davis believes the therapeutic relationship is key. This is supported by couple and family therapy outcome research that indicates that the therapeutic relationship for clients is highly predictive of positive treatment outcomes (Duncan, 2019; Sparks & Duncan, 2010; Sprenkle, Davis, & Lebow, 2009). According to Weiner-Davis, what couples get is the person she is outside the therapy arena, which consists of: being authentic, warm, passionate, enthusiastic, engendering hope, being playful, and using lots of humor (Weiner-Davis, personal communication, May 25, 2022).

It has been Weiner-Davis's experience working with these troubled and stuck couples that they had been desperate to learn helpful tools and strategies and just get plain "advice," none of which they had received in their multiple past couple therapy experiences. With the advice-giving, Weiner-Davis might begin with qualifiers like: "Have you considered trying X?" or "I wonder if X might be helpful?" Most of the advice she shares with couples are strategies she and her husband found useful and other couples she worked with (Weiner-Davis, personal communication, May 25, 2022).

Weiner-Davis also finds it useful to send letters to couples between sessions to check-in to see how they are doing with implementing new change strategies, to further underscore their progress, and to just see how they are doing in general. She has found that this further deepens her therapeutic alliances with each couple partner and that they appreciate the extra attention and care she devotes to them (Weiner-Davis, personal communication, May 25, 2022).

To help normalize couples' struggles and intuitively she thinks it can benefit her clients, she purposefully shares her own personal individual and marital stories, which offer wisdom and potential solutions for the clients. Clients often appreciate hearing these stories knowing that Weiner-Davis has experienced trials and tribulations and suffered at times individually and in her marital relationship and how these life experiences make us more resilient and can strengthen our couple relationship bonds. After sharing her stories, she carefully listens to and observes the nonverbal feedback to make sure this was useful to the couple (Weiner-Davis, personal communication, May 25, 2022).

Signature Techniques and Strategies

When working with high-conflict couples, Weiner-Davis has developed a very effective strategy for disrupting their blame-counter-blame or "I'm right, you're wrong" destructive patterns of interaction they are stuck in. She first invites each partner to share his or her primary complaint. While one has the floor, the other partner has to listen to the other. After each partner shares his or her concerns, Weiner-Davis responds with, "I so get the way you feel the way you do." She further shares, "This is the case of 'two rights' and it is really possible to hold both true and at the same time, you are both 'right.'" Finally, she points out, "You have probably been spending years arguing about who's 'right' and who's wrong, rather than trying to figure out together about what to do about it." Next, she teaches the partners how to hold in one's mind two opposing views or truths, getting each partner to honor what each one brings to the table, rather than having to prove him or her wrong (Weiner-Davis, personal communication, May 25, 2022).

With demoralized couples that have experienced multiple treatment failures and seeing Weiner-Davis is their last ditched effort to see if they can save their marriage, she engenders hope through underscoring past successes the couple have had and makes use of presuppositional language to help the partners anticipate a brighter future ahead for their relationship. For example, with couple that experienced an extra-marital crisis situation, Weiner-Davis likes to share the following:

> I know you won't believe me with what I am about to tell you but I imagine you are going to feel this way the rest of your life and it is absolutely not true. There's going to come a time, a month or two from now, or maybe a year from now, that you will look back and say, "That really was awful but look at where we are now." I promise you that there will be certain triggers that may happen but the time between these triggers will be wider and wider and wider, and when they do happen, you will not feel the same kind of sting that you feel right now and I GUARANTEE THAT!
>
> (Weiner-Davis, personal communication, May 25, 2022)

Weiner-Davis does a masterful job of using presuppositional language to empower couples to envision and expect the kind of future realities they would like to have, which includes possible "triggers" that may occur, but will be manageable for them.

Another way Weiner-Davis engenders hope with couples hanging on by a thread with their marriages is to have them take her back in time to where and how they met, positive courting experiences, how they decided to marry, and any challenges that they had faced and overcame with great teamwork. By doing so, this triggers positive emotions and memories for the couple partners, which helps with the hope-building and with the solution construction process. There often are bits and pieces of the couple's past positive experiences together (loving moments and fun times) that can be utilized in the here and now to improve their relationship. Weiner-Davis contends that when these couple partners enter therapy their individual narratives about what their marriage is and what it will be in the future is quite pessimistic, are rigidified, and like carved in stone for them. By having the partners reminisce and relive the best moments of their past relationship, it changes their problem-saturated stories and opens up space for the co-authoring of a new more preferred future marital story.

John H. Weakland

Weakland had joined the Mental Research Institute's (MRI) core team in 1967. The original MRI core team consisted of the co-founders Don Jackson and Virginia Satir, Paul Watzlawick, Richard Fisch, and Janet Beavin. For years, they regularly consulted with Milton H. Erickson and the cultural anthropologist Gregory Bateson and both the MRI team and Jay Haley who had spent a great deal of time with this group, were greatly inspired by these two brilliant thinkers and heavily based their therapy approaches on the therapeutic techniques and strategies and the theoretical ideas of Erickson and Bateson respectfully. Although Weakland came to the psychotherapy world as a second career, he made good use of his chemical engineering background to be a skillful observer for redundant problem-maintaining patterns of interaction in couples and families, listening for narrow and fixed client beliefs that were contributing to perpetuating their difficulties, and discovered by introducing novelty or something different to clients' problem situations had the potential to trigger second order long-lasting changes (Watzlawick, Weakland, & Fisch, 1974). Weakland and his colleagues co-authored three groundbreaking books, they are: *Change: Principles of Problem Formation and Problem Resolution* (1974); *The Tactics of Change: Doing Therapy Briefly* (1982); and *Pragmatics of Human Communication: A Study of Interactional Patterns, Pathologies, and Paradoxes* (1967).

My first exposure to Weakland and the MRI team's innovative therapeutic work was back in 1978 as an undergraduate student at Cleveland State University. I had analyzed couple communication patterns for Frank and Edna Millar's research study on couple communications in the university's communication department. At the time, they were affiliated with the MRI team and were studying both adaptive and problematic couple communication patterns. Our research team were using both *Pragmatics of Human Communication: A Study of Interactional Patterns, Pathologies, and Paradoxes* and *Change: Principles of Problem Formation and Problem Resolution* books to help guide us in our work and make sense of our research findings.

Eight years later, I got to meet Weakland when he was serving as a consultant at our youth and family service agency. He was a great storyteller, very warm and friendly, had a wonderful sense of humor, and offered my colleagues and I valuable input on our tougher family cases.

One of Weakland and the MRI team's core assumptions they built their whole model around is that it is the clients' attempted solutions that is the problem. They are stuck doing *more-of-the-same*, which is further perpetuating their difficulties. Often clients' attempted solutions are well-intended or would be considered loving acts, such as: the wife's finding and emptying out her alcohol-abusing husband's liquor and beer bottles or parents who rescue their son from experiencing the serious consequences of their actions by bailing him out of trouble at school or with the police. Not only do clients get stuck doing *more-of-the same* but so do the treatment professionals they had been involved with past and present. For example, there are many traditional private practitioners working from a psychodynamic perspective that would gladly see a child or adolescent individually for two or more years and exclude the parents from the treatment process. It is often recommended by these therapists that the parents see a separate therapist. Meanwhile, the child or adolescent's acting out behaviors continue to occur at school and/or at home and problem-maintaining patterns of interaction between them and their parents are left intact. A utopian or grand solution that a lot of parents and treatment providers pursue with children, adolescents, and young adults with serious DSM-V diagnoses and extreme and provocative behaviors is to load them up with multiple treatment modalities, have them medicated, and/or have them placed in psychiatric hospital-based programs or residential treatment facilities. The belief is that big problems require equally big solutions, but often times the positive results of treatment over-kill is short-lived and after a brief honeymoon period, treatment relapses occur, and clients are back to square one. Finally, it is important to explore in great detail all of the clients' and current and past treatment providers' attempted solutions, so as not to replicate what has not worked (Fisch, Weakland, & Segal, 1982; Watzlawick, Weakland, & Fisch, 1974). As part of the clients' attempted solution inquiry, find out about their and past treatment providers' successes with them. Any past successes our clients have had can serve as blueprints for future successes.

Position on the Use of Self

When beginning with new clients, Weakland in a highly disciplined way, practiced *not-doing*, which he had learned from his marriage to a Chinese woman and having had ample opportunities to be with her immediate and extended families and discovering culturally about the benefits of taking this stance as a way to keep things calm and not make waves with anyone. Steve de Shazer, the father of the solution-focused brief therapy approach, had spent years studying with the MRI core team and became good friends with Weakland. In fact, de Shazer regularly invited him to the Brief Family Therapy Center in Milwaukee to spend time with his team, exchange ideas, and observe Weakland work with their clients. De Shazer was intrigued by Weakland's use of himself in the therapeutic process with clients and began to micro-analyze videotapes of his consultations at his training center, looking for patterns in what he does, what he avoids doing, and how he thinks. De Shazer (1999, p. 30) identified three steps that Weakland typically takes in his therapy sessions with clients, they are:

1 not-doing;
2 getting ready to do something; and
3 doing something.

By *not-doing*, Weakland from a position of curiosity, would ask the couple partners or family members information about what they thought the problem was and what they had attempted to do to solve it. He uses this inquiry to listen intently and observe the clients' interactions in the room, to their beliefs about the problem and the words they use to describe it, which helps him to decide what to explore more with them about and deciding what not to do, and avoid it all costs. Weakland would argue that it is better to do nothing when stuck or confused then do something that may not work, can further exacerbate the couple or family's problem situation, or lead to their losing faith and confidence in the therapist's ability to help them. He would go to great lengths to negotiate a solvable problem with clients, such as: having the clients define the problem into behavioral terms (actions or doings), something we can see and measure; break the problem down further into bite-size pieces and find out from the couple or family what piece of the problem situation they wished to change first. For example, the mother defines her husband's "depression" as the family problem. When asked what piece of the "depression" she and the kids would like to see changed first, she responds with, "He'll stop isolating in our bedroom and mingle with the family more." Weakland might explore how that would make a difference for the family members. By gathering this important information, he may learn that the bonuses of having father mingling with the family members more often were that they enjoyed spending time with him and the father would appear "happier." Weakland would make a mental note of this positive exception pattern and in the getting ready to do something phase, explore if the family would like this to become their initial treatment goal, by having them increase doing what's working.

With *getting ready to do something*, Weakland needed to have a clear sense of how the couple or family will know that they are making progress with the problem situation over the next week. He would inquire about what the concrete behavioral signs or indicators of change would look like to the couple partners or family members. Weakland would secure this important information by asking the following type of questions:

* "What will be a small sign of progress happening over the next week?"
* "What will be the first sign of improvement?"
* "What will have to begin to change over the next week that will tell you that you are making good headway?"
* "How will you know that you are really succeeding in counseling?"

Once Weakland discovered this important information, both he and the clients will know what to look for that will serve as indicators that change is really happening and more specifically, what is working that he wanted to have clients do more of.

With *doing something*, once it is clear what the central problem-maintaining attempted solution pattern of interaction is between the couple partners or the parents and identified client child or adolescent, Weakland would let the couple partner or parent(s) know that they have become too predictable with their yelling, lecturing, threats, and so forth that his or her partner or child or adolescent knows what's coming and will rebel against their wishes and dig in more. He would then coach the couple partner or parent(s) to experiment with doing-something-different that would be surprising and the identified client had never experienced from them before. When the timing is right for this therapeutic experiment and it produces positive results, not only does it disrupt the central problem-maintaining pattern but the couple partner or child or adolescent change as well to accommodate to their changes.

Weakland believed that therapeutic maneuverability is a must. The timing and pacing of what the therapist chooses to do is important. During the do something phase, the therapist is much more active and directive. Like Erickson, Weakland and his colleagues were free to meet alone with individual couple partners and family members when they thought it might be useful, to further strengthen their alliances with them, to ask specific questions, and offer therapeutic experiments when they felt the clients were ready to try them out. Often, Weakland would get the clients on the edge of their seats about a therapeutic experiment he thought would be useful to them and would "test the waters" to see if they were ready for it. Sometimes he would perk the clients' interest by prefacing that the experiment he is thinking about offering them may sound absurd at first but could make sense after they test it out. Similar to Erickson, Weakland would work in a more indirect way with couples and families that are grappling with rigidified and longstanding problem-maintaining patterns of interaction, narrow and fixed beliefs, and had already experienced multiple treatment failures. With these situations, he would use reframing and pattern intervention strategies. With clinical situations where the clients would respond to his reframing or their therapeutic experiments offered or tried out with confusion, feeling misunderstood, or angry with him, Weakland would do a *U-turn*, that is, shift gears and try something else (Segal, 1991; Fisch, Weakland, & Segal, 1982).

When faced with involuntary status clients who are court-ordered to see him or a couple partner or the parents who are making the identified client go for treatment, Weakland would take a *one-down position*, gather information about the referral process, and try and position himself as an ally of the couple partner or family member being forced to go see him. In trying to better understand the reason for the referral to him, Weakland would ask the following questions:

- "What is your understanding of why Mr. Smith (the referring professional) had referred you to me?"
- "What do you think Mr. Smith would need to see happen here, that would make him less concerned about you?"
- "Anything else that you can think of that we could do together that could help get Mr. Smith off your back?"
- "Can you think of one step your wife/parents would need to see you take over the next week that could make her/them less concerned about you?"
- "By taking that step, what other positive effects could that have on your relationship with her/them?"
- "Is there something your parents are doing that really ticks you off that you would like me to work on changing?"
- "How would that change make a big difference to you?"

Once the couple partner or adolescent would feel more comfortable with Weakland and perceive him as an ally, he or she will move from being a window-shopper for counseling to becoming a potential customer for change.

Signature Techniques and Strategies

Weakland and his MRI team have developed many signature techniques and strategies that were designed to rapidly disrupt couple and family problem-maintaining patterns and alter their narrow and fixed beliefs. Below, I present seven pattern intervention and change strategies. They are: (i) *go slow/restraint from immediate change*, (ii) *reframing behaviors and patterns*, (iii) *prescribing the symptom/problem behavior/problem-maintaining pattern*, (iv) *harnessing self-fulfilling prophecies*, (v) *benevolent sabotage/other ordeals*, (vi) *the negative consequences of change*, and (vii) *the illusion of alternatives* (Segal, 1991; Fisch, Weakland, & Segal, 1982; Watzlawick, Weakland, & Fisch, 1974).

Go slow! messages and *restraint from immediate change* are actually empathic therapeutic actions in that, clients who have had longstanding and seemingly intractable problems have become acclimatized to having these difficulties present in their lives. Any sudden change could be uncomfortable, increase the clients' anxiety levels, and be a threat to their couple or family relationships. Therefore, recommending that clients go slowly with making any sudden changes too quickly can be comforting to them. This therapeutic strategy also can inspire the clients to want to prove their therapist wrong that they do desperately want relief from their oppressive difficulties and are ready to take action.

Reframing behaviors and patterns, consists of normalizing or relabeling negative behaviors and patterns into positive behaviors and patterns. For example, a couple who argue all of the time are "fighting to improve their marriage" and it is a sign of "emotional love and commitment to their relationship." By changing the meaning of problematic behaviors and patterns, this can lead to a new way of viewing their problem situations and to new more adaptive patterns of interactions.

Once couple and family behaviors and patterns are reframed, *prescribing the symptom/problem behavior/problem-maintaining pattern* could be most fitting to try. With the aforementioned chronically arguing couple example above, the therapist could prescribe a *structured couple fighting experiment*. The couple are to come up with a daily 10-minute fighting time schedule each day at different times over the next week. An important rule is that when one partner has the floor, the other partner has to give him or her all eyes and ears. They are to flip a coin and the heads partner goes first. For 5 minutes, the first partner is to complain at the other partner. When the iPhone alarm or kitchen timer goes off, he or she is to say, "Thank you dear!" Anything left over to complain about is to be written on a piece paper and brought to the next scheduled fighting session. The other partner takes his or her 5 minutes and is to do exactly what the other partner did. The rules are that they are not allowed to complain at or argue with their partners outside of the scheduled fighting session times. What typically happens with couples doing this experiment is that they abandon their incessant arguing, start treating each other in a more respectful way, and identify something they would like to work on together to further improve their relationships.

Similar to the work of Weiner-Davis and other Solution-Focused practitioners, Weakland and his colleagues have their clients be on the lookout for *exceptions*, that is the times when the problematic behavior or patterns of interaction did not occur. Weakland and his team referred to this as *harnessing self-fulfilling prophecies*. Couple partners and family members are asked to catch each other at their best. Once they discovered what works, Weakland would prescribe for them to do more of what works and co-create with them positive self-fulfilling prophecies (Bodin, 1981). In fact, this therapeutic strategy had played a role in inspiring Steve de Shazer's later research on how solutions develop, which paved the way for the creation of his Solution-Focused Brief Therapy model (de Shazer, 1988, 1985).

Benevolent sabotage and other ordeals are particularly useful when couples and families are deeply entrenched in such problem-maintaining interactions as: "My way or the highway!" The more super-responsible the couple partner or parents are, the more super-irresponsible the other partner or child or adolescent behaves. Ordeals in general are more of a last resort pattern intervention strategy. They make it extremely uncomfortable for the couple partner or child or adolescent to engage in their problematic behaviors. For example, with a highly oppositional adolescent who is constantly breaking the parents' rules and has dethroned them and they are ready and willing to try anything to turn the situation with their son or daughter, benevolent sabotage can be in order (Watzlawick, Weakland, & Fisch, 1974). The parents are to pick one specific behavior they wish to change with their adolescent. If it is the daughter's constantly breaking her curfew time and coming home at 1 or 2 a.m., the parents instead of waiting up all night for her can chain and lock all of the doors and turn out all of the lights in the home. When the daughter eventually comes home and they hear her trying to enter one of the chained doors, they can take their time with letting her in. When it is cold outside, this can be a very uncomfortable experience for adolescents. Eventually, one of the parents can come to the door in his or her bathrobe looking sleepy-eyed and confused and let her in. When she lashes out at the parent with obscenities, the parent does not react and simply says, "I can't believe I chained the doors … I have not been myself lately." After this happens repeatedly to the daughter with curfew violation and with other oppositional behaviors, she will eventually learn that her behaviors are making her parents crazy and it may be better to cooperate (Segal, 1991; Watzlawick, Weakland, & Fisch, 1974).

When working with stuck couple and family case situations, Weakland might wonder aloud with them about the dangers or *negative consequences of change*. For example, he might wonder aloud with the clients if the adolescent identified client changes, would the parents argue more, or if the younger daughter will develop symptoms or difficulties once her brother changes. This therapeutic strategy challenges the family to prove the therapist wrong. However, if the parents start arguing more or the younger daughter develops difficulties, they will perceive the therapist as being very competent and accurate with his or her predictions. It also holds the clients accountable for the change effort and any negative repercussions that may crop up as a result of it (Fisch, Weakland, & Segal, 1982).

The *illusion of alternatives* is very effective at getting the couple partner or identified child or adolescent client to choose what small change he or she would be willing to make (Watzlawick, Weakland, & Fisch, 1974). For example, with a

16-year-old's messy bedroom situation that his parents have been trying to get him straighten up for the past year, he can be asked, "What part of the bedroom do you wish to straighten up first, under the bed, your desktop, or your clothing closet?" By putting the son in charge of deciding where he begins with straightening up his bedroom, it will be difficult for him to oppose doing this since it was his choice. Once he straightens up a portion of his bedroom, he can choose what the next part will be, and so forth. The parents are not to put time constraints on when each portion of the bedroom is to be cleaned and refrain from reminders and nagging behaviors. This strategy helps parents sidestep power struggles and abandon their incessant nagging.

Harry Goolishian

My first exposure to the work of Harry Goolishian was back in 1988 at an American Family Therapy Association Conference with his co-presenter and close colleague Harlene Anderson. I was most impressed with their highly respectful and effective therapeutic work with families that had had longstanding and severe mental health and substance-abusing difficulties and extensive treatment histories. Many of the families they had worked with at the Houston-Galveston Family Institute had multiple helping professionals from larger systems involved with them for several years. In many cases, the helping professionals had become the privileged experts in determining what they thought was best for the family members. To help illustrate this point, Goolishian showed us a video of a family he had been involved with that had been recycled through the mental health system several times around, each family member was carrying multiple DSM diagnoses, had been deemed noncompliant, and there had been an army of helping professionals involved with them for years. From a position of respectful curiosity, Goolishian explored with each family member if there had been anything that their current and past therapists or treatment program staff had overlooked or missed with their family situation that would be important for him to know. Each family member took risks and shared ways they had felt misunderstood and mishandled by these treatment providers and how their family situation had gotten worse. Next, the family members shared what they really needed from their treatment providers that could make a big difference to them. It was amazing to observe the power of putting families in charge as the experts of their stories, voicing their needs, expectations for the treatment providers, and inviting them to share their best hopes for the kind of treatment outcomes they wished to have.

The added bonus with the consultation Goolishian had conducted was that some of the involved helping professionals were in the audience listening to the individual family members' feedback and recommendations for what they needed to do differently with them, which appeared to mesmerize them to such a high degree that the family members were capable of transcending the various DSM labels they had been given and assert their needs and wishes in a healthy and adaptive way. When some of the helping professionals were interviewed, they reported that their former ways of viewing the family members had changed and they were not only hopeful that the family would have a better future but with their guidance as the lead authors of their new story, they could better meet their needs in their work together. Goolishian showed the same high level of respect with larger systems professionals that are involved with his couple and family clients. He wants to come to know their stories of involvement, sincerely listens to their questions and concerns, is interested in their expectations and goals for the clients, and avoids at all costs passing judgement or blaming the professionals for mishandling his clients' situations. Goolishian would argue that helping professionals can get stuck just like clients and do appreciate having opportunities to collaborate with therapists. He conveys every which way to these helping professionals that "we are in this together" and "I value your concerns, wisdom, and expertise."

Another excellent and transformative training experience I had had with Goolishian and Anderson was when I had brought them to Chicago, IL in 1988 to provide a weekend intensive live supervision training with a small group of social workers and psychologists. Each day of the weekend families were brought in for live consultations and Goolishian and Anderson took turns teaming one another. I brought in a family I had been working with where the identified client Bill had just gotten out of the hospital after his first psychotic breakdown at the age of 18. I had seen the family four times after Bill had gotten out of the hospital and he had made progress with self-care and not isolating in his bedroom. However, these changes were differences that did not seem to make a difference to family members, in that they continued to talk about Bill when he would be present in their company, as if he was invisible. The only other things I knew about this family was that Bill's mother was deceased and had a history of schizophrenia and made his 24-year-old sister Isabella go with her out on the city streets with her looking for Jesus Christ. Bill had a 17-year-old brother David who was high functioning. Bill's father was a Bulgarian immigrant and factory worker and had not participated in our family meetings but agreed to come to our consultation with Goolishian.

In Goolishian's trademark fashion, he used his warmth and inviting demeanor to create a safe sacred conversational space. It felt like we were all sitting by the fireplace with the loving and caring grandfather you always wanted to have. Goolishian began by asking me how long I had been seeing the family and the work we had been doing together. He then invited family members to reflect on what I had shared and how they wished to use our time together. Draw bridges started lowering left and right, where family members began sharing stories about past chapters in their lives that I had never heard before. I learned that there were two older sisters, one who had schizophrenia and killed herself by throwing herself in front of commuter train and another sister who had Down's Syndrome and lived in a residential program out-of-state. Isabella disclosed that her father used to discipline her with their dog's chain. The father admitted to his harsh discipline but felt it had worked because Isabella stopped her acting out behaviors as a teenager. The most dramatic change that had occurred in this consultation was Bill's confronting his father about not going to his high school graduation. Up to this point, Bill had been quiet for most of the session and looking heavily doped up on anti-psychotic medication. It was this huge disappointment and critical life event that had triggered Bill's first psychotic episode and psychiatric hospitalization. I was blown away by all of the family members' disclosures which were highly important and painful family story material that I had inadvertently been blocking them from talking about by focusing too sharply on small behavioral goals with them. After the family left our consultation session, Goolishian offered to stay in touch with me via written correspondence to offer follow-up free consultation because he sincerely cared about the family and I and wanted to optimize for our treatment success. I gladly took him up on this kind offer. Unlike other trainers or gurus who work their magic and leave the therapists and families they consult with high and dry after their workshops, Goolishian demonstrated to me that he was the epitome of what a trainer should be all about and as ethically responsible as you can get. Bill's family also greatly appreciated Goolishian taking the time long distance to help them out.

Much to my pleasant surprise with this family in our future sessions together, they would come into my office and immediately launch into sharing other chapters of the family's story like historians, some sad and some positive. As a family group, the communications changed dramatically where they talked with Bill and listened to him and respected his voice for the first time, rather than talk about him in his company. Bill appeared happier and had become more spontaneous. He also had landed a job working in a grocery store. The family did all of the work and I became an engaged and curious listener occasionally asking open-ended questions to learn more about their past and present evolving family story.

In reflecting back on this Goolishian consultation, there were a number of important takeaways. Families who have had lots of treatment and have experienced painful traumatic life events have long stories to tell. We have to be careful not to do them a terrible disservice by becoming narrative editors. Instead, therapists should operate from a position of *not-knowing* and respectful curiosity and stay close to the family's story. By creating a safe and sacred conversational space, family members can feel compelled to share the *not-yet-said*, that is what they really need from one another or never shared before, and disclosing painful secrets and other undiscussables. As a result of Goolishian's consultation, the family members not only changed the way they viewed Bill but their interactions with him as well, which led to his functioning better as a competent young adult with a respected voice in the family.

Both Goolishian and Anderson have been outspoken critics of the deficiency language that has been used in our mental health field for decades and how it can create a black hole situation in which our clients and us cannot escape into other realities (Goolishian, 1991). In 1991, they sponsored in San Antonio, Texas one of the most incredible two-day conferences I ever attended called *The Dis-Diseasing of Mental Health*. Not only were there many national and international family therapy pioneers attending the conference but some of them were facilitating small discussion groups with the participants on a wide range of topics regarding the conference theme, such as abandoning DSM labels and deficiency language altogether focusing much more attention on clients' strengths and wellness and creative ways to keep our clients out of psychiatric hospitals and residential treatment centers by sustaining them in the community through the help of key resource people from their social networks and building cooperative partnerships with involved larger systems professionals. At the end of each day of the conference, a small group representative would share the cutting-edge ideas his or her group came up with the larger group. Larger group participants than would reflect on the smaller groups' contributions and rich dialogue would take place further evolving the ideas presented. Fascinating and innovative ideas were co-generated in this wonderful conference.

Position on the Use of Self

Unlike the other pioneers mentioned earlier in the chapter, Goolishian's therapeutic stance is more non-directive and he operates from a position of not-knowing, rather than entering a couple or family therapy session *pre-knowing* about how to view the family's situation armed with known questions and therapeutic interventions. Goolishian allows couple partners and family members to take the lead in determining what they wish to share and what topics they wish to discuss. He uses respectful curiosity and responsive listening to come to know the couple or family's story. Goolishian's primary therapeutic tool was the use of open-ended *conversational questions*, which were designed to learn more about the various chapters of the family's story. As a way to keep the conversation going, he would ask more questions in a Socratic questioning manner, providing plenty of space for client reflection and responses between questions. According to Goolishian, "Knowledge is always on the way," that is, there is always more to learn about the family's story" (Goolishian & Anderson, 1988). Goolishian goes to great lengths to create a safe conversational space where both couple partners' and family members' voices are honored and respected. It is in the telling and retelling of their stories that new meaning is co-generated and their narratives change, which in turn can lead to new more positive interactions in their couple and family relationships (Anderson, 1997).

For Goolishian, the therapist's ability to tolerate and embrace uncertainty and ambiguity when conversing with couples and families in initial and subsequent sessions, can be a great opportunity for co-creating a context for endless possibilities. The same is true when Goolishian collaborates with involved helping professionals, he enters the meeting operating from a true Buddhist mindset of "Don't Know Mind," sincerely curious to learn more about their stories of involvement, their unique perspectives, best hopes, and attempted solutions. He had the ability to hold in his mind multiple perspectives from the helping professionals without latching onto any one way of viewing the couple or family's problem situation or privileging his own perspective.

Signature Techniques and Strategies

One of Goolishian's signature techniques was the use of *multi-partiality*, which is siding simultaneously in the room with both couple partners, all family members, and with involved helping professionals in collaborative meetings. By doing so, he is celebrating a multiplicity of viewpoints and honors everyone's right to their own unique perspectives or truths (Goolishian & Anderson, 1988). This can be a novel experience for some couples and families who had felt misunderstood or invalidated by their former therapists who had operated from privileged expert positions with them. For helping professionals, it can be a novel experience to have their different viewpoints respectfully listened to and honored by Goolishian, particularly if their past interactions with therapists had been quite negative where they had tried to dictate how they should both view the clients' problem situations and what actions they needed to take to help them.

For Goolishian, the *therapeutic conversation* and *conversational questions* are the primary vehicles for co-generating new meanings and narrative change with couples and families. It is the mutual search and exploration through dialogue, a two-way exchange, a crisscrossing of ideas in which new meanings are continually evolving toward the dis-solving of problems (linguistic constructions). Change is the evolution of new meaning through narratives created in the therapeutic conversation and dialogue. New narratives have the transformational power to result in changed behaviors, beliefs, and feelings in couple and family relationships (Anderson, 1997; Goolishian & Anderson, 1988).

Michael White

My first exposure to Michael White and his narrative therapy approach was at the AAMFT Annual Conference in 1987 in Chicago, IL with Karl Tomm, who was showcasing White's innovative work. It was my first introduction to one of White's signature therapeutic strategies of *externalizing the problem*, which was a major contribution to the couple and family therapy fields. Based on clients' descriptions of or beliefs about their oppressive presenting problems would determine what White would attempt to co-construct their problems into (Tomm & White, 1987). Oppressive DSM-V disorders, problems, habits, patriarchal assumptions, lifestyles, and couple or family intergenerational patterns can be externalized, depending on what the clients want to change and liberate themselves from. Once White received nonverbal or verbal feedback from the clients that the new externalized objectified problem was acceptable to their belief systems, like a coach he would inspire them as a couple or family team to conquer the problem. So, the identified client is not the problem but the problem is the problem (White, 2007). Not only is the is the identified client being victimized by the problem but so are the couple partner or family members, concerned relatives, and involved helping professionals from larger systems. When couples and families have been oppressed by their difficulties for a long time, a problem life support system develops which becomes rigidified by the partners' and family members' narrow and fixed beliefs; the professionals that have been involved with their situations; unsuccessful attempted solutions to resolve their difficulties; and dominant problem-saturated stories about their predicaments; which have become self-perpetuating by both their limiting views and those of concerned others. Any sparkling moments or unique outcomes when couple partners or family members are temporarily free from the problem's grip on them or when they take a stand against it, often go unnoticed because they don't fit with the dominant story about them and their situation. Through his use of externalizing and other questions, rituals, and letters exchanged with clients between sessions underscoring their strengths and resilience, White attempted to co-author with couples and families' new stories of freedom from the shackles of their former problems and the kind of future realities they would like to have (White, 2007; White & Epston, 1990b).

After my first exposure to White's work, I participated in longer trainings with him in 1988 and in 2000 with his colleague and the co-developer of the narrative therapy approach David Epston (White, 1988b; Epston, 2000). I began to incorporate into my strengths-based couple and family therapy approach some of the best elements of his Narrative approach and particularly found externalizing the problem as a useful strategy and pathway to pursue with couples and families that had been oppressed by their problems for years and had had extensive treatment histories. I found that the narrative approach was quite compatible with the Solution-Focused and other family therapy approaches. For example, I began to include in the miracle question inquiry with families the absence of the externalized problem, as a way to co-author with them solution-determined stories.

In 1996, I attended the highly informative *Narrative Solutions/Solution Narratives Conference* in Milwaukee where Steve de Shazer and Michael White spent three-days comparing and contrasting their approaches. There were more similarities than differences with their models. Both approaches were heavily based on the theoretical ideas of Gregory Bateson and I would argue, the therapeutic ideas of Milton H. Erickson, particularly utilizing stories, metaphors, clients' strengths, and exceptions (unique outcomes), and rituals to co-author with them more preferred future realities. As far as differences go, White's approach was more problem-focused and heavily influenced by the philosophical ideas of Foucault, while de Shazer's approach utilized client self-generated changes (exceptions) as building blocks for solution construction and philosophically influenced by William of Ockham (Ockham's razor) and Wittgenstein (de Shazer, 1991, 1985). Another major difference was their thoughts on how change occurs. For de Shazer, like Erickson, the key is to get clients to do something different, no matter how small that has the potential to ripple into bigger changes. So, new ways of viewing, follows behavior change. While for White, new ways of viewing or knowing leads to new ways of thinking, feeling, and doing. Finally, another major difference with their approaches was White's taking a stand for and empowering his clients in terms of social injustice issues and gender power imbalances in couple and family relationships (de Shazer & White, 1996; White, 1988a, 1988b).

Position on the Use of Self

White would argue that the narrative therapist is flexible, active, and uses a variety of relationship styles, which reflect different roles and strategies that he or she can carry out in relationship to the client-as-storyteller. The therapist can be an *audience*, in the sense of being there to listen, giving couple partners or family members the right to tell. The therapist can go further and be a *witness*, to affirm the validity or reality of the client's experience. The therapist can be a *director*, assisting clients in finding the most effective ways of telling their stories and conquering their difficulties. The therapist may be an *interpreter* of their stories translating them into another way of viewing them, such as by externalizing their problems and underscoring their sparkling moments and unique outcomes. Finally, the therapist can be a *co-author* engaging in a mutual process of new storytelling and co-creating workable realities (White, 1988a, 1988b; McLeod, 1997). White (1995) had the following to say about how he uses himself with clients in the therapeutic process:

> I cry with the people that consult me, and I also laugh with them. I join them in outrage, and also in joy. As I walk for a while with these people, I experience all of the emotions that on experiences in bearing witness to testimony. As well, there are contexts in which I find myself celebrating with people – contexts in which the alternative stories of their lives are being honored, when the other accounts of their identity are being fully authenticated.
>
> (White, 1995, pp. 86–87)

In a given session, clients get the full range of personhood that White brings to them. By doing so, he equaled the playing field with clients and strongly conveyed that he genuinely and deeply cared about them and their plight. White often used humor and playfulness with his clients, particularly with children and adolescents (White, 1985). I will never forget the video he had shown us at his 1988 workshop empowering a child who had been pushed around by "fears" for a long time. White had the child draw pictures of what the "fears" looked like, create a "Monster Box" with her parents, and lock up the externalized "fears" pictures in the box every night, which helped her to eventually conquer them. In a later family session, he had the girl bring in the "Monster Box" so he could take a peek at what the "fears" looked like. After slightly opening the box top, White started shaking and fell out of his chair on to the floor in his office. The girl walked over not only to comfort White but helped him up again back into his office chair. He complimented her for being so brave and for rescuing him from the "fears" powers (White, 1988b). Both White and Epston further empower their clients by inducting them into their expert consultants' associations, where they call upon them to help them to share their expertise with other clients being presently pushed around by the same problems they had conquered (White & Epston, 1990a).

Unlike the other pioneers showcased in this and in the next chapter, White used himself as a crusader against the social injustices his clients' experienced, on local community, state, and governmental levels. He took a political stand against the historical trauma and mistreatment of the Aboriginal First Nation People in Australia. With his female clients being pushed around by eating-distressed behaviors, he also was quite passionate about challenging traditional patriarchal assumptions about how women should look and act to help liberate them from these powerful familial and societal forces (White, 1988a, 1988b, 1987). Additionally, with couples and families where there were gender power imbalances and violence occurring, White would actively challenge these dynamics by not only making sure partners and family members were safe but by externalizing intergenerational patterns and male dominant socialization practices that were being perpetuated in their relationships (White, 1986).

Signature Techniques and Strategies

As part of the externalization of the problem process and co-authoring with his clients alternative more preferred future stories, he conducted two different types of conversations with them, which are: *externalizing conversations* and *re-storying conversations* (White, 2007). With externalizing conversations, there is a 4-step process of questioning. The four steps are as follows:

1 Co-constructing with the couple or family an objectified or externalized new description of the problem which is based on the language they use to describe it or their beliefs about it.
2 Mapping the effects of the problem on individual couple partners or family members and their relationships. This can be extended to how the problem impacts on their relationships with involved key resource people from their social networks and larger system professionals.
3 Exploring with couple partners and family members how the problem brainwashes or coaches them to do certain things that get them into trouble with others, limit their life pursuits, and fuel hopelessness and despair.
4 Exploring with couple partners and family members their theories about the "why" the problem chose to invade their couple relationship or family and what has been holding them back or constraining them from taking a stand against it and not allowing it to reign over them.

Some examples of externalizing questions are as follows:

• "What contributed to your becoming vulnerable prey to and being pushed around by the Anorexia?"

- "Which would you prefer, a self-erasing (anorectic) or a self-embracing lifestyle?"
- "In what settings or situations is 'cutting' (self-injury) most likely to prey on you?"
- "What kind of things happen that you think lead to 'cutting' taking over?"
- "What has Bipolar brainwashed you to do that goes against your better judgment?"
- "What effect does Depression have on your relationships and life pursuits?"
- "Does Depression put up a smokescreen that prevents you from seeing all of your strengths and resourcefulness, or can you see through it?"
- "Why do you think 'arguing' chose to invade your couple relationship and how does it get the best of you?"
- "I'm curious, did 'arguing' get the best of your relationship with you and your parents when you were growing up?"
- "In what ways is 'arguing' wreaking havoc in your relationship with your daughter?"
- "Which would you prefer, a self-erasing (anorectic) or a self-embracing lifestyle?"

Unique outcomes and *sparkling moments*, which are the times when couple partners and family members stand up to the problem and don't allow it to get the best of them by tapping into their useful self-talk and resourcefulness with creative problem-solving. This useful couple and family re-storying information helps White to thicken the counter-plot or evolving alternative story that they have been successful at outsmarting and not allowing the problem to push them around. It is the unique outcomes and sparkling moments that serve as the scaffolding for the re-storying process and development of an alternative client preferred story of pioneering a new direction with their lives free of the problem. Some examples of re-storying questions are as follows:

- "What do you tell yourself to avoid accepting invitations from 'anger' to lock horns with your wife?"
- "Have there been any times lately where you have been able to outsmart or stand up to the ADD and did not allow it to push you around when it was lurking about?"
- "Any other times you can think of where you courageously stood up to ADD and put it in its place?"
- "How about your partner, can you think of any times lately where 'coke' (cocaine) tried to seduce you into using but your wife thwarted its hold on you?"
- "What kinds of things have you been telling yourself lately to frustrate 'coke' and take back control of your life and your marriage from it?"
- "As you continue to trailblaze a more positive direction with your marriage, how are you viewing each other and your relationship differently now, as opposed to how you used to view your situation when we first starting working together?"

As part of the re-storying process, White amplifies and consolidates the positive effects of the couple and family's unique outcomes and sparkling moments on their new views of themselves, changes in relationship interactions, new hopes, dreams, and future possibilities. White contends that the most rewarding aspect of the therapeutic process is to contribute to rich story development with his clients. Once liberated from the clutches of the problem and the dominate narratives that had been oppressing them, clients' personal agency returns and they can pioneer the kind of future reality they would like to have (White, 2007).

Letter-writing is used by White and Epston to further underscore new and positive developing themes of their evolving alternative story, to highlight and thicken *news of a difference* (client changes and new ways of viewing their situation), and to offer after session reflections and questions for the couple or family to ponder between sessions (Maisel, Epston, & Borden, 2004; Epston, 2000). The use of letter-writing in therapy conveys to the clients your investment in and how much you care about them. It also can help strengthen the therapist's alliances with both couple partners and family members.

The next two *pioneers* presented in this chapter Virginia Satir and Peggy Papp co-authored with families and couples more preferred future stories for themselves through the use of drama, ritual, metaphor, movement, and space. They are the creators of *family sculpting* and *couple choreography* respectively (Satir, 1988; Papp, 1983). Both of these therapeutic strategies help families and couples temporarily step outside of their systems and gain a meta-perspective of their family and couple relationships to see how they get stuck, fuel relationship conflicts with one another, and what they do that contributes to emotional and physical disconnection in their family and couple relationships. Both the use of family sculpting and couple choreography provide insight and teachable moments for changing problem-maintaining interactions in their relationships and learning more positive ways of interacting with one another. Next, I provide further discussion about how and when Satir and Papp used these powerful strategies.

Virginia Satir

Many would argue that Virginia Satir was the mother of family therapy. Having studied her work through watching her videos of her family consultations and having participated in workshops by her colleagues, Satir was warm, empathic, charismatic, had a great sense of humor, was playful with families, was a masterful choreographer, and both a skillful observer and listener. With a given family, she celebrated and honored all family members' voices. She published three seminal books: *Conjoint Family Therapy* (1967, 3rd edition 1983), *People-Making* (1972), and *The New People-Making* (1988).

Satir was the co-founder of the Mental Research Institute (MRI) in Palo Alto, California with Don Jackson, MD and was greatly influenced by the work of Milton H. Erickson. One of her first major contributions to the field of family therapy was that the identified client's presenting problem was not the real problem but rather was a coping strategy or attempted solution for the issue or event that had created it, which fits nicely with the MRI team's view of how problems are attempted solutions (Watzlawick, Weakland, & Fisch, 1974). Regarding the identified client's presenting problem, Satir would often think about after observing her interacting with her family and hearing their stories about their situation what she thought she could contribute to her life so that engaging in the problem behaviors would no longer be necessary (Andreas, 1991).

Satir adopted a normative view of families and rather than searching for individual and family pathology she was much more interested in identifying and accentuating her clients' strengths and resources and empowering them to become all that they could possibly become. For Satir (1972, 1988) healthy high functioning families presented with the following features:

1 Family members had high self-esteem and self-worth.
2 Communication was direct, clear, specific, and honest.
3 The family rules were known, flexible, humane, appropriate, and were changeable when necessary.
4 The family's connection with the community and society in general was open and hopeful, and was based on choice.

Families who present with opposite dynamics of the above are struggling to adapt to environmental, family life cycle, crises, and other unexpected changes. Satir believed that all families were unique and experienced trials and tribulations, which can lead to their getting stuck. She saw her primary role as being the catalyst for healing and growth.

Satir developed the *Process of Change Stage Model*, which is a family adaptation framework to help therapists assess how well a family is adapting to its individual members' and as a group's changes both within and in its interactions with the outside world (Satir, 1972, 1983; Satir, Banmen, Gerber, & Gomori, 2006). There are four stages to her model:

1 Late Status Quo;
2 Chaos;
3 Practice and Integration; and
4 New Status Quo.

With the *Late Status Quo* stage, it is all about familiarity and predictability for family members. All family members know the rules and routines, may have certain roles and established behaviors, and have fixed views about the world.

In the *Chaos* stage, a change in an individual family member or in the environment can spark discomfort and a sense of instability reverberating throughout the family system. This can lead to the family system becoming unstable and fueling such strong feelings as anxiety, fear, confusion, and a high level of stress. For Satir, the therapist must help family members constructively manage their emotions and reframe this change or crisis situation as an opportunity to come up with creative solutions to help stabilize the situation.

The *Practice and Integration* stage consists of family members trying out their co-constructed solutions and new ways of responding to inevitable changes occurring with individual family members and in the environment. With the guidance of the therapist, he or she can help the family identify what works and can amplify and consolidate their gains.

Finally, in the *New Status Quo* stage, the creative solutions the family came up with to better adapt to members' and environmental changes in the practice and integration stage are no longer new and may need modifications. During this stage, the therapist needs to assist the family with helping them to modify their coping and problem-solving skills that are not working so well and offer them some new tools and strategies to experiment with that may work better. The therapist also needs to amplify and consolidate the family's positive solution-maintaining patterns of interaction. By this stage, family members have often become much more skilled at working together to better cope with changes and constructively diffuse crises that may occur.

Position on the Use of Self

Satir uses the metaphor of a musical instrument when she thinks of the therapist's use of self. She said the following:

> How it is made, how it is cared for, its fine-tuning, and the ability, experience, sensitivity, and the creativity of the player will determine how the music will sound. A competent player with a fine instrument can play well almost any music designed for the instrument. The music is the client's presenting problem. How that music is heard and understood by the therapist can greatly contribute to determining the treatment outcome.
>
> (Satir, 2013, p. 25)

Satir believed that the stronger the therapist's relationships are with the couple partners or family members, the more we can take more risks with our therapeutic moves in sessions. For Satir, the therapist is responsible for providing emotional safety in sessions where couple partners or family members can be vulnerable with one another, and everyone's voices should be respected and honored. She believed that the therapeutic process must be aimed at opening up space for healing and growth for each couple partner and family member. According to Satir (2013), "How that happens is when the deepest self of the therapist meets the deepest self of the client" (p. 26). Satir believed that in order to be fully present and be clinically effective with one's clients we must do our own work on our inner emotional world and have made peace with our family-of-origin dramas. To help achieve this end with her supervisees and trainees, she used a powerful experiential exercise called *family reconstruction* (Satir, Banmen, Gerber, & Gomori, 2006; Lum, 2002). This consisted of having the therapist bring to life his or her own family of origin experience in the form of sculpting drama work, carefully examining his or her role in the family, reliving troubling family dynamics and how to better handle them, and the impact of the family politics on his or her therapeutic work. Family reconstruction personal work often has a liberating effect on the therapist in that it increases his or her self-awareness, be more objective and less emotionally reactive to similar families he or she may see in their offices, reclaim their freedom of choice and self-worth, and reawaken their emotions and passions (Satir, Banmen, Gerber, & Gomori, 2006; Lum, 2002).

Satir used a lot of humor and playfulness in her sessions to help family members loosen up, see the absurdities in their difficulties, to take the sting out of their problems, and gain a new perspective or way of viewing their problems. She found that by providing a playful and fun therapeutic context clients' creative problem-solving capacities are greatly enhanced (Satir, 2013; Andreas, 1991).

Signature Techniques and Strategies

Throughout her long and illustrious family therapy career, Satir contributed many major therapeutic techniques and strategies to our field, too numerous to cover in this chapter. Therefore, I present some of her major therapeutic techniques and strategies Satir regularly employed in her family therapy sessions. As mentioned earlier, Satir was heavily influenced by the therapeutic wizardry of Milton H. Erickson and incorporated a lot of his techniques and strategies in work, such as the use of *presuppositional language and questions, embedded commands, positively relabeling negative behaviors and reframing, striving to help her clients achieve their desired treatment outcomes* (Andreas, 1991).

Presuppositional language is embedding in one's questions with words like: *when, will, going to, used to,* which is known as *change talk* in Solution-Focused Brief Therapy circles (Gingerich, de Shazer, & Weiner-Davis, 1988). Satir would ask family members the following:

- "When the three of you are communicating better what *will* that look like?"
- "What are you *going to* do over the next week to further improve your communications?"
- "How *will* you know that you are really succeeding in counseling?"

By conveying with confidence that the clients will change and it is only a matter of *when,* can greatly influence their behavior and compel them to take action.

Embedded commands are designed to indirectly instruct a client to do something without making it an obvious order or command. For example, with a couple that argue a lot, "I think it would be very interesting to see how your wife will respond to you *when you refuse to argue* with her the next time you get into it."

No matter how extreme, problematic, or negative a family member's behavior was, Satir was quite skilled at relabeling or reframing it into something positive. For example, an angry parent is a *concerned* and *committed* parent. By pointing out the positive intentions of negative behaviors of a particular family member or a destructive family interaction, offers family members a new way of viewing them, which can dramatically change their beliefs about them. Satir used positive relabeling and reframing as a way to begin co-authoring alternative more preferred stories with her clients.

Like Erickson and Weiner-Davis, Satir was present and future-oriented and strived to empower her clients to achieve their desired future outcomes (Andreas, 1991). She used the following questions for goal-setting:

- "What do you want to change?"
- "How will you know when it happened?"
- "What stops you now from achieving it?"
- "What do you need to achieve it?"

Satir believed that clients should take the lead in determining the goals for therapy. She believed the therapist's job was to negotiate solvable treatment goals with his or her clients to optimize for their success at achieving them.

Out of all of her signature techniques and strategies, *family sculpting* is what Satir is most well-known for. Family sculpting is a versatile in-session therapeutic strategy that can be used at any stage of treatment for helping family members temporarily step outside of their family system to gain a meta-perspective of their family dynamics, such as: problem-maintaining interactions, power and control unbalances in their relationships, closeness and distance in relationships, and rigid role behaviors. Although the family sculptures are static, they offer family members valuable insight into how their negative interactions are maintained and what specifically would have to change to improve their relationships and overall family functioning. For example, Satir would invite the identified client daughter to sculpt her family in terms of closeness and distance to other family members and use herself as an emotional barometer as Satir moved her closer to more distant members. The daughter would let her know when to stop. Satir would then ask what specifically would have to change with a distant family member and in their relationship that would make it more comfortable to get closer to him or her. The daughter is also to choreograph how family members' facial expressions and postures look to her. Satir sometimes would use props like ropes to highlight rigid family rules, role behaviors, and expectations. Family sculpting can be quite helpful to use early in family therapy for learning about problem-maintaining family dynamics, which can offer several locus points for intervention. At times, Satir would have family members add movement to their sculptures to increase their awareness about their problem-maintaining interactions that may be occurring in a given session and as an opportunity to learn how to interact differently with one another (Satir, 1988; Satir & Baldwin, 1984).

Peggy Papp

Peggy Papp brought to her therapeutic work with couples and families an integrative systemic family therapy approach that incorporated the therapeutic ideas of Nathan Ackerman, advancements of the Bowenian approach by Philip Guerin and Thomas Fogarty, the MRI Brief Strategic model, and the innovative work of the Milan Systemic Therapy team (Guerin et al., 1987; Fogarty, 1976a, 1976b; Watzlawick, Weakland, & Fisch, 1974; Palazzoli et al., 1978; Papp, 1983). While on the faculty at the Ackerman Institute for the Family, Papp spearheaded four major projects with her colleagues, they were: The Brief Therapy Project, Adolescents and their Families Project, The Women's Project, and the Depression and Gender Project. She edited, authored, and co-authored four seminal couple and family therapy books, they are: *Couples on the Fault Line: New Directions for Therapists* (2000); *Family Therapy: Full-Length Case Studies* (1977); *The Process of Change* (1983); and (with Marianne Walters, Betty Carter, and Olga Silverstein) *The Invisible Web: Gender Patterns in Family Relationships* (1988).

In addition to helping to advance the feminist family therapy movement through the Women's Project, her Depression and Gender Project research findings not only demonstrated the efficacy of couple therapy with a depressed partner but it sparked new insights on how men and women get depressed for different reasons, cope with depressive symptoms differently, and are responded to differently by their partners (Papp, 2000b). Her *couple choreography* strategy was one of her most important contributions to the couple therapy field. This highly creative and powerful therapeutic strategy can help couples to transcend their usual unproductive and destructive words and ways of mishandling disagreements and longstanding conflicts through the use of dreaming, fantasy, metaphors, drama, and movement. I discuss in more detail the mechanics of couple choreography later in this chapter.

When working with couples and families, Papp was particularly interested in assessing what function the symptom or problem serves in stabilizing the couple or family, determining in what ways does the couple or family functioning maintains the symptom or presenting problem, and trying to assess what is the *central theme* that the couple partners and family members organize themselves around. Papp believes that symptoms or problems develop in couple relationships and families in response to some major change or anticipated change around family life cycle transitions and crises, such as: the birth of the first child, higher parental stress in the adolescent stage, leaving home, parental divorce, serious illnesses, deaths, and so forth. These major changes can shake up the couple relationship and family equilibrium, which can lead to symptom or problem development as a result. The changes also can fuel anxiety and the surfacing of unresolved longstanding conflicts, in which symptom or problem development can be protective and defocus everyone's attention on the symptom-bearer rather than the threatening change. It also can be a valiant effort by a couple partner or family member to prevent the change (Papp, 1983, 2000a, 2000b).

There are three major levels of functioning that Papp assesses for with new couple and family clients, they are: the *behavioral, emotional,* and *ideational* levels (Papp, 1983). In order to get a clear picture of how the couple partners or family members organize themselves around the presenting problem when it occurs, Papp recruits one of the partners or a family member to give her a videotape description of how things look when the identified client is symptomatic or engaging problematic behavior, that is what specifically do they do (their attempted solutions) and how does the identified client respond, tracking the whole circular process. By doing so, Papp can learn about their unproductive attempted solutions and how the symptom or problems is being maintained behaviorally.

On the emotional level, Papp assesses how feelings are expressed and what functions they play in the couple relationship or family. For Papp the expression of feelings and how they are expressed can be triggering to a couple partner or family members, and they in turn may express feelings that can trigger an escalation of intense feelings and highly emotional exchanges. She tries to determine with the couple partners and family members in what specific situations or contexts are strong feelings aroused or expressed.

With the ideational level, Papp wants to learn from the couple partners or family members their perceptions or beliefs about why the problem exists and how they respond to each other's unique perspectives. Papp also listens carefully to the couple partners' or family members' metaphors and attitudinal statements, such as a mother telling her launching son, "I know that you want to go out-of-state for college but family is the most important thing in life, so I would prefer that you live closer to us." Often, these beliefs and attitudes are rooted in one's family-of-origin experiences and Papp would explore this with the mother. More than likely, Papp will discover that a similar message was given to her by her mother and that her family was also quite enmeshed and the launching of a member was perceived as a threat to status quo. Papp (1983) has found that by gathering this historical information it may uncover the central theme that ties the behavioral, emotional, and ideational levels of family functioning together.

With couples, Papp contends that we need to observe for *reciprocity* in their relationships and the central theme which organizes it. Some common examples of reciprocity in a couple relationships are as follows: pursuer-distancer, over-adequate-under-adequate, and super-responsible-super-irresponsible. For Papp, she is most interested in the central emotional theme in the couple relationship and how it is connected to and maintained by their reciprocal positioning (Papp, 1983, 2000a, 2000b).

Position on the Use of Self

Similar to Satir, Papp used her natural charisma, warmth, compassion, empathy, and great sense of humor to quickly foster cooperative partnerships with couples and families. She used curiosity and generous listening as a way to learn what a couple or family's central theme was, what repetitive patterns of interaction and beliefs were maintaining their presenting symptoms or problems, and empathically explored with them any fears or concerns they may have about the consequences of change.

When working with couples and families, Papp believed that it is critical that we are gender and culturally sensitive and be aware of our own biases and unhelpful beliefs about gender role behaviors and how marital relationships and families should function. In couple therapy, Papp gave the couple partners the lead voice in not only determining their goals but what issues were worth fighting for or should be ignored, how much involvement should one or both spouses have with their ex-partners, and what the boundaries will be with their relationships with their in-laws (Papp, 2000a).

Like Satir, Papp was a master choreographer and her office became a Broadway theater production with her use of couple choreography. It empowered couples to transcend their usual verbal jousting with one another and tap their imagination powers through the use of metaphors, dreaming, fantasizing to find their own unique creative solutions to their presenting difficulties.

Signature Techniques and Strategies

In her Brief Therapy Project, Papp and her colleagues used paradoxical interventions with families inspired by the Milan Systemic therapy team (Papp, 1983). They found that paradoxical interventions worked particularly well with couples and families that have had longstanding difficulties presenting with rigidly entrenched patterns of interactions and belief systems. One type of paradoxical intervention they used were *defiance-based*. This consisted of sharing with the family a double message simultaneously albeit sounding contradictory: the first message implied that changing would be a good thing, while the other message would indicate that there may be negative costs to changing. The hope here is the family will rebel against the second message and prove to the therapist and his team that they can change without repercussions. Papp and her colleagues use a similar strategy with an observing consultation team, which is called the *therapeutic debate* (Sheinberg, 1985). The therapist takes the pro-change position with the family while her colleagues are skeptical about this being good for the family and take the stability position about the dangers of changing. Sometimes a team member will take the side of the parents and another team member takes the side of the adolescent or whoever is the identified client and encourages them to dig in more and resist change.

Papp also used *compliance-based* interventions like *reversals* with couples and families. A couple partner or family member is instructed to do the opposite of how he or she typically interacts with the other partner or family members as an experiment to see how they respond (Papp, 1983). This pattern intervention strategy is similar to the *do something different* therapeutic experiment Weakland and the MRI team used, as well as de Shazer and his colleagues (de Shazer, 1999; de Shazer et al., 2007).

Since Papp was influenced by the MRI team, she used *reframing* and *restraint from immediate change* regularly with couples and families. With reframing it offered couples and families a new way of viewing their presenting symptoms or problems. Restraint from immediate change was used with couples and families with longstanding difficulties to encourage them to go slow with the change process to help lower their anxiety levels and better adjust to symptom reduction or changes with the presenting problem that they have been organized around.

Finally, it is Papp's couple choreography therapeutic strategy that is one of her greatest contributions to the couple therapy field. Although she typically would use this strategy in a couple group therapeutic context, it can be used with individual couples. There are five steps that the therapist guides the couple to take when using this strategy, they are:

1 The couple partners are to close their eyes and have a dream or fantasy about their partner and visualize him or her in whatever symbolic form he or she would take in the dream or fantasy.
2 They are then asked to visualize what form they themselves would take in relation to his or her partner's form to assure that the dream or fantasy will be systemic as well as symbolic.
3 They are asked to imagine what movement or dance would take place between these two forms, given the presenting problems they described to you.
4 Next, they are to enact the dream or fantasy physically with one another.
5 The therapist guides them through the enactment, asking them to provide the details of time, setting, mood, and movement (Papp, 1983, p. 142).

While observing the couple's dramatization, the therapist needs to reflect on the following four questions:

• "What is the central theme in which the problem is organized?"
• "What are the reciprocal perceptions and positions of each partner?"
• "What is the pattern of interaction that results from their negotiations to maintain their reciprocal positions?"
• "What will be the negative consequences of change for this couple?"

The power in couple choreography is that it shuts down the typical problem-maintaining interactions and words change to images, movements, space, and physical positioning. According to Papp, "What emerges is a living, moving picture in which complex relationships are condensed into simple, eloquent images uncensored by logic." (Papp, 1983, p. 143). Changes in the couple's interactions, beliefs, and reciprocal positioning can dramatically occur quite rapidly using couple choreography. Like family sculpting, couple choreography is a versatile therapeutic strategy that can be used in the first session as part of the couple assessment process and used throughout the course of therapy as a measurement of change.

The Co-authors: A Comparative Analysis

In this section of the chapter, I present a comparative analysis of how each of the master therapists used themselves as the catalysts for change in the therapeutic process with couples and families. In addition, I attempt to extract the key ingredients and techniques that the masters' brought to their clients for co-creating a therapeutic climate ripe for change and ultimately, compelling future realities with them. Important findings from psychotherapy process research on the role *therapist effects* play in building strong therapeutic alliances and contributing to positive treatment outcomes are presented to help provide some empirical support for what made the masters so effective with their clients.

All of the masters possessed strong *facilitative interpersonal skills*, which consists of the following: empathy, warmth, genuineness, validation, exhibited a high level of presence and active responsiveness, excellent listening and observation skills, intuitive understanding, established both strong emotional connections with and emotional safety with their clients in sessions, engendered hope, were transparent and used self-disclosure in a purposeful way, used humor and playfulness, were collaborative with goal consensus and purposeful focused work with their clients, and had gentle persuasive skills (Duncan, 2019; Barkham, Lutz, Lambert, & Saxon, 2017; Wampold, Baldwin, Holtforth, & Imel, 2017; Anderson & Hill, 2017; Knox et al., 2017; Anderson, Crowley, Himawan, Holmberg, & Uhlin, 2016; Hansen, Lambert, & Vlass, 2015; Pereira & Barkham, 2015; Friedlander, Escudero, Heatherington, & Diamond, 2011). The masters possessed charisma, that is their passion, compelling attractiveness, likability, magnetic charm, wisdom, and high levels of compassion and commitment conveyed to their clients was infectious and paved the way for rapid alliance-building, and raised their hope, optimism, and expectancy levels that they were going to have a positive treatment outcome. Duncan (2019) found in his large Norwegian couple therapy research study that therapist's effects contributed to 57% of the positive treatment outcomes of the participants. According to Duncan (2019), "Clients remember us, not our techniques. They remember what they liked about us and our work together." Bacon (2018) contends that many of the masters of family therapy, including Erickson possessed a perfect balance of wisdom and compassion that were important elements of their charisma.

The masters believed that their clients were the true experts on their lives and possessed the necessary strengths and resources and self-healing capacities for change. Bohart and Tallman (2022), Greaves (2022), and Rennie (1994, 1992) found in their qualitative research that the client is the true hero in making therapy work, while the therapist's expertise is identifying and utilizing to maximum degree their clients' expertise and in igniting their self-healing capacities.

Another characteristic the masters shared was therapeutic flexibility with attempting to find *fit* with both what couple partners and family members needed from them in their therapeutic relationships with them and with tailor-fitting their treatment approaches to the unique needs, characteristics, and goals of their clients. In the therapeutic process, the masters were very attuned and responsive to providing what the clients needed in their relationships with them in any given moment in sessions, such as being more conversational, more or less active, listening and reflecting, using more humor and playfulness, and carefully selecting the right therapeutic questions to ask or interventions to try that they thought might benefit their clients, or even held off on trying certain therapeutic interventions after determining that the clients may not be ready for them (Stiles & Horvath, 2017; Fluckiger, Del Re, Wampold, Symonds, & Horvath, 2012). Erickson was quite outspoken against therapists who rigidly adhered to their choice therapy approaches and routinely tried to fit their clients into the box of their therapy models. He believed that therapists should be flexible and tailor-fit their approaches to the unique needs of their clients (Short, 2020; Havens, 1996; O'Hanlon, 1987).

Schon (1983) has identified two operations that therapists can use to stay therapeutically flexible and keep an open mind in the therapeutic process, they are: *reflection-in-action* and *reflection-on-action*. Reflection-in-action is therapists' ability to step outside of themselves, like double vision in their moment-to-moment interactions with their clients and observe how their clients are responding to what they say or do, and adjust their therapeutic stances accordingly to provide better fit in their relationships with them. Reflection-on-action is asking oneself, "If I could conduct this session all over again, what would I have done differently?" By taking the time to incubate and reflect on this question, helps us to stay therapeutically flexible, hold in our minds and play with multiple ways of viewing our clients' situations, and entertain new ways we can improve upon our therapeutic approach with the clients in future sessions. All of the masters presented in this chapter relied on some form of these therapeutic operations to better find fit with their clients in terms of the relationships of choice that would best meet their needs and with therapeutic decision-making with them.

The masters possessed *extraordinary presence* with their clients (Hayes & Vinca, 2017). Extraordinary presence consists of being fully and deeply centered, relaxed, open, and alert. Therapists with extraordinary presence are interested in both their inner and outer experiences without losing their attentional focus with the client. According to Hayes and Vinca:

> In a state of extraordinary presence, the therapist is likely to facilitate change, irrespective of theoretical orientation or specific interventions; the quality of extraordinary presence is therapeutic in and of itself.
>
> (Hayes & Vinca, 2017, p. 96)

Since both Weiner-Davis's solution-focused brief therapy and Weakland's MRI brief problem-focused approaches are heavily based on Erickson's therapeutic work, there are more similarities than differences in how they used themselves as the catalysts for change. Like a super sleuth detective, Weiner-Davis skillfully sifts through clients' *problem talk* and listens for and seizes their past successes at coping and problem-solving, self-generated pretreatment changes, and exceptions occurring in sessions to utilize as building blocks for co-constructing solutions with them (Weiner-Davis, personal communication, May 22, 2022; O'Hanlon & Weiner-Davis, 1989; Gingerich, de Shazer, & Weiner-Davis, 1988). Weiner-Davis's high levels of optimism, passion, presence, great sense of humor, and use of personal marital storytelling has successfully ignited hope in and provided a context ripe for change for the many couples she had worked with hanging on by a thread with their marriages and dead-locked and entrenched in conflict (Weiner-Davis, personal communication, May 25, 2022). Although Weakland would keep his ears open for client exceptions and encourage clients to do more of what works, he was much more interested in finding out about clients' unsuccessful attempted solutions that were perpetuating their difficulties and like Erickson, getting them to do something different. Erickson, Weiner-Davis, and Weakland go to great lengths to negotiate realistic and solvable behavioral goals with their clients to pave the way for co-constructing with them blueprints for change. Even Satir, incorporated into her experiential family treatment approach many of Erickson's therapeutic techniques and strategies for goal-setting and co-creating compelling future realities with her clients. Papp also integrated into her experiential and systemic family therapy approach strategic techniques from Erickson and MRI, such as determining the negative consequences of change with clients and working strategically in an indirect way with more challenging couples and families entrenched in their rigid problem-maintaining patterns by using compliance and defiance-based paradoxical interventions. One can argue that White's narrative therapy approach and extensive use of metaphors, stories, and rituals had been inspired by Erickson's therapeutic work as well.

Out of all the masters presented in this chapter, Goolishian's use of self and unique collaborative language systems therapy approach stands alone. Although Goolishian possesses many of the aforementioned facilitative interpersonal skills, particularly a high level of warmth, emotional sensitivity, and charisma, his way of using himself in the therapeutic process was very different than the other masters showcased in this chapter. For example, the questions he asked were from a position of not-knowing and respectful curiosity. He never entered a session pre-knowing what categories of questions he would ask based on particular therapeutic models and clients' responses or armed with a toolkit of therapeutic techniques and strategies to try to change and move the clients in a particular direction that he thought might be helpful to them. Instead, like Erickson, Weiner-Davis, Satir, and White, he believed clients were the experts on their stories and new what they needed and what was best for them. Similar to White, Goolishian believed that it is in the context of therapeutic conversations where new meanings and narratives are co-generated with the therapist, that it is the telling and retelling of important chapters and key events of clients' stories which can be transformative. Although some of these chapters and key events in the clients' stories may have involved trauma and other painful life experiences, both Goolishian and White would listen for themes of resilience and perseverance to underscore and from positions of respectful curiosity, want to come to know more about how they bounced back from adversity and not given up. Goolishian's collaborative language systems therapy approach is particularly useful with therapy-veteran clients, clients that have trauma and extensive loss histories, and with couples and families who have had a long history of involvement with multiple helping professionals from larger systems. They have long stories to tell which we need to honor. From a position of respectful curiosity, asking open-ended conversational questions can be helpful to use when detecting family secrets or other undiscussables, or when feeling stuck or confused by clients' problem presentations.

White also possessed excellent facilitative interpersonal skills and was quite charismatic. One of White's major contributions to the family therapy field was *externalization of the problem* (White, 2007; Tomm & White, 1987). He believed that the problem was the problem. Based on couples and families' descriptions of the problem or beliefs about it, he would externalize or co-construct the presenting problem into an external oppressive tyrant. He would than through the use of rituals organize and fire up like a coach the couple or family team to conquer it. By changing the viewing of the problem as being the true culprit in the couple or family story, problem-maintaining interactions and narrow or fixed ways of viewing the identified client couple partner or family member can dramatically change. Unlike Erickson, Weiner-Davis, and Weakland's belief that insight follows behavior change, White's position is that new ways of viewing or knowing leads to behavior change. I have found White's Narrative Therapy approach to be a great therapeutic option to pursue with therapy-veteran clients that have been oppressed by their presenting problems for a long time. Additionally, with clients that rigidly cling to their DSM-V labels, externalizing them can be a viable therapeutic option (Selekman, 1996). Some clients naturally externalize their problems, such as by saying, "Depression has been getting the best of me lately" or "I feel like Alcohol is in control of me and calling the shots." We can seize these opportunities by asking both externalizing and re-storying questions with these clients. The re-storying questions can help pave the way for liberating the clients from the clutches of their oppressive problems and dominant stories.

Finally, both Satir and Papp possessed excellent facilitative interpersonal skills and were quite charismatic. However, what differentiated their approaches from the other masters covered in this chapter, was their use of *family sculpting* and *couple choreography* respectively. These powerful techniques helped families and couples to step outside of their systems and gain a meta-perspective to see how they had gotten stuck and how their difficulties are being perpetuated. Through the use of drama, ritual, metaphor, movement, and space, families and couples can learn how to communicate better, abandon rigid role behaviors, and strengthen their relationship bonds. Family sculpting and couple choreography are great therapeutic options to pursue for both couple and family assessment purposes and to use as novel in-session techniques for producing family and couple changes throughout the course of therapy, particularly if straightforward change efforts are going nowhere.

Masters of the Use of Self

Couple and Family Therapy Pioneers that Perfected the Craft of Being the Catalysts for Change – Part II

In this chapter, I present the last three masters of the use of self, the family therapy pioneers: Salvador Minuchin, Harry Aponte, and Carl Whitaker. I refer to them as *the directors*, in that their therapeutic moves in sessions were often quite provocative, bold, daring, surprising, theatrical, and transformative for couples and families entrenched in rigid problem-maintaining relationship interactions, belief systems, and role behaviors. Unlike the more collaborative and strengths-based pioneers described in Chapter 1, they assumed a leadership role early in the couple and family treatment process and actively challenged their clients' maladaptive ways of communicating and functioning, which would often result in a crisis occurring in sessions, such as the identified client becoming symptomatic and acting out or the couple or family engaging in their destructive interactions. Once observing how the couple or family handles crisis and stress, they would begin to disrupt their negative interactions, challenge the symptom-bearer, tighten up diffuse generational boundaries or help them to be less disconnected from one another, move couple partners or family members out of their rigid roles, and help them to function in a more adaptive way together.

Although Minuchin and Aponte use a structural family therapy approach, they have very different styles as therapists. When I think of Minuchin, President Theodore Roosevelt and his Big Stick Policy no-nonsense approach comes to mind. Minuchin wastes no time in a first family session challenging boundary issues, problem-maintaining transactional patterns, and going after the symptom-bearer in very powerful and creative ways. He becomes the director and producer of a new and more adaptive family drama. While Aponte could be forceful at times and take charge like Minuchin, he tends to adopt a softer touch with his adaptation of the structural family therapy approach. He is a master at connecting at the heart with family members.

Out of the three pioneers, Whitaker was probably the most provocative and regularly tapped into his primary process to unleash and share his random thoughts, crazy and absurd ideas, and make other surprise moves that the couple partners and family members had never before experienced with other therapists. This would raise their anxiety and confusion levels, making them ripe for Whitaker's moving

DOI: 10.4324/9781003334460-2

them into a better functional state. Whitaker's office became the theater of the absurd and he could outperform the most troubled or craziest of clients. According to Whitaker:

> Why is the theater of the absurd so popular? The attraction derives from its relation to our general problem with living—our world is absurd, our culture is absurd, my life is absurd, my reasoning is absurd. Psychotherapy is like this drama, a microcosm of our living. The drama of the absurd says, "This is not the life I express, this is a work of art about life."
>
> (Whitaker, 1975, p. 9)

The Directors

I begin with showcasing the father of the structural family therapy model Salvador Minuchin. Next, I will cover his long-term colleague, Harry Aponte. This will be followed by the presentation of Carl Whitaker's unique and difficult to classify family therapy approach. Using a similar format as the first chapter, I cover each pioneer's position on the use of self and signature techniques and strategies. Finally, I compare and contrast the pioneers and present practical guidelines for when to incorporate their therapeutic tools and strategies into one's couple and family therapy approach.

Salvador Minuchin

One of the best all time family therapy training experiences I had ever had was my week of videotape and live supervision with Minuchin, albeit anxiety-provoking (Minuchin, 1986). In addition to bearing witness in observing several live couple and family consultations with him, his therapeutic wizardry, and he had the amazing ability to transform tough couple and family cases in less than an hour. I will never forget what he had shared with me on a walk we had together during a coffee break, he said, "Matt you've got to have fun in there. You need to dance with the family!" I found Sal's words of wisdom to be both liberating and inspiring. In fact, after this training experience I had become more daring, taking more risks outside my comfort zone, and being much more playful with the couples and families I worked with. Out of all of the pioneers presented in the first two chapters, Minuchin had one of the widest ranges of the use of self as being the catalyst for change. He could be highly provocative, funny, compassionate, mesmerizing, transparent, make skillful use of reframing, weave powerful and vivid tapestries of metaphors, and hypnotic with his careful use of language, such as trance-inducing specific words and themes he was trying to seed in the minds of couple partners or family members.

In addition to being the father of Structural Family Therapy, he was the author and co-author of the following classics in the family therapy field: *Families and*

Family Therapy (1974); (with H.C. Fishman) *Family Therapy Techniques* (1981); (with Braulio Montalvo, Bernard Guerney, Bernice Rosman, and Florence Schumer) *Families of the Slums: An Exploration of their Structure and Treatment* (1967); (with Bernice Rosman and Lester Baker) *Psychosomatic Families: Anorexia Nervosa in Context* (1978); (with Patricia Minuchin and Jorge Colapinto) *Working with Families of the Poor* (1998). Minuchin was the first family therapy pioneer to create an ecological systemic family therapy approach that was quite effective with inner city delinquent and emotionally troubled youth and their families, which is described in his *Families of the Slums* book. Minuchin and his team not only intervened with the family but with other involved larger systems like: the school, mental health, Juvenile justice, and child protection systems. He further developed his structural family therapy approach with his colleagues at the Philadelphia Child Guidance Center and at the Children's Hospital of Philadelphia.

Later, Minuchin conducted treatment outcome research with Rosman and Baker at the Children's Hospital of Philadelphia with what they called *psychosomatic families*, which were families with children and youth presenting with anorexia, asthma, and diabetes to demonstrate that symptoms can be both triggered by and maintained by particular types of family interactions and dynamics. Minuchin and his team successfully demonstrated that structural family therapy could be quite effective with psychosomatic illnesses by changing their family problem-maintaining interactions, beliefs, and rigid role behaviors. One common finding and family dynamic across the three psychosomatic illnesses found in their study was the role of parental *conflict-detouring*, which consisted of parents detouring their conflicts through the child or adolescent rather than deal with them directly. This is the catastrophic fear of the illness-bearing child or adolescent, so in a heroic way with noble intent he or she becomes both at home and in sessions extremely symptomatic or stages a health-related crisis to demand that their parents focus on him or her, rather than each other. Minuchin and his team also discovered that another common family dynamic was a pattern of rigid and redundant power struggles between the parents and the child or youth around eating, self-care, and taking their medications as prescribed (Minuchin, Rosman, & Baker, 1978).

Later in his career, Minuchin, his wife Patricia, Jorge Colapinto, and their other colleagues received a federal grant to use Structural Family Therapy on a macrolevel with attempting to revamp the archaic foster care system in New York City. This was quite an enormous undertaking and the work that Minuchin and his colleagues did was both innovative and revolutionary. In working closely with foster parents, all the larger systems involved, and involving the children's and youths' biological parents in the treatment process, they were eventually able to reunify many of these kids with their biological parents again (Minuchin, Colapinto, & Minuchin, 1998).

For the sake of brevity, I provide a very brief overview of Minuchin's structural family therapy approach. Minuchin believed that symptoms or problems develop in children and adolescents when there are extremes in family structure, ranging from *enmeshment* or diffuse generational boundaries when autonomy is perceived as a threat to status quo, to *disengagement* where the parents are disconnected emotionally or physically from their kids. With the latter these kids often gravitate towards a *second family* of other disconnected kids where they may learn and develop self-destructive behaviors or engage in delinquent behavior (Minuchin, 1974; Taffel & Blau, 2001; Selekman, 2017). In some cases, kids are *parentified* and overburdened or in a *cross-generational coalition* with one parent or a grandparent, which can lead to children and adolescents developing difficulties. Another family dynamic that can lead to kids developing substance-abusing and delinquent behaviors is that the parents may never agree on anything and adolescents in particular will exploit their lack of parental unification (Minuchin, 1974; Selekman, 2017; Selekman & Beyebach, 2013; Stanton & Todd, 1982; Todd & Selekman, 1991a).

When working with couples, Minuchin assesses the power and control dynamic and rigid role reciprocity patterns in the relationship. He will attempt to rebalance the relationship if there is a disparity in who yields the most power and control in the relationship, so that they function in a more adaptive way. He uses a technique called *unbalancing*, which can create a crisis in the session when the symptomatic or disempowered partner is empowered and supported. Sometimes one of the partners becomes symptomatic or disempowered in the couple relationship because one of the partners allows one or both of their own parents to become involved in their private relationship affairs. Minuchin would actively disrupt these problem-maintaining transactional patterns of interaction and tighten up their relationship boundaries. Finally, he believed that couples and families are most amenable to change at the highest point of crisis (Minuchin, 1986; Minuchin & Fishman, 1981).

Position on the Use of Self

According to Minuchin, he liked to pretend that he had sitting on his left shoulder an invisible companion, a *homunculus*, which was a mythological being that looks and thinks like the therapist and can observe and reflect on every therapeutic move he made (Minuchin, Reiter, & Borda, 2021). In support of this helpful strategy, Schon (1983) found in his research with expert practitioners from a wide range of professional disciplines that they used *reflection-in-action*, that is, stepping outside of themselves and observing the effects of their decision-making and their actions taken on the task at hand, which helped them to keep an open mind and stay flexible while trying to master the task.

Another important dimension of the use of self in structural family therapy is determining in the therapeutic process how and when to position oneself closer or more distant from particular family members. Both of these positions have advantages and disadvantages. When in closer proximity, it is harder to step back and reflect and quickly determine your next therapeutic moves. If we are too distant to family members, we may lose our connection with them. Based on family members' nonverbal and verbal feedback and how they respond to our in-session therapeutic moves should help the therapist determine how best to position him or herself with each family member (Minuchin, Reiter, & Borda, 2021; Minuchin, 1986).

According to Colapinto (1991), the structural family therapist needs to use himself or herself in three different ways, they are: *stage director*, *protagonist*, and *narrator*. As the stage director, he or she challenges and pushes the family members toward more functional and novel ways of interacting. When playing the protagonist role, he or she intervenes directly in the problem-maintaining transactional patterns by interrupting, pushing, and supporting family members selectively. In the narrator role, he or she is a co-author with the family in revising their old transactional scripts. This can lead to changing their beliefs, unhelpful assumptions about the motivations, capabilities, and limitations of certain family members, particularly the symptom-bearer. The therapist can highlight old and new family members' views of their situation, which can lead to the co-generation of new meanings and possibilities.

After establishing rapport with each family member or couple partner, Minuchin (1986) would conduct three major operations in a given session, they are:

1   challenge key problem-maintaining transactional patterns;
2   challenge the couple or family structure; and
3   challenge the symptom-bearer.

When disrupting the key problem-maintaining transactional patterns, Minuchin might use *physical boundary making* (physically positioning his seat between the parents and daughter) to block or prevent an anorexic daughter from using her symptoms or emotional meltdown in the session to distract the parents from directly addressing a surfacing longstanding conflict in their relationship. Minuchin would instruct family members to talk directly with one another rather than through a family member playing a switchboard operating role in the family. In order to prevent couple partners and family members from looking at him, he would look at his left foot, let them know that he was listening, and that they needed to talk to one another. According to Minuchin, this is how the therapist can become temporarily invisible in the session (Minuchin, 1986; Minuchin & Fishman, 1981).

When challenging both the enmeshed or disengaged family structure or the symptom-bearer, Minuchin would *kick and stroke* couple partners or family members. This consisted of first being provocative or challenging them directly and then compliment them on their skillful use of their protective and dramatic use of their symptoms or extreme behaviors. Sometimes he would weave together a tapestry of metaphors to provide the couple partners or family members with provocative, new, and vivid ways of viewing their situations, which could lead to dramatic changes in couple partners or family members' beliefs and behaviors. For example, with my family of Roger and Tim described at the beginning of Chapter 1, in challenging both their enmeshed family structure and Tim as the symptom-bearer, he used the metaphors of Corsican twins and how Tim was like *Zelig*, the lead character in Woody Allen's movie *Zelig*, who was a human chameleon and could turn into a woman, a Latino person, a movie star, and so forth in an effort to find an identity (Minuchin, 1986; Allen, 1983). Minuchin also made good *use of props* to be provocative and challenge clients. With Roger and Tim, Minuchin found a palmistry hand on a coffee table in the same room we were doing our consultation together. He then held the Tim's hand right next to the palmistry hand and pointed out to him in a highly provocative way that he lacked the "separate line of life and would not be able to separate from his father." Tim reacted in an angry way indicating that he disagreed with Minuchin's prediction. Minuchin then jokingly shared with us that he had no idea that "palmistry hands could be a useful psychiatric tool!" (Minuchin, 1986)

Colapinto (1991), a long-time associate of Minuchin's, believed that it is the therapist's behavior that helps families to change not his or her therapeutic techniques and strategies. Sprenkle, Davis, and Lebow (2009) have adopted a similar view that the therapist's use of self could be considered as a common factor in that the qualities and capabilities of the therapist are more important than one's chosen therapeutic approach. Minuchin believed that therapists should adopt a leadership role, knowing when to work with subsystems (seeing parents and kids separately), having good timing with trying out specific interventions, engendering hope, and eschew competence and confidence with their clients. What Minuchin is referring to are therapist *structuring skills*, which have been highly rated in family treatment outcome studies by clients as what contributed to their success in therapy (Alexander et al., 2013; Minuchin, 1986; Minuchin & Fishman, 1981).

Signature Techniques and Strategies

Since Minuchin had developed across his long illustrious career many effective therapeutic techniques and strategies for changing couples and families, I limit my coverage to six of his major interventions, they are: *restructuring, creating intensity, enactments, complementarity, reframing*, and *defiance-based paradoxical interventions*. In any given session, Minuchin may use all or some of these interventions depending on what the unique needs and goals of a given couple or family dictates.

Restructuring is a major therapeutic strategy for either tightening up generational boundaries or creating closer proximity between a disengaged parent and the identified client child or adolescent. Minuchin would have family members change their seats in the session either creating more space in relationships or more intimacy in terms of emotional and physical closeness. He also would use himself physically as a boundary marker to block interference from the mother or a sibling while he worked on strengthening the relationship between an adolescent and his distant father. With enmeshed families where an adolescent or young adult is having their autonomy squelched, Minuchin would support the young person's wish for more independence and have the over-involved parent lean on the shoulders of his or her partner while they struggled with the letting go process. He also worked with subsystems in the family to better unify the parental teamwork and to support the young person's attempts to become more independent and self-sufficient.

In clinical situations where it appears that the parents are too laissez-faire or disengaged from their severely acting out daredevil adolescent, Minuchin would *create intensity* with the parents to get them to step up and take charge before something dire happened with their daredevil son or daughter (Minuchin & Fishman, 1981). He would share with the parents the following: "Your son is signing his death sentence if you don't act now! Parents rarely recover from losing their kids. Their marital relationships often crash and burn." Minuchin would often repeat such provocative messages until it would begin to sink in with the parents that they need to step up more and take charge of the situation. If in spite of more direct attempts, the parents are not budging, that is when Minuchin would be more strategic and restrain them from changing or use *positioning* (exaggerating a key problem-maintaining transactional pattern with a dire consequence attached to it) with them, that is, providing the following tragic scenario and asking them:

- "Let's say it is 3:00 a.m. Saturday morning, and a police officer rings your front doorbell, and tells you your son is no longer with us."
- "What effect would his loss have on your marital relationship?"
- "What effect would his loss have on each of you individually?"
- What will each of you miss the most not having your son around anymore?"
- "Who will attend his funeral?"
- "What will the eulogies be?"

Most parents often respond to this tragic scenario with, "Oh my God! We can't let that happen!" Often parents begin to step up and partner with the therapist to prevent dire situations like this from happening to their adolescents.

Enactments are a useful therapeutic strategy for disrupting problem-maintaining couple and family transactional patterns and offer teachable moments for the couple and family to learn new dance steps with one another. The therapist can ask for the couple or family to dramatize or re-enact a recent unproductive interaction they had in the session. The therapist can then disrupt the pattern by having them experiment with new ways of interacting with one another. This can include changing the order of involvement, moving people around, and practicing in the session new more adaptive and positive patterns of interaction.

With *complementarity*, Minuchin carefully observes for the reciprocal role positioning or coupling in couple or family relationships that are contributing to the maintenance of the presenting problem. Some common reciprocal positioning or coupling patterns that fuel relationship difficulties are: pursuer/distancer, over-adequate/under-adequate, super-responsible/super-irresponsible, overprotective-permissive parent/authoritarian heavy parent, and so forth. Once Minuchin assesses these rigid reciprocal role positions in the couple or family relationships, he will use *unbalancing* as a powerful strategy to rebalance these relationships in a more functional way minus the extremes. In order for unbalancing to be successful, the therapist must have built trust and therapeutic alliances with both partners and family members when side-taking to rebalance the power and control dynamics in their relationships and changing their rigid role behaviors. When using unbalancing, timing and skill are a must. Ultimately, unbalancing can lead to more equity in the couple partners' or parents' relationships and unify their teamwork (Minuchin, 1986; Minuchin & Fishman, 1981).

Like Erickson, Weakland, and Papp, Minuchin used *reframing* and sometimes *defiance-based paradoxical interventions* (Papp, 1983; Watzlawick, Weakland, & Fisch, 1974). Reframing offers couple partners and families a new way of looking at their problem situations in more positive terms. For example, Minuchin might say to a mother who repeatedly spoke for her daughter in the session, "That was marvelous! You are the ventriloquist and she is your puppet! Can you show me that again?"

By the end of my consultation session with Roger and Tim, Tim was much more motivated and inspired to transform his situation and set goals for himself over the next week. Minuchin who had stepped behind the one-way mirror phoned into me with the following message: "Tell Tim that he will probably write down his father's goals for him, not his own." This therapeutic move is known as a defiance-based paradoxical intervention, in that Minuchin adopted the stability or don't change position with the hope that Tim would rebel against him and prove him wrong. Not only did Tim react with anger in response to Minuchin's phone-in message but he achieved two of his goals over the next week: getting extra help with two of his classes that he was failing and secured a job.

Harry Aponte

Harry Aponte, a structural Family therapist, had grown up in Spanish Harlem, and because of his background growing up in New York City had true empathy and deep compassion for the economically disadvantaged families of color he and Minuchin worked with at the Philadelphia Child Guidance Center. Although Aponte has spent most of his career practicing structural family therapy, his original training was in Psychoanalysis and at the Menninger Foundation in Topeka, Kansas, which exposed him to other Psychodynamic ideas and to the pioneering family therapy work of Murray Bowen (Bowen, 1978). Aponte is the author of the excellent book *Bread and Spirit: Therapy with the New Poor: Diversity of Race, Culture, and Values* (1994). He is the co-editor (along with Karni Kissil) of *The Person of the Therapist Training Model: Mastering the Use of Self* (2016). Aponte is a highly skilled family therapist, teacher, trainer, and wise and true master of the use of self. I have seen Aponte present workshops and conduct live family therapy consultations several times. I was most impressed with his high level of empathy and compassion for clients and his tremendous ability to make heart-felt connections with them. Aponte has a real knack for getting in the door with reluctant and tough adolescents and gaining the leverage he needs to not lose them when he supports their parents' position of authority in their families. He contends that we have to be *intergenerational negotiators* and work both sides of the generational fence simultaneously supporting the adolescents bottom up and the parents top down. Although this is like walking a tightrope, Aponte has mastered this ability without losing either the adolescents or the parents (Aponte & Van Deusen, 1981).

In addition to Aponte's major contributions to the Philadelphia Child Guidance Center with training and the advancement of the Structural Family Therapy approach, in the 1980's Aponte and his colleague Joan Winter developed the innovative *The-Person-and-Practice-of-the-Therapist* (POTT) training model (Aponte & Winter, 2013; Aponte, 2016; Aponte et al., 2009). Their POTT training model is not affiliated with any one family therapy or psychotherapy approach and cannot only be incorporated into any therapist's choice way of working but can greatly enhance one's use of self and lead to better treatment outcomes. There are four skill areas that therapists need to achieve mastery with:

1 theoretical/conceptual skills;
2 collaborative skills;
3 external/technical skills; and
4 internal skills.

Theoretical or conceptual skills are the therapists' ability of applying a particular treatment approach or approaches to a client case situation in an effort to gain more understanding of what is contributing to and maintaining the family's presenting problems and how and where to intervene in the family system. Aponte and Winter contend that therapists must be grounded in some theoretical bases like developmental theories, structural family therapy, and so forth.

Collaborative skills are the therapist's ability to establish cooperative partnerships with the referring person and other involved helping professionals from larger systems. Therapists need to be mindful of the fact that the involved helping professions are not only part of the problem system but can be valuable resources in the co-construction of solutions. Therapists need to avoid being privileged experts with the involved helping professionals and adopt a *both/and* mindset when collaborating with them.

External or *technical skills* are therapists' in-session therapy skills. This consists of the following: the use of self in the therapeutic process, knowing when and what therapeutic techniques and strategies to use, negotiating realistic treatment goals and a treatment plan, and being effective at producing client changes and best meeting their needs.

Internal skills involve not only therapists' own inner emotional work but making attempts to resolve past family of origin conflicts that may be gravely affecting their therapeutic work with their clients. Bowen (1978), Aponte (2016), and Aponte and Winter (2013) have their trainees and supervisees "take a voyage home" and construct a three-generational family genogram with their own parents. This family of origin exercise helps the trainees or supervisees gain more self-awareness of their roles in their families and problematic family dynamics, and be less emotionally reactive and more objective with the families they work with, particularly families that look very much like their own. They believe that most therapists rarely leave their families of origins unscathed from the family dynamics and politics. Aponte and Winter (2013) contend that once therapists have done sufficient work on themselves in identifying their blind-spots, vulnerabilities, and any unfinished business from their families of origin, will help them to be much more present with their clients and more effective clinicians.

Position on the Use of Self

Aponte believes structural family therapists should be highly active, courageous with their risk-taking in sessions, and bring their full range of strengths and resources to their clients. According to Aponte (2016), there are three aspects of the use of self that therapists need to continually work on, they are:

1 Knowledge of self
2 Access of self
3 Management of self

Knowledge of self consists of being keenly aware of one's worldviews, personal biases, values, and morality and how this colors our vision of our clients, their issues, and our positions human problems and change. We must gain insight into how these factors play out individually and in our relationships.

Access to self occurs in the therapeutic process while interacting with our clients when certain emotions, thoughts, or memories are triggered in us. We need to figure out what the sources are for our reactions. We can self-reflect, "In listening to the client's story or difficulty does it remind me of my own experience in my family?" It is critical that we are in touch with what belongs to us.

Management of self consists of determining in the therapeutic process what might be useful to take a risk and share with the client from our own past experiences to help normalize their situation and equalize the therapy playing field. What we choose to share must be in line with the client's dilemma and used in a purposeful way.

Two ways Aponte and other structural family therapists use themselves in the therapeutic process are: *facilitating engagement* and *centralizing engagement* (Aponte & Van Deusen, 1981). With facilitating engagement, the therapist encourages family members to talk directly to one another rather than through a particular family member or to the therapist. When the therapist uses centralizing engagement, he or she discourages or blocks unproductive negative interactions and has the family members instead talk to him or her.

Signature Techniques and Strategies

Having observed Aponte conduct live family therapy consultations and observed video examples of his work, he does a masterful job of the timing of when to work with family subsystems and make it rewarding for all parties involved. Not only does he use this separate time with the parents, adolescent or sibling subsystem to strengthen his alliances with them but he gains their cooperation when negotiating realistic goals, rules, consequences, and privileges. He is like an intergenerational labor relations arbitrator successfully negotiating a win-win outcome for all parties involved.

Similar to Minuchin and other Structural family therapists, Aponte regularly uses *reframing, enactments, creating* intensity, *unbalancing,* and *facilitating complementarity in family relationships.*

One of the most powerful exercises Aponte uses with his POTT model is to have therapists identify their *signature themes* (Aponte & Winter, 2013; Aponte et al., 2009). When doing a deep dive into one's signature themes, therapists need to think about a personal issue they have struggled with all of their lives and continues to be a problem for them to the present day. They need to look at how they both constructively and poorly manage their signature themes and who in their lives have been most helpful with support and advice and least helpful in dealing with them. Zeytinoglu (2016) has identified some common characteristics of signature themes:

- The biggest source of anxiety or fear, such as: being abandoned, rejected, not being good enough, or failing at something.
- Something private about oneself you don't want anybody to know about it and how you try and conceal it.
- A characteristic or idiosyncrasy of oneself that limits your functioning in relationships.
- A reoccurring pattern in one's life that impinges on your functioning individually, in relationships, and in your work with clients.
- Determining how well or poorly does one manage stress and what strategies do they use to cope (Zeytinoglu, 2016, p. 16).

In a similar way Satir uses family reconstruction, Aponte will have trainees or supervisees identify their signature themes and do some deep work on them, tracing the family of origin sources for them or how the roles they played in their families scripted their signature themes. The therapists' work on themselves becomes a great opportunity to increase their self-awareness levels and self-consciously and purposefully, they then can make fuller use of themselves to connect to and intervene more effectively with their clients (Aponte & Winter, 2013).

Carl Whitaker

Long-time professional colleague and friend David Keith (2015) offers one of the best descriptions of the many sides of Carl Whitaker that he brought to both his clients, colleagues, and trainees alike:

> He was a change agent, or what I like to think of as a metamorphosis. He was simultaneously an accessible and elusive metamorphosis. He was a founder, master therapist, pioneer, innovator, artist, intuitive genius, and superb clinician. He was a role model not only for how to survive personally and professionally, but also for how to do so with vigor and creativity.
>
> (Keith, 2015, p. 3)

Like Minuchin, Whitaker brought the full range of his inner resources and personhood to his clients to catalyze second-order and long-lasting changes with their challenging problem situations. Having worked for decades with schizophrenics and other clients with severe mental health issues and their families, Whitaker mastered the ability to reach many of these therapy veteran clients on a deep primary process level and tap into his own "craziness" and use it as a resource for change. Whitaker turned on its head the importance of proper therapeutic etiquette and operating by traditional psychotherapy rules and beliefs about how best to interact with clients and work with them to solve their difficulties (Keith, 2015; Whitaker, 1975).

Whitaker first started working in psychiatric hospitals back in 1938. He was the first family therapy pioneer to observe the family's role in contributing to and maintaining schizophrenics' symptoms. This led to his treating schizophrenics in a family therapy context. In 1946, he ran the department of psychiatry at Emory University where he mainly focused on research and working with schizophrenics and their families. In the early sixties, Whitaker spent time in residence with Salvador Minuchin and Jay Haley at the Philadelphia Child Guidance Center. Whitaker and Minuchin became close friends and highly respected colleagues after their time working together. From 1965-1982, he served as a professor of psychiatry at the University of Wisconsin School of Medicine. It was here that he developed his symbolic-experiential family therapy approach (Keith, 2015; Whitaker & Keith, 1981a).

Whitaker is the author and co-author of three seminal family therapy books: (co-edited with Margaret Ryan) *Midnight Musings of a Family Therapist* (1989), (co-authored with Thomas Malone) *The Roots of Psychotherapy* (1981), and (co-authored with Augustus Napier) *The Family Crucible* (1978). He also authored and co-authored several outstanding articles in the *Family Process* and *Journal of Marital and Family Therapy* journals.

It is difficult to classify Whitaker's unique symbolic-experiential family therapy approach. However, when I had had the opportunity to see him do live family therapy consultations in the context of workshops, looked at many of his training videos, and read both his description of his clinical thinking and methods, as well as his close colleagues' clinical work, one can see elements of Milton H. Erickson, strategic, structural, narrative, Virginia Satir, Murray Bowen's approaches, and of course, many of his own creative and innovative ideas. Although there appears to be a logical flow to the five stages of Whitaker's symbolic-experiential family therapy approach, he gives himself plenty of room to take risks and improvise at any stage of the family treatment process by using humor, doing or saying something absurd or provocative, and like a magician, pull out of his hat surprises to spark laughter or shake things up with the family. Unlike strategic and other systemic family therapists, Whitaker focused and intervened on the emotional level of family members, using symbolism, real life experiences, storytelling, humor, play, absurdity, and affective confrontation to promote family change (Keith, 2015).

As part of the human condition and one's rich fantasy life, Whitaker believed that at some point in our lives we may have had fleeting thoughts of committing suicide during the darkest moments of our lives and homicidal thoughts when wronged by or extremely angry at somebody who hurt us emotionally or physically. He believed that when you marry someone you also marry his or her family. Furthermore, he contended that both partners vie for whose family of origin dynamics will dictate the marital system's reality (Whitaker, 1975; Whitaker & Ryan, 1989). Below, I briefly discuss the five stages of Whitaker's symbolic-experiential family therapy approach.

Joining

Whitaker would often begin with a new family coming to know them by their strengths, interests, and work roles. He often would present a playful demeanor and use humor to lighten up the therapeutic climate and eschew warmth and concern regarding the family presenting problems. He loved having grandparents and other relatives participate in sessions, but welcomed young children participating as well. With young children, Whitaker would get on the floor and join the child or children in their play activities. When the child would exclude Whitaker from the play activity, he would pretend to cry and say, "I'm going to tell my mommy on you!" The child and family would often respond to Whitaker's surprise move with laughter. This is what he would call *switching generations* (Whitaker & Keith, 1981b). The other advantages of observing and joining children's play activities is that it models for the parents the importance of being more playful and less serious with their kids and the nature of the children's play activity may be rich in metaphors or symbolic of their family drama situation. While conducting the family therapy session from the floor, Whitaker would tap into the expertise of the children as their parents' consultants and ask, "Do you have any advice for your parents so that they can argue less?" Parents are often quite impressed by their children's advice and it begins to challenge their narrow views, particularly of the identified client child as being "always problematic and difficult." Children and adolescents often have creative ideas about how their parents can both improve their parenting and their relationship, they are like shaman (Whitaker & Keith, 1981b; Selekman, 2017, 2010).

Whitaker and Napier (1977) contend that it is important to establish at the beginning of the treatment process with the family what they call the *battle for structure* or establishing the integrity of the therapist. This consisted of them making it clear to the family that they ran the show, determined who participates in sessions, how the treatment process is conducted, and not interrupting the therapist when he or she is conversing with a particular family member. Once the structure of therapy process is established with the family, they felt it was extremely important that families need to be allowed to win the *battle for initiative*, that is they are completely in charge of determining their goals, any major life decision-making, and taking responsibility for the change effort throughout the treatment process.

Expanding and Redefining the Presenting Symptom or Problem

In the next stage of family therapy, Whitaker redefines for the family the presenting problems and symptoms of the identified client as being a family system's problem. He looked for what has contributed to the maintenance of the symptom-bearer's difficulties and how as a family they have gotten stuck in resolving his or her difficulties. Whitaker also looked for ways to spread around all family members' responsibility in changing destructive problem-maintaining interactions and their outmoded beliefs about the symptom-bearer. Another way Whitaker broadened the view of the family's presenting problems was expand the treatment system to include grandparents and other involved relatives. By doing so, it afforded Whitaker and the family to make connections between the current symptom-bearer's and other family difficulties to intergenerational patterns and role behaviors. It helps them to not only gain insight into how certain patterns and role behaviors are perpetuated throughout family history but it can have a liberating effect for both the symptom-bearer and family members when they decide to mobilize their efforts to rewrite history and break-free from the intergenerational patterns together. Whitaker also redefined or reframed the "craziness" of the symptom-bearer's behavior and "crazy" family interactions as attempted solutions to grow but are both costing them and not working (Connell, Mitten, & Burberry, 1999; Roberto, 1991; Whitaker & Keith, 1981a; Whitaker, 1975).

Whitaker was intrigued by the language families used when describing their story and would communicate in a similar way with them. It was not what they said that Whitaker paid attention to but how they said it, such as paying attention to inferred meanings, the descriptors and metaphors they used, and the tone and mood of the speaker. Whitaker strived to broaden the family's symbolic descriptions of their issues. This led to his gaining a deeper understanding of the symptom-bearer's perspective and how it is connected to the family system and other contexts they interface with. He also paid close attention to nonverbal gestures of family members (Connell, Mitten, & Burberry, 1999).

Stimulating a Symbolic Context

In this stage of therapy, Whitaker uses the therapeutic operation of *stimulating a symbolic context*, which is analogous to the beloved *Alice in Wonderland* story (Carroll, 2018; originally published 1865). Whitaker strives to create a context in which the family invited him into their fantasy or symbolic world. He wanted to gain access to the family's primary process, their inner world of fantasies, impulses, and dreams. Whitaker wanted to infiltrate the family's infrastructure, to go underground and engage the family in uncensored spontaneity. The therapy takes on a dream-like state, the defensive wall between family and therapist comes down, and they can converse on a deeper level and take more mutual risks with one another. Both entering the family's looking glass and participating in the family's symbolic world intensifies the therapeutic experience. The family begins to share more of their inner life with the therapist and with one another. By engaging in joint fantasies, the therapist and family may co-author a fairy tale that reorganizes their experience of living (Connell, Mitten, & Burberry, 1999; Roberto, 1991; Whitaker & Keith, 1981a, 1981b). Once inside the family system, the process between the therapist and family is like play therapy. Connell, Mitten, and Burberry (1999) share a great quote from Whitaker on the importance of the therapist's use of play, humor, and absurdity:

> The freedom to be non-rational is an important part of human experience. For deeper satisfaction, we want the capacity to be silly, to be humorous, and to laugh at jokes. We want to experience those aspects of our self not ordinarily experienced when we are responsible doing our everyday jobs. Our dreams, intuitions, unique momentary sensations, temper outbursts, mediation, fantasy, and prayer connote a freedom to move beyond the experience of everyday life into a recognition of the creative interior of each person. For this deeper satisfaction in living, we need a rich feeling life as a foundation for a rich idea life.
>
> (Quoted in Connell, Mitten, & Burberry, 1999, p. 93)

The use of play, humor, and absurdity helped Whitaker to move families temporarily out of their rigid role structure and into a dream-like "as if" world where anything is possible. Whitaker believed that by this stage of family treatment family members are more congruent with their communications and open to taking in new experiences, and ripe for growth and change (Whitaker & Keith, 1981b; Connell, Mitten, & Burberry, 1999).

Activating Stress and Anxiety in the Family

In this stage of the family treatment process, Whitaker would activate stress within the family, which increases members' anxiety levels. He would push family members hard outside of their comfort zones so that they can become more resilient and cope better with life challenges and being in new territory as a family group. Whitaker believed that there are no secrets in families, only denials of what everybody knows. He strived to create positive anxiety experiences for family members, which would trigger feelings of positive expectancy and hopefulness that their situation is going to get better and that their changes were going to be long-lasting. When negative anxiety is triggered, family members will tend to cling to their familiar patterns of living and to status quo. As family members resist change and their anxiety levels are high, the therapist needs to be able to tolerate this without getting frustrated or defensive. Another way that Whitaker increased anxiety and stress in the family system was to use silence or *active waiting*. This deliberate therapeutic move compels family members to look inward and self-reflect what is important to talk about and resolve. When therapists are too active, talk too much, and can't handle family members' high anxiety levels about the threat of change, it robs the family of the opportunity to be in the driver's seat of setting session agendas, their own growth, and strive for the kind of outcome picture they desire. Like Minuchin and Aponte, Whitaker challenged rigid role behaviors family members had been locked into, which often fueled an increase in family members' anxiety and stress levels. At times, in an attempt to liberate the symptom-bearer or family scapegoat out of his or her role, Whitaker would upstage him or her by exaggerating his or her symptoms or behaviors, not listening to him or her, not talk about him or her, or outdo his or her so-called "craziness" in sessions. Moving the symptom-bearer or scapegoat out of his or her role would often spark increased family stress and anxiety (Connell, Mitten, & Burberry, 1999; Whitaker & Ryan, 1989; Whitaker & Keith, 1981a, 1981b).

Termination

In the termination stage, Whitaker uses these sessions to consolidate family's gains by amplifying their changes and highlighting differences. By this time, family anxiety and stress has greatly diminished and there has been much individual growth among family members. Whitaker left it up to the families to decide when they were done with therapy (Connell, Mitten, & Burberry, 1999; Whitaker & Keith, 1981a).

Position on the Use of Self

According to Whitaker and Keith (1981a), the family therapist is both a coach and surrogate grandparent. At times providing structure and focus, and at other times being caring and building strong connections with family members. The therapist is very active and makes strategic use of silence, or *active waiting*. For Whitaker and Keith, active waiting serves multiple purposes, such as:

1 respectfully waiting for family members to take risks and share anxiety-laden material or whatever they wish to talk about;
2 increasing the family's anxiety level and opening up space for them to gain access to family secrets and other undiscussables;

3 to underscore certain events that occur in sessions; redirect a focus back on something that had been said or was important to revisit;
4 a way to encourage the family to work for achieving their goals and improving their family functioning; or
5 a time to reflect and incubate on what was shared or what the next therapeutic move might be.

Whitaker made purposeful use of self-disclosure, which consisted of sharing personal reflections, fantasies, stories and his responses to the family's dysfunctional dynamics occurring in sessions. Stierlin and his colleagues (1980) refer to this participant observer therapist behavior as "healing by encounter," which can induce family change by producing shifts in their viewing of their problem situation and in their interactions. Whitaker's personal storytelling gave family members permission to take risks and share their own subjective experiences for study and elaboration, particularly critical life events, conflicts, desires, and needs that they have been keeping a lid on (Connell, Mitten, & Burberry, 1999; Roberto, 1991). At times, Whitaker would share with the family random off-the-wall, absurd, and humorous thoughts that spontaneously popped into his mind to inject an element of surprise in sessions (Keith, 2015; Whitaker & Ryan, 1989).

Similar to Satir, Minuchin, and Aponte, Whitaker believed that therapists need to be free of any emotionally unresolved issues from their families of origin in order to be truly present and be effective healers with families. Therapists need to be aware of their blind spots and not get in the ways of their clients' growth (Whitaker & Ryan, 1989; Whitaker & Keith, 1981a). Additionally, like Aponte's position on making purposeful use of sharing some element of one's signature theme to normalize what a family member is struggling with, Whitaker believed that identifying with and sharing a fragment or piece of one's own pain or challenging life experiences with clients can not only strengthen our therapeutic alliances with them but can instill hope and help with the healing process (Roberto, 1991).

Signature Techniques and Strategies

What Whitaker was most well-known for was not only unleashing his own "craziness" in sessions but redefining it as the ability to be unique, spontaneous, and playful. He taught families to accept their craziness and absurd ways of being with one another and how to channel it creatively both within the family and in other contexts to add spice to their lives. Connell and colleagues share what Whitaker often told the families he worked with:

> It's okay to be crazy as long as you're smart about it. If you're stupid you'll end up eating frozen peas in a mental institution. You need to be smart about it, being selective about how and where you choose to express your craziness. The trick is to learn how to make a living of it.
>
> (Connell, Mitten, & Burberry, 1999, p. 65)

By reframing craziness, Whitaker removed the stigma of the labels his clients had been given by other treatment providers, normalized it as an attempt at personal growth, and it helped loosen up narrow and fixed beliefs family members had held about the symptom-bearer in the family.

Whitaker believed that *creating a crisis* in sessions is like a psychological orgasm, which produces a *meta-event* and powerful orgasmic release that can lead to a second-order change. By second-order change, Whitaker meant transformation of the family's problem-maintaining family dynamics into a higher level of family functioning (Whitaker & Ryan, 1989).

Like Erickson, Whitaker made strategic *use of confusion* with clients. However, Whitaker used confusion to increase the family's anxiety level, particularly if they were vague or clearly avoiding addressing their emotionally laden issues. He believed that confusion stimulated connections in the brains of family members with their thinking process and helped them to begin to make sense of how they got into their current predicament. Whitaker also found that confusion helped better ground clients in the present and confront and address their issues, rather than living in the past or fantasizing about a better future (Whitaker & Ryan, 1989).

Sometimes Whitaker would *laugh at or verbally tickle* family members about their irrational and absurd ways of interacting and living together. When Whitaker would have in his office an emotionally disconnected husband and a wife and mother who worries too much, he would chuckle and say to the wife, "You know, men can be stupid. I don't think they know anything about change and they don't know anything about feelings (Whitaker & Keith, 1981b, p.249)." This provocative therapeutic move can propel the husband into action and getting more involved in his marital and family life.

Another playful strategy Whitaker and Keith (1981b) used with the symptom-bearer in the family is called *teaching acting out*. For example, with a child who had severe temper tantrums they would have the child teach her mother the necessary skills to throw severe temper tantrums. They could have a training session in the family meeting and be instructed to practice over the next week daily so the daughter could demonstrate that she was a great coach and the mother can master the fine art of throwing severe temper tantrums and perform for them in the next session. Often, both family members rebel against the therapist's directive and by doing so, the frequency of the temper tantrums is greatly reduced or eliminated altogether.

With children and adolescents, Whitaker and Keith (1981b) like to use *talking silly* as a way to both build playful relationships with them. You can use silly made up words, share riddles, and jokes. If the child is engaging in some annoying behaviors like burping loudly or farting, the therapist can have a contest in the session to determine who is the most skilled at engaging in these bad habits.

The therapist can engage in *absurd and strange behaviors* as a way to make the session less humdrum and shake things up (Whitaker & Keith, 1981b). When asked by family members why he or she is behaving this way, he or she could respond in an arbitrary way: "I just felt like it," "I just wanted to entertain myself," or "I felt like

I needed a break" (Whitaker sometimes would spontaneously get up and leave the session and the clients would be left wondering if he was coming back).

The Directors: A Comparative Analysis

In this section of the chapter, I compare and contrast the therapeutic work and use of themselves of Minuchin, Aponte, and Whitaker. This will be followed by offering guidelines for when to use their treatment approaches. All three of these master therapists possess strong facilitative interpersonal skills and are like charismatic leaders with how they took charge in sessions and gained their clients' trust to follow them on their journeys to possibility land, or in Whitaker's case, through the looking glass of *Alice in Wonderland* (Carroll, 2018). They all believed that how entrenched and stuck couples and families change is that the therapist by challenging their problem-maintaining transactional patterns, rigid role behaviors and beliefs, and the symptom-bearer will induce a crisis response from the couple or family, making them most amenable for change and restructuring into a more adaptive way of functioning. Whitaker did all of the above and went even deeper with couples and families' emotional lives, probing, pushing, and provoking the partners and family members to express how they truly think and felt about certain life events and in their present relationship interactions with one another, including tabooed topics and fantasies about wanting to harm others or themselves. Whitaker, Minuchin, and Aponte all saw eye-to-eye about the shortcomings of Solution-Focused and other behavioral approaches to change, in that these approaches fail to make room for the open exploration of unresolved conflicts with couples and families, which will leave them ill-equipped skill-wise to resolve future conflicts and disagreements (Fishman, 2022; Minuchin, Colapinto, & Minuchin, 1998; Whitaker & Ryan, 1989; Aponte, 2016). Minuchin and Aponte would use enactments with couples and families in sessions to help teach them new skills for resolving their conflicts and disagreements and improving their communications.

Both Whitaker and Minuchin were masters at outperforming and exaggerating to an absurd level the symptomatic couple partner's or family member's behaviors. Operating from his theater of the absurd mindset, Whitaker was known to put on impromptu Tony Award performances in sessions with his couples and families either by exaggerating the symptom-bearer's behavior to an absurd level, being highly provocative, or unleashing his own craziness in response to negative interactions that occurred in the sessions. Minuchin would weave together vivid tapestries of metaphors to help change family members' views of and interactions with the symptom-bearer, and attempt to liberate him or her out of this family role. Both Minuchin and Whitaker also would reframe and prescribe for the symptom-bearer to practice his or her arsenal of provocative and problematic behaviors with family members until behaving this way became irrelevant and he or she rebelled against the therapist by changing.

Whitaker and Aponte, more so than Minuchin believed that the therapist's purposeful use of self-disclosure should be used in an effort to benefit the clients. Minuchin, on the other hand, limited his self-disclosure to when he would kick (challenge) and stroke (compliment) family members when challenging them about their problematic behaviors and interactions. He felt that self-disclosing personal material from one's life distracts the clients from focusing on the task at hand, which was to help them to resolve their presenting difficulties (Minuchin, 1986). Both Whitaker and Aponte freely share their thoughts and feelings with their clients. Whitaker would spontaneously share his fantasies and absurd thoughts with his clients, which in some cases led to their coming up with some novel ideas for change together. Aponte encourages therapists to make purposeful use of their own signature themes from their family of origin experiences if they paralleled what their clients were currently struggling with to both normalize and convey empathy.

What I appreciate with all three of these masters was their high level of courage and confidence to take big time risks with their clients. Many of the couples and families they had seen, had had extensive unsuccessful treatment histories, were presenting with serious DSM-V disorders, and entrenched in rigid problem-maintaining interactions, role behaviors, and fixed belief systems. The individual couple partners and family members often have had lengthy individual therapy experiences, couple or family therapy where the therapists had not been active enough disrupting destructive in-session interactions, the treatment goals were vague, too big, or were the therapists' goals for them, and they were not given weekly therapeutic change strategies to implement. Therefore, the clients' problem situations became further compounded and they became demoralized. These couple and families are desperate for clinical leadership to guide them into a higher functional state and help them to once-and-for-all conquer their longstanding difficulties. The family therapy approaches of Minuchin, Aponte, and Whitaker can provide this and more.

As far as other clinical situations that respond best to the structural family therapy approach of Minuchin and Aponte, they have found that highly enmeshed, disengaged, chaotic, and conflict -avoidant families have had positive treatment outcomes with their approach (Fishman, 2022; Minuchin, Reiter, & Borda, 2021; Minuchin, 1986; Minuchin, Rosman, & Baker, 1978). Additionally, structural family therapy combined with strategic therapy methods has shown excellent results with substance-abusing families (Todd & Selekman, 1991a; Stanton & Todd, 1982). Whitaker's symbolic-experiential family therapy approach also has had great clinical results with specific types of client problem presentations. According to Whitaker and Keith (1981a, p. 202) the symbolic-experiential family approach can work well with the following types of families:

1 families with a schizophrenic or other serious mental health disorder member who serves as the scapegoat;
2 families with young children;
3 families presenting with multiple problems;

4 families in crisis;
5 crazy therapy-veteran families who are in for fun and/or involved in a dilemma which is multi-faceted and there are multiple people involved with the problem situation; and
6 families who are at the mercy of larger systems professionals who are over-involved and calling the shots for how they should lead their lives.

Once couples and families can be pried out of their stuck positions and see how absurd their ways of living have become by the help of the more provocative therapeutic approaches of Minuchin, Aponte, and Whitaker, their situations can become dramatically transformed into more workable realities.

Practice Evidence-Based Wisdom

A Resource for Informing Our Therapeutic Decision-Making

In this chapter, I discuss the strengths and limitations of how practice evidence-based wisdom can be used as a resource for informing our therapeutic decision-making. Throughout our professional careers, we have developed skill at and have had positive outcomes with applying certain couple and family therapy approaches and sets of therapeutic tools and strategies to particular couple and family presenting problems and as a way to offer them alternative ways of viewing their problem situations, to disrupt their problem-maintaining patterns of interactions, and change their narrow and fix belief systems to help them to function in a more adaptive way. Our brains are hardwired to recognize patterns we have seen before, which is known as *pattern recognition* as a way to aid us in making sense of what we are observing with our clients' clinical presentations and guide us with determining what treatment regimen would be a good fit for them, almost like a lock and key (Klein, 2013, 1998). Back in 1986, when I had trained with Minuchin, I had heard him say both in the company of couples and families and from behind the one-way mirror with the other trainees, "I have seen this before." In his long and illustrious family therapy career, Minuchin had seen almost every type of presenting problem and the family dynamics they were embedded in and perfected matching sets of therapeutic tools and strategies and ways to use himself as the catalyst for change that best fit their clinical presentations.

There also is a growing body of fascinating research on psychotherapists and other individuals deemed wise and how they made thoughtful and effective decisions even when faced with highly complex problem situations, which can be of great benefit to therapists in our therapeutic decision-making with intervention selection and/or co-constructing novel high-quality solutions with our clients. Some of the key findings from research on wisdom are presented in this chapter. To help counter-balance the dangers of relying too heavily on particular treatment approaches or solely on practice evidence-based wisdom with therapeutic decision-making alone, I cover the importance of critical-thinking in examining our mental traps and cognitive biases to help us make better decisions in what we choose to do both in our in-session micro-interactions with our clients, and with deciding what therapeutic tools and strategies are the best fit for helping them to resolve their difficulties. Finally, two

DOI: 10.4324/9781003334460-3

case examples are presented in this chapter that illustrate respectively the advantages and disadvantages of relying on practice evidenced-based experience and wisdom alone to guide our couple and family assessments and therapeutic decision-making.

Pattern Recognition and Wisdom: Resources for Informing Our Clinical Practices

In this section of the chapter, I cover important research on pattern recognition and on wise psychotherapists and individuals. The findings from these important studies can help inform our therapeutic formulations, how we use ourselves in our interactions with our clients and others involved with their case situations, and decision-making with intervention selection and design.

Pattern Recognition

Gary Klein and his colleagues, using naturalistic research methodology, have done some of the most ground-breaking studies on the use of pattern recognition for rapid decision-making when faced with time constraints (Klein, 2013, 1998). They studied firefighters, emergency room nurses and doctors, military and naval servicemen and women, oil-rig managers, airport air controllers and luggage screeners, and other professionals that had jobs that demanded that they be able to make quick decisions to help determine their decision-making processes. They found that the more experienced professionals relied on their past successes with resolving specific types of problem situations or crises, the patterns they had acquired over years and decades of experience, to quickly assess situations and recognize the options most likely to work. For example, Klein (2013) found that firefighters made decisions by recognizing how the situations they encountered (different types of fires and their root causes) fit the patterns they had learned. The pattern-matching part of their decisions was rapid and automatic. This is how they used their intuitions or insights to quickly identify a problem-solving strategy that was likely to succeed. Next, they would critically evaluate their intuitions, by consciously and deliberately conduct mental simulations or visualizations in their minds how it would fare if they carried them out. If in their mental simulation of the chosen strategy seemed to have potential loopholes or could potentially miss the mark with the outcome they were hoping for, they would shift gears and come up with an option B or C that may have a better shot at succeeding. Klein later referred to this mental thought exercise as conducting a *premortem* (Klein, 2002).

Through their rigorous research efforts, Klein and his team developed what they call the *Recognition-Primed Decision Model* (Klein, 2002, 1998). By carefully studying the decision-making processes of the experienced professionals mentioned above, they identified different scenarios and courses of action to pursue when faced with challenging problems with limited time for problem-solving. Below, I summarize three different types of problem scenarios Klein and his colleagues have identified with matching action steps that decision-makers should follow, they are:

1 The decision-makers recognize the problem situation as being typical and familiar. They understand what types of *goals* make sense to pursue, which *cues* are important (so as to avoid information overload), what to expect next (so they can prepare themselves and notice any anomalies or surprises), and the typical ways of responding with this given situation. By recognizing a problem situation as typical, they also recognize a matching course of action, based on past experiences solving similar problem situations.

2 With more challenging problem situations, the decision-makers need to spend more time assessing the situation, since the problem situation may not clearly match a typical case or may overlap onto more than one typical case. Another complication is that the decision-makers may have misinterpreted the problem situation but do not realize it until some expectancies have been violated. When this occurs, the decision-makers will respond to the anomaly or ambiguity by reviewing what other potential interpretations they had come up with as back-ups earlier in the process may better match the features of the problem situation.

3 The third problem scenario involves problem-solving in an unpredictable or volatile environment and/or being in unfamiliar territory with recognizing patterns for the problem situation. In these situations, the decision-makers need to rapidly experiment and evaluate single options by imagining how a chosen course of action will play out using mental simulation. If the decision-makers anticipate potential difficulties occurring or they do happen with a chosen strategy, they may need to adjust the course of action, or maybe reject it and look for better options.

In applying this research to clinical practice, it offers therapists practical methods for making sense of their clients' problem situations and determining which matching courses of action (particular approaches or sets of therapeutic tools and strategies) make the most sense to pursue, and to use mental simulation or conduct premortems to critically evaluate particular courses of action selected. Recognitional decision-making accuracy depends on decades of experience to build up hundreds and thousands of patterns and matching courses of action, such is the case for Minuchin, Satir, Whitaker, Erickson, and the other master therapists presented in chapters 1 and 2. Being a skilled creative problem-solver requires pattern recognition. We need to regularly add to our pattern recognition system new information so that our brains have a vast mental storehouse of patterns it needs to make connections between ideas (Klein, 2013).

Wise Psychotherapists

There is a growing body of research on psychotherapists and individuals who are deemed wise with how they solve even the most complex client problem situations

(Levitt & Grabowski, 2019; Levitt & Piazza-Bonin, 2016; Levitt & Williams, 2010; Roffman, 2014; Jennings & Skovholt, 1999; Jennings et al., 2008; Gluck & Weststrate, 2022; Weststrate, 2019; Sternberg, 2019; Gluck, 2019; Grossman & Kross, 2014). Research indicates that "openness to experience," that wise therapists can embrace ambiguity and unpredictability with challenging client situations and give themselves time to reflect on the unique aspects of clients' presentations and try and make sense of their problem situations before trying out specific interventions, which may not be a good fit or are too premature to try out (Jennings & Skovholt, 1999; Jennings et al., 2008). Wise therapists deliver interventions when the timing is right in the therapeutic process and carefully assess for what system level(s) or contexts to target specific interventions. They have comfort with and appreciation for emotional exploration with clients, which is strongly associated with wisdom. Their self-knowledge allows them to be free and comfortable with being vulnerable and authentic with their clients, to make purposeful use of self-disclosure to normalize their clients' difficulties. In fact, wise therapists relied on their emotional wisdom, which was grounded in their own difficult life experiences. They drew upon these experiences to better understand how to work through painful and emotional experiences of their clients (Levitt & Piazza-Bonin, 2016). According to Jennings and Skovholt (1999), wise therapists recognize the crucial importance of establishing and maintaining strong therapeutic alliances with their clients and how by doing so, it can optimize for positive treatment outcomes. They prioritize their clients' emotional safety and are remarkably attuned to their needs, they are compassionate, regularly solicit feedback from them about the quality of their relationships and perceptions of the change process, and immediately address any complaints or ruptures in their alliances with them (Levitt & Piazza-Bonin, 2016; Roffman, 2014; Duncan, 2019). Wise therapists are highly flexible, integrate therapeutic tools and strategies from a wide range of treatment approaches, and tailor-fit what they do based on their clients' theories of change, unique needs, goals, and characteristics of their clients, including adapting their therapeutic approaches to clients from different cultural backgrounds than them (Levitt & Williams, 2010; Levitt & Piazza-Bonin, 2016). Wise therapists believe that challenging client problem situations that require wisdom do not have easy answers or simple solutions, so learning how to craft and pose questions that could lead to greater understanding was considered a to be a much more valuable skill than the ability to memorize the facts of clients' problem stories or offer some quick fix solution strategies. Clinical wisdom was relied upon by these therapists when they were experiencing vulnerability and ambiguity in sessions to better understand the complexities of their clients' problem situations and to find solutions together that could work. Finally, wise therapists approached their therapeutic work with humility and did not seek to know the answers to change but rather could sit with calm optimism that they and their clients will eventually find some useful ideas to co-create new narratives and solutions with them (Levitt & Piazza-Bonin, 2016; Roffman, 2014).

Wise Individuals

Wisdom researchers and pioneers Gluck and Weststrate (2022) have done extensive meta-analysis on the existing research and literature on wise individuals and have developed an integrative model of wise behavior based on these publications and their own research. I present below some of the key empirically supported thinking and behavior of wise individuals which can inform our clinical practices. Wise individuals take the time with complex problem situations to gather as much information as possible so as to gain a good grasp of the factual, emotional, and social aspects of the problems. They "take a step back" to gain a mental and objective picture of both the larger context or contexts the problem is embedded in and to learn more in-depth details about it. Using respectful curiosity wise individuals listen generously to all the people involved with the problem situation, no matter how different their perspectives are from their own views, and remain calm, have an open-mind, and are empathic. In fact, they consider perspectives that differ from their own as interesting and informative, not as challenging or threatening (Grossman & Kross, 2014; Itzchakov et al., 2018). Once wise individuals have a clear picture of complex problem situations, they draw upon their wisdom-related knowledge and expertise to consider ways to balance the involved others' concerns and work together to co-generate solutions that maximize the common good for all parties involved. With complex problem situations, the first goal may not be to identify a solution, but to come up with workable pathways toward a solution, taking into consideration both short-term and long-term consequences into account (Sternberg, 2019). In some cases, more time may be needed with highly complex problem situations where the outcomes of selected solutions are uncertain or a solution cannot be found initially. In these situations, wise individuals will encourage all parties involved to brainstorm with them, co-generate new solution strategies, critically evaluate them, look for obstacles that may prevent implementation or any other shortcomings of the selected solutions, modify or further refine them (Montgomery et al., 2002).

Wise individuals are deeply curious about life and oriented toward learning and growth, and they are open to new ideas, inner and outer experiences, which allows them to react to challenging situations in an understanding-oriented and open-minded way (Gluck & Weststrate, 2022). Along with being highly curious, they are empathically attuned to others in such a way that they feel felt and understood by them. They are highly skilled at regulating their emotions and maintain their emotional balance even when faced highly stressful and challenging life situations (Kunzmann & Gluck, 2019). According to Weststrate (2019), wise individuals rely on self-reflection to examine their feelings, thoughts, behaviors, aiming to overcome their blind spots and biases and gain self-insight and self-knowledge. Wise individuals know their limitations, reflect on their intuitions, and are able to learn from their mistakes and failures (Grossmann, 2017). In summary, wise individuals' "wisdom state of mind" enables them to use their life experiences and self-knowledge in reasoning about life challenges or problems they encounter, to consider different perspectives and contextual factors, and not to overestimate their knowledge or control over what happens (Gluck & Weststrate, 2022).

Case Example: "You Look Old but Talk Young"

Charlie, a Caucasian 16-year-old, had been referred to me by his high school social worker for poor grades, being disruptive in some of his classes, and reports of his substance use and possible dealing. According to the school social worker, the mother had been very laissez-faire when she had contacted her about Charlie's poor grades, disruptive class behavior, and suspected substance use and dealing. She also had learned from the mother that her husband, Charlie's biological father, traveled a lot with his work and when he was around, he and Charlie were "like pals," rather than like father and son. I asked the school social worker to elaborate more on what the mother had meant by how they were "like pals." Apparently, they would disappear for a whole weekend day and do their own thing and when they would return, they would treat the mother with disrespect and not listen to her wishes. There also was a long history of the father undermining the mother's attempts to enforce consequences on Charlie by letting him off the hook. So, in structural family therapy terms Charlie was sitting on his father's shoulders in a cross-generational coalition (Minuchin, 1974). I recognized these problem-maintaining patterns that I had seen before with other adolescent substance abusers and their families. At times, the father would get angry with Charlie and yell at him when he would hear reports from the mother that he was failing some of his classes and was ending up in his dean's office for "clowning around in class." During these times, the mother would also express her disappointment with Charlie and compare him to his 22-year-old angelic brother who just got into law school. In my first family session, I had learned from the parents that Charlie had had seven treatment experiences, some outpatient individual and family therapy, participation in two intensive outpatient programs and one outward bound residential program for adolescent substance abusers. The parents opened up our session by blasting Charlie verbally for all of his behavioral difficulties and how they were seriously considering sending him to a long-term residential treatment program and remain there until he graduated high school. I could tell that Charlie was not handling the parental attack and plans for him well by his being slumped low in his chair, with his head down, and looking sad. At this point, I decided to meet alone with the parents. Immediately, they launched into a blame-counter-blame exchange about the father's feeling that the mother does a poor job as a parent when he was not around and caused Charlie's difficulties. The mother accused the father of being like "a big kid" with Charlie, rather than a father and authority figure with him. I disrupted their destructive interaction by creating intensity with the parents around the need for them to be a unified and dynamic duo parenting team in order to prevent Charlie from failing out of school, escalating his drug use into harder drugs, and possibly getting arrested for drug dealing. The parents became silent and finally agreed to stop the blaming and try and work together as a team. I encouraged the father to step up more as the captain of the ship and guide his son into becoming a responsible young man. Neither parent wanted to see Charlie fail out of school and become a passenger in life abusing drugs and possibly ending up in jail. I impressed upon them that they needed consistently to enforce their rules, expectations, and consequences for Charlie and establish a no drug use policy with him. They did agree to provide random hair follicle analyses to help Charlie be accountable for staying drug-free. Clean hair follicle analyses and other signs of being drug-free, academic and behavioral improvements, would be rewarded with privileges Charlie had wished for. Out of all the privileges the parents were aware of that Charlie really wanted was being able to get his driver's license. We agreed that we could work on this longer-term reward with Charlie once we saw visible signs and heard reports from the school that he was making a concerted effort to turn things around. I encouraged the parents over the next week to firm up the rules, expectations, and consequences they wished to enforce with Charlie. I did predict since this was new territory for the parents to be a unified team that over the next week they may disagree or clash but that these slips can be great opportunities for comeback practice and being a dynamic duo together. Finally, as part of their parental teamwork they needed to abandon negative and destructive interactions with Charlie that could compel him to want to use drugs to eliminate triggered negative emotions, thoughts, and stress. Instead, I encouraged them to play detectives and capture him at his best and praise him when he was taking responsibility and being respectful. I met alone with Charlie and asked him about his life passions and talents. I learned that he played a Fender Stratocaster, which was the same guitar the great rock guitarist Jimi Hendrix had played and that he had a band. Charlie shared with me that he loved the same rock music that I still listen to, such as Jimi Hendrix, Led Zeppelin, Santana, the Who, and Pink Floyd. I acknowledged that those were my favorite groups too. Charlie smiled. I shared with him that when I was in high school, I sang in my friend's garage band. I also shared with him that I loved percussion instruments and liked to jam on my djembe drum. Charlie responded with, "sweet" (cool) and he became more animated. We talked about his new girlfriend and how he wished his parents would let him get his driver's license so he could take her out. I had shared with him that his parents are well aware of his desired privilege and would like to see him earn it by trying to achieve drug abstinence and do better academically and behaviorally in school. I told him that we could make this happen together by turning things around in these areas and really blowing his parents' minds beginning this upcoming week by his taking positive steps in that direction. We discussed steps he could take both at home and school to help get him on the road to earning the driving privilege. By this time in the session, I captured Charlie in heart and spirit and felt like an alliance was building. After reconvening the family, I complimented both the parents and Charlie for being committed to the change effort and having consensus around what they wanted to have happen to achieve their ideal treatment outcomes. I solicited feedback from all parties about our initial session, both their likes and dislikes, and how our meeting was different than other therapy experiences they had had in the past. When it came to Charlie's turn, he said, "You look old but you talk young." I asked if this was a good thing and he said, "Yes." He explained that former therapists who "talked old" with him had lectured him about the dangers of drug use, violated his confidentiality, sided with his parents against him, and were not really interested in what he wanted to get out of counseling. Charlie went on to say that he liked that we got into the same music and that I was really interested in him as a person. I thanked him for all of his positive feedback and letting me know what I need to avoid doing with him at all costs as a therapist.

In reflecting back on my first family session with Charlie, there were some family patterns that I had seen before with other adolescent substance abusers and their families. Often, the parents are not a unified team, rarely agree on how best to manage their substance abusing adolescent, and he or she may be in a cross-generational coalition with one parent who either protects him or her from the other parent or relates to him or her like a peer rather than an authority figure. In some cases, the "pal" parent may smoke marijuana or drink with the adolescent even though the latter is being adversely affected in multiple areas of his or her life by their substance abuse. This same parent might express that he or she wants his or her son to stop using but the parent continues to drink and do drugs, which is a double standard and serves as the green light for the adolescent to keep using. Thank goodness this was not an issue with Charlie's parents, since this adds another layer of complexity. With Charlie and other adolescents, I find the purposeful use of self-disclosure, taking a deep interest in their strengths and life passions, the use of humor, and not engaging in *problem talk* to be great ways to build alliances with them. I loved Charlie's famous line, "You look old but you talk young." By exploring with him both what he liked about my "talking young" and what "talking old" looked like, I learned what to do more of and what to avoid at all costs doing with him. The other thing that is critical to do as a therapist working with adolescents and their families is to serve as an intergenerational labor relations arbitrator working both sides of the generational fence striving to best meet both parties' needs. Where there was consensus was that Charlie really wanted to earn the privilege of getting his driver's license and the parents also wanted this for him once he achieved drug abstinence and improved his academic performance and behavior at school. This provided the perfect opportunity to establish a *something-for-something* contract between the parents and Charlie that we could work on to make happen. I ended up seeing Charlie and his family five more times with longer time intervals between sessions two and six as a vote of confidence and due to their tremendous progress. The parents made great strides as a unified team, they stopped their destructive blame-counter-blame pattern, the cross-generational coalition with the father and Charlie was eliminated, and they were able to consistently enforce their rules, expectations, and consequences with Charlie. They also started to be more positive and encouraging in their interactions with Charlie, which had worked with his older brother. It is helpful to find out what parents had done with older siblings that worked that could be potentially utilized with the current sibling that is having difficulties. As Charlie grew more serious in his relationship with his girlfriend, he earned the privilege to get his driver's license. Charlie was able to achieve abstinence from his marijuana use and give up drug dealing, secure a part-time job, and with a lot of close collaboration with his teachers, we came up with a catch-up plan at school to help him to pull up his grades. During the course of the treatment process, I consolidated the family's gains and predicted that there might be slips but indicated that if they should occur that I was totally confident that they would bounce back quickly and stronger. Charlie was also thrilled that I checked out his band at his high school annual talent show. I was most impressed with his guitar playing and told him that Hendrix would have been proud of him. He responded with a big smile. Finally, I followed up with the family at six and twelve months and not only was Charlie still drug-free but he and his family were planning to tour colleges that he was interested in.

Practical Strategies for Becoming Wiser

In addition to accruing more experience working with a wide range of client presenting problems and patterns and clients from different cultural backgrounds from our own, there are some daily and weekly practices we can engage in that can increase our capacities for becoming wiser as therapists, become better at regulating are emotions, increase are self-awareness, be more empathically-attuned to and compassionate with our clients, be more open-minded and curious about novel experiences, better tolerate uncertainty and unpredictable situations, and use self-reflection to critically evaluate our thinking and therapeutic decision-making. The six wisdom boosting practices are: *institute a daily mindfulness practice, explore what sparks your curiosity and ask more questions, practice self-reflecting, try something new outside of your comfort zone, engage in service work,* and *keep a gratitude log.* Below, I describe each one of these wisdom boosters.

Institute a Daily Mindfulness Practice

By instituting a daily mindfulness meditation practice, therapists will find over time that they will start to notice the following in their sessions: they will start to notice, hear, and get better at seizing important in-session anomalies, exceptions, and sparkling moments occurring and more present with their clients due to their increase in their self-awareness levels; they will find that their concentration and focusing abilities will become much sharper; and they will be better able to sit with and tolerate listening to painful and emotionally laden client self-disclosures and stories and be less emotionally reactive to hostile and provocative interactions towards their partners or family members or towards them. Additionally, with the increased ability to maintain our emotional center or balance, we will be better able to tolerate unpredictability, uncertainty, and not knowing what to do with more challenging and complex client situations. Our capacity to self-reflect, step back and look at the big picture, and determine what the best therapeutic options to pursue when stuck will be enhanced as well. Finally, aside from all of the benefits described above, mindfulness meditation psychologically and physically can provide the following medicinal benefits: an increase in positive emotions, such as being happier, optimistic, present with others, and savor the miraculous moment; it lowers are breathing and heart rates and blood pressure level; it strengthens our immune systems, we sleep better, and it enhances our creative problem-solving capacities (Fredrickson, 2009; Hanson, 2013; Hanson & Mendius, 2009; Moffit, 2012; Pollak et al., 2014).

Being mindful is embracing all that comes in the miraculous moment, both positive and negative. Over time by engaging in a daily mindfulness meditation practice, therapists will discover that they will get better at observing their thoughts and feelings, even powerful negative thoughts and emotions without flinching, and knowing that they are temporary visitors like hiccups that will come and go on their own. So, knowing this, there will be no need to be emotionally reactive, panic, or try and flee from these negative thoughts or feelings.

We do not have to pursue a formal mindfulness meditation training class in order to know how to meditate. One can simply practice carefully observing an object or objects, paying close attention to one's natural breathing or other bodily sensations, or listen to different sounds for fifteen minutes or longer per day or twice a day as their mindfulness practice. Since I daily engage in some form of cardio workout per day when I am outside jogging, bicycling, or walking, I like to pay close attention to all that I observe, hear, and smell to help strengthen my mindfulness abilities and better enjoy the workout experience. Over the years, I have found that by doing so, I have gotten better at noticing aspects of nature that I had missed or taken for granite and have discovered how much beauty exists in the world.

Explore What Sparks Your Curiosity and Ask More Questions

We all have those special moments where something we have seen or heard sparked our curiosity to want to learn more about what intrigued, interested, or inspired us. However, many of us get caught up in the rat race of our lives and do not devote enough time to allow our curiosity to run wild and seize these great opportunities to expand our knowledge bases or to master new skills. For some of us, we have lost our sense of child-like wonder, strong desire for discovery, and undying curiosity, which used to take the form of deep diving into books and asking lots of questions. By bringing back the child-like wonder, strong desire for discovery, allowing our curiosity to run wild, and asking lots of questions we can enhance our creative problem-solving capacities and add more meaning and purpose to our lives. Two joys in my life that stimulate my curiosity, are to go to art museums and discover new artists I had never heard of before and to go to jazz concerts with top players and allow myself to be surprised by their brilliant improvisational moves either quoting lines from other tunes and be curious about how each of the musicians are going to build off of the previous soloing player with something new and inventive. With both the discovery of new artists and top jazz players that moved me in concert, I am inspired to learn more about them as people, what and who influenced them, and check out more of their work. By setting aside time to do this, we can make these positive life experiences richer for us.

Curiosity is a wonderful therapeutic tool to use when we are feeling stuck and suspect that there are important missing pieces to the couple or family problem story or secrets that we need to explore for, and to help remedy these treatment dilemmas, we should ask ourselves and the clients the following questions:

- "Do I have enough information about the couple or family's presenting difficulties to support how I am viewing their situation and where best to intervene first?"
- "Do we have a well-formulated and realistic treatment goal or is it too big or vague?"
- "Do we have a customer for change present with us or do we need to expand the couple or family system and explore with the clients if there are others in their social network that are highly concerned and may need to be recruited for future sessions?"
- "Do I need to better strengthen my alliance with the male partner or father to get him to participate more in sessions and to follow through with the implementation of change strategies at home?"
- "It seemed like we got off to a great start in our first few sessions. Now, and I don't know if others feel this way, but it feels like we have run into a brick wall and things are at a standstill. What's not being talked about that you think we need to talk about?"
- "Did any of you before you came in here for the first time tell yourselves that there was something that you were not going to bring up in our meetings together?"
- "If there was one question any of you were hoping I would ask you about your situation while we are working together, what might that be?"
- "If you were my supervising consultation team and I was to work with another family just like you, what advice would you have for me about what questions about their difficulties I should ask them, and what else should I do differently with them that might work?"
- "Anything else you would recommend that I try with that family that you think could help?"

Questions like these can help redirect us back to the basics of having a clear picture of what the clients deem to be the *right problem* to work on first, as well as making sure their problems and goals have been negotiated into solvable terms, that we have strong alliances with both partners and the family members, and that we have a customer for change present and actively participating in the treatment process. The questions above also can aid us in unsticking the treatment system by removing constraints or opening up space for the revelation of secrets that may be blocking the change process.

One therapeutic strategy I use with couples and families when I am picking up on innuendos of secrets or some other unpleasant undiscussables the couple partners or family members are avoiding talking about or when I am feeling stuck, I will use *question-storming* with them (Selekman, 2018, 2017). The couple or family are to respond to the following question: "What are the essential questions we have not yet asked ourselves about our couple/family situation?" Next, using qualifiers like *what, what if, how*, or *why*, the couple partners and family members are to separately come up with 4–5 questions in response to the central question. They are to allow their curiosity to run wild with crafting bold and intriguing questions. I usually give them about 20 minutes to craft their questions. The couple partners and family members are to take turns sharing their questions with one another. Often the question-storming exercise leads to some meaningful discussions and couple partners and family members sharing things that they had never talked about before, which can have a liberating effect on them and help strengthen their relationship bonds. Additionally, the exercise can help remove constraints and move the treatment process in a more positive direction. An added bonus for us is that couples and families often want to continue to share and discuss their questions in subsequent sessions and work on further improving the quality of their relationships and as a more unified team, resolve their presenting difficulties.

Practice Self-Reflecting

When faced with challenging situations or having to make a big decision, it is in our best interest to step back and away from the situation or decision, incubate, and reflect on your options and the potential advantages and costs of each choice. In some cases, when we are not feeling totally confident with any of the possible options, we should involve others who can offer their unique perspectives, which can either help us to improve upon our options, point out the potential costs that we missed with pursuing the options we came up, make us aware of our blind-spots, or offer us fresh and novel options that may have a better shot at working or benefitting us and everyone involved. Unfortunately, for many of us with large caseloads, we don't allow ourselves to have a mini in-session break within the hour to take the time to reflect on our own inner and outer experiences in our interactions with the clients, questions that may be useful to pose, and determine what therapeutic experiments have the best shot at working with empowering our clients to achieve their goals. Furthermore, we may not leave a window of time between each client session to reflect on our actions, and ask ourselves the question, "If I had another shot at conducting this session all over again, what could I have done differently?" Based on your answers to this question, you can prepare a checklist of what you need to do differently in your next session with the clients, such as: certain subjects to pose more questions about;

who you need to build a stronger alliance with; exploring with the clients if they thought it would be useful to involve a concerned grandparent or other relative or other key resource person from their social network in a future session(s); or trying out some other therapeutic experiment(s) that the clients may be in a better place to implement. This form of reflection-on-action can help us to keep an open mind and not lock down on one or two particular formulations about clients' presenting problem situations and be therapeutically flexible. Another form of self-reflection to use in our sessions is reflection-in-action, that is like double-vision, stepping outside of ourselves to carefully notice the effects what we choose to say or do has on each couple partner or family member both by their nonverbal and verbal responses. This helps us to find *fit* in terms of what works based on the clients' feedback.

Try Something New Outside of Your Comfort Zone

Most of us have grave difficulty sitting with not knowing, not having control, and avoid at all costs venturing outside of our comfort zones. A powerful and potentially life changing way for us to build up more resilience and grit is to once a week try something outside of your comfort zone. Whatever we choose to do, must be challenging and something we have never done before. Some examples might be: taking up a glass-blowing class, learning how to play an instrument, learning a new language, doing something more physically challenging like a long bicycle trip or hiking up or running on a mountain trail, the sky's the limits in terms of what we do outside of our comfort zones. Once we achieve mastery of the selected outside of the comfort zone activity, it will dramatically boost our self-confidence, resilience, and grit when faced with future challenging life situations. In their therapy sessions, therapists will find that having achieved mastery and success with the outside their comfort zone experiences will help liberate them to take more risks and be more daring with their clients. Finally, as the research on wisdom has indicated *open-mindedness* is an important characteristic of both wise psychotherapists and individuals in general (Gluck & Weststrate, 2022).

Be a Generalist and See Clients with a Wide Range of Presenting Problems and from Different Cultural Backgrounds

The more clinical experience we accrue working with couples and families presenting with a wide range of problems and from different cultural backgrounds, can increase are pattern recognition capacities, skill development, knowledge base, and wisdom about what works. By doing so, we will be able to keep an open mind, be more curious, culturally sensitive, therapeutically flexible, and better tailor-fit what we do to best meet the unique needs of our clients. The danger of becoming specialists with particular types of client problems can lead us to falling prey to overconfidence and one-size-fits-all thinking and treatment approaches, which loses sight of the uniqueness of each client's presenting problem situation.

Engage in Service Work

At least once a month or more frequently, doing some form of service work in the community can help us to become even more empathically attuned to and compassionate in our work with our clients. When doing service work with one's partner or family, increases more positive emotions in us and in our relationships. We feel good about doing good in the world. When my family and I used to volunteer in a church preparing dinner for 40 homeless men and women and coming to know their stories, we would leave experiencing many positive emotions and feel closer as a family. Post and Niemark (2007) found that adolescents who do volunteer work and regularly engage in altruistic acts in their communities are least likely to engage in self-destructive behaviors, are less likely to get depressed, have higher self-esteem, have higher grades in school, greatly enhanced their social skills, and have continued involvement in service work well into their adulthoods.

Keep a Gratitude Log

Research indicates that by keeping a *gratitude log* and adding a few entries per week, increases our optimism and happiness levels, decreases negative emotions, increases our positive emotions, helps us to be more empathic with our partners, family members, and more socially connected to others, can calm our nervous systems, can serve as a resiliency protective factor, and improves sleep quality, particularly when writing new entries into the log right before going to bed (Emmons, 2007; Emmons & McCullough, 2004). I regularly recommend to couples and families that they keep a gratitude log and strive to regularly express their deep appreciation and love for one another. After instituting the gratitude log, both couple partners and family members often share in my sessions how the communications and couple or family mood has changed for the better. The gratitude log is a constant reminder of how much all of us are blessed to have each other in our lives. Finally, during the darkest moments, we can review our gratitude logs for a good dose of positive emotions.

Mental Traps and the Limitations of Relying Solely on Practice Evidence-Based Wisdom

How do we know what we know? How can we be absolutely certain that our selected couple or family therapy approach has a great shot of working just because you have had past success with using the same approach with similar couples and families? In what ways does this new couple or family client differ? Asking oneself these critical types of questions can help us to not fall prey to our brains' mental traps, cognitive biases, and one-size-fits-all thinking in terms of what we choose to do with our clients therapeutically. Below, I present eight mental traps and biases we need to be mindful of with our client therapeutic formulations and intervention selection and design decision-making. I describe each one and then offer action steps we can take to not fall prey to them. They are: *salient analogies and bias, confirmation bias, availability bias, representative bias, anchoring bias, halo effect, overconfidence,* and *predictive bias.*

Salient Analogies Bias

Our treatment formulations and therapeutic decision-making is based on past experiences we have had identifying similar patterns and characteristics connected to specific types of clients' presenting problems. We may have a long track record of successfully treating specific types of couple and family problems and even view ourselves as experts in these client problem areas. However, each couple and family are unique and not a carbon copy of other couples and families, even if they are presenting with similar types of problems and dynamics that we have seen before. Therefore, to help us to not fall prey to salient analogies bias, we can first ask ourselves, "In what ways is this couple or family I am currently working with different then past similar couples and families I have treated?" We can take it a step further and do a deep dive into the past and think of as many similar couples and families you have worked with and do a critical analysis to identify how they all were different in some ways from your current couple or family. By doing this deep dive, we will not only discover these important case differences but we can learn about other therapeutic options that may be more useful to pursue with the current couple or family then what we had been presently planning to try with them (Kahneman, Sibony, & Sunstein, 2021; Kahneman, Lovallo, & Sibony, 2015; Mudd, 2015).

Confirmation Bias

In some cases, we prematurely lock down onto a particular problem explanation, strategy, intervention, or treatment approach without gathering enough client information or considering any other problem explanations or alternative ways of viewing the couple or family's presenting problem situation, and/or considering other therapeutic options (Kahneman, Sibony, & Sunstein, 2021; Kahneman, 2011; Nisbett, 2015; Mudd, 2015). When we find ourselves locking down too quickly with our problem explanations and matching change strategies, we need to turn to Emile Chartier, the nineteenth century French existentialist's valuable words of wisdom, "There is nothing more dangerous than an idea when it is the only one you have" (cited by Goolishian & Anderson, 1988). We can use our curiosity to help determine if our treatment focus is too narrow, wonder about missing pieces of the couple or family's problem story that might be worthwhile exploring, and in what ways could the treatment approach, strategy, or each therapeutic experiment you were planning to pursue and offer the couple or family could fail and possibly further exacerbate their difficulties.

Availability Bias

Kahneman (2011) describes the mind-set of when we fall prey to the availability bias as being, "what you see is all there is." We too quickly sift through the complexities of a couple or family case to try and make sense of what we are seeing, hearing, and experiencing with them. Our minds have a tendency to construct for us a coherent and limiting narrative about the client's problem story based on the evidence we have (Kahneman, Sibony, & Sunstein, 2021; Nisbett, 2015). As Mauboussin (2009) has pointed out, this bias can get us into trouble because we have a tendency to put too much weight into something occurring if we have seen it recently with a similar client or if it is vivid in our minds. We tend to overlook that there are important pieces or elements of the client's problem story that we have missed or failed to ask about in order to keep things simple or we think we know enough to begin implementing change strategies.

Representative Bias

With the representative bias, we often leap to conclusions based on representative categories in our minds, discounting any other possible explanations for what might be contributing to the maintenance of the couple or family's difficulties (Nisbett, 2015; Mauboussin, 2009). At times, we all fall prey to observing a particular symptom or behavior occurring with our clients and too quickly, often due to insurance coverage purposes and time constraints with our caseloads, leads us to thinking of a matching DSM-V disorder label that best fits their problem presentations. We don't give ourselves enough time to be curious about or to gather other important information about our clients' problem stories and consider what the best course of therapeutic action would be based on their clinical presentations. It also can be helpful to ask ourselves, "Did I too quickly discard other ways of viewing the client's situation or alternative treatment approaches because I thought they were bad ideas or because of my salient analogies, confirmation, availability biases?" Research indicates that when people think more than once about a problem, they often come at it from a different perspective, which adds valuable information (Soll et al., 2015). Spetzler, Winter, and Meyer (2016) recommend that we use *system 3* thinking to help counter our representative bias, which consists of imagining how professionals from different fields and skill sets would view and try to solve your client's problem situation. They also found that when it comes to complex problems and decision-making involving colleagues' input and having one colleague playing the role of devil's advocate who can challenge our narrow assumptions and unmerited confidence. With the colleagues' help, we can recognize the limitations that our mind can impose on us and consciously step outside of that box.

Anchoring Bias

The anchoring bias involves are tendency to buy into our clinical hunches, problem explanations, hypotheses, and associations like they are the truth. Since we think we have come up with the best therapeutic formulations and course of action for a client's problem situation, we don't put forth any extra time to gather hard facts to support our hypotheses nor explore for alternative therapeutic actions to take. According to Kahneman (2011), we have a tendency to start with a specific piece of information (the anchor) about a client situation and adjust as necessary to come up with a final explanation about it. Therefore, our therapeutic approach will be off the mark because our case formulations are too close to the anchor and we still do not have enough information about our client's problem story and based on this additional information, what therapeutic approach may be a better fit. Popper (1965) believed that intellectual honesty meant trying to refute, rather than prove a theory about the world. It was his contention that a scientist could never know with absolute certainty whether his or her research findings are true, but he or she may be able sometimes establish with reasonable certainty that a theory is false through rigorous testing.

Halo Effect

Sometimes we view our clients' stories and presenting difficulties as simpler than they really are. We stop gathering more information and we fail to be sensitive to the complexities of their problem stories and situations. By doing so, our approach may lead to making mistakes, treatment impasses, and possible treatment failure. With complex problem situations in general the halo effect compels us to simplify, pursue mental short-cuts, and be satisfied with good enough decisions (Kahneman, Sibony, & Sunstein, 2021; Spetzler, Winter, & Meyer, 2016). We need to gather more information and ask ourselves, "How can I be absolutely certain that my case formulation is totally accurate and using my choice therapy approach is a good fit for this family?" Kanter (2023) recommends that we *zoom out* and gain a big picture aerial type of view of the problem situation at hand to see what important information we might be missing and need to take into consideration with solution-finding.

Overconfidence

This mental trap occurs when therapists view their clinical formulations as accurate based on their past experiences of working with similar clients. Furthermore, they have matched their treatment approach with what they have done before that seemed to work. They believe what they are thinking and doing clinically with their clients is full proof. Because of this way of thinking, they see no need to cover the back door once client changes start to happen by providing relapse prevention work to empower their clients to constructively manage slips and stay on track with their gains. They have become the privileged experts for their clients. Tetlock and Gardner (2015) would contend that therapists need to strike the right balance between over- and under-confidence when it comes to solving complex client problems and with predicting the outcome of the change strategies that are implemented with them. They also believe that we should step back, incubate, and defer judgment without locking down on any one particular problem explanation or treatment approach when it comes to making sense of and resolving complex problem situations. Another way we can keep our tendency to fall prey to overconfidence in check is to carefully analyze our positive treatment outcomes with our clients. We have a tendency to believe that our past successes are due to evidence that not only that our existing skills and approaches work but also that we have the knowledge base and information we need to be successful with a wide range of clients. We over-inflate our abilities. With careful case analysis, we may discover that some positive good luck or random events occurred in our clients' lives or their own creative self-generated coping and problem-solving had contributed to their treatment success and held more weight for them than our skills or treatment approach. We need to try to come to understand the *why* of our treatment successes. The flip-side of being successful is that we may minimize the need for learning and further professional growth and that we become less reflective in our day-to-day work with our clients (Gino & Pisano, 2022). By regularly soliciting from our clients' session-by-session feedback from them on the quality of our therapeutic relationships and their perceptions of the change process, we can counter the overconfidence mental trap and ensure we are delivering what works for them (Duncan, 2019, 2010).

Predictive Bias

Although we may be highly seasoned couple and family therapists, have trained with leading pioneers in the field, and have had a great deal of success with particular types of presenting problems, this does not mean that we can forecast the future with 100% accuracy in terms of our treatment outcomes with our clients. As Mudd (2015) has pointed out, "Deep expertise leads us to assume that we can predict the future. It's the confusion between expertise and the ability to see tomorrow that we need to avoid" (p. 195). Kahneman (2011) has found in his research that we have a tendency to overestimate our performances and the outcomes of others. Furthermore, Gilbert (2007) contends that we also have a tendency to imagine future success based on our past emotionally memorable successes at solving particular types of problems, which are illusions about our ability to predict the future. When we become aware of our falling prey to the predictive bias, we need to remind ourselves that learning is a life-long process and there is always more to know, be willing to open ourselves up to our colleagues' fresh and novel ideas, and remember that there are many ways to view our clients' difficulties, with no one view more correct than the others. The bottom line is that our clients know what is best for them in terms of the kind of treatment outcomes they would like to have. Our job should be to empower our clients by having them determine their goals and deciding what proposed therapeutic tools and strategies they think could best pave the way for them to achieve their preferred future realities, not what we think is best for them.

Case Example: "He Never Stands Up for Me!"

Ron and Stella, a Caucasian couple in their forties, sought marital therapy for conflicts with his mother and his going out after work and drink and smoke marijuana too much with friends and work colleagues. Stella found Ron's mother to be "too controlling and difficult" ever since she had been involved in planning their wedding. Since the wedding, Stella contended that her mother-in-law continued to be difficult in terms of giving her parenting advice about their two children (12 and 10 years old), coming over to their home uninvited, and making family vacation plans without Stella's input. Stella was furious with Ron and shared with me in our first session, "He never stands up for me!" I had discovered that this was a long-standing pattern that was fueling a great deal of anger and conflict in their relationship. Although Ron would admit that he had a hard time standing up to and setting limits on his mother, I learned that he was her favorite sibling and the prodigal son and this is what made it hard for him to assert himself with her, he also knew that for many years she was unhappy in her marriage with his father and did not want to upset her. Apparently, there had been many incidents where Ron would know that his mother was planning to come by their home or had made future plans with his parents to go on a family vacation with them, including Stella and the kids without telling her. The couple had seen four other marital therapists before me and Stella had felt that Ron and the mother-in-law conflict situation had not changed. I also had discovered that none of the former therapists had attempted one or more sessions with Stella and her mother-in-law. As far as Stella's concerns about Ron's drinking and smoking a lot of marijuana goes, I had discovered that her biological father used to drink a lot and they were not close because of it. In fact, she no longer communicated with him after her parents divorced. Learning about Stella's father's drinking problem helped me to better understand why she was being highly emotionally reactive to Ron's drinking and smoking marijuana. She felt at times that Ron would get carried away with his drinking after going to Happy Hours at restaurants after work with colleagues or get together with his close friends to smoke marijuana. Stella would not know how to plan dinners because she never knew when Ron would be coming home some weeknights. Ron openly admitted that when it would get more heated and negative in their relationship that he would want to avoid coming home and instead, drinking, smoking marijuana, and hanging out with his friends. Stella pointed out how this was Ron's pattern of running away from conflict with her and not standing up to his mother because he would feel guilty and not loyal to her.

In our second and third sessions, there were some reported improvements with Ron's taking a break from his drinking, coming home right after work, helping out with the kids more, and setting limits on his mother. Stella was encouraged by Ron's changes, but she was still fearful that these changes would be short-lived and her mother-in-law would work on Ron in private conversations with him to get him to cave into her wishes. I used unbalancing (Minuchin & Fishman, 1981) to help support and empower Stella in the marital relationship and predicted that although Ron was making some changes that she had appreciated, the powerful emotional grip his mother had on him might lead him to going backwards and falling prey to the old patterns that upset Stella. We discussed the possibility of Stella's meeting alone with Ron's mother to attempt to resolve her conflicts with her. Both Stella and Ron agreed that if they could resolve this conflict situation that it would greatly improve their marital relationship. We discussed what the plan B, C, and D would be if Stella was struggling to gain her mother-in-law's cooperation and support with the conflict-resolution process. I also shared with Stella that sometimes in spite of one's best and most respectful efforts to resolve issues with in-laws, they cling to their take on reality and see no need to change their problematic behaviors. Stella voiced with confidence to give it her best shot and still meet with her mother-in-law Sonia. Ron set up the meeting with his mother for one week later.

For our fourth session, Stella courageously and with confidence met with Sonia to attempt to resolve her conflicts with her. Stella did a great job of sharing some past events that had occurred that had been upsetting to her and what she needed from Sonia so they could get along better. As part of the past negative events she had experienced, Stella shared for the first time with Sonia and I that she had been bullied in high school and was mistreated by a former boss in her last job. Hearing about Stella's past traumatic experiences, helped me to better understand why she was having such a strong negative emotional reaction to Sonia and why she was being perceived by her as a threat, which further amplified the emotional impact of Sonia's repeated boundary invasions. Stella then brought up how she had felt that Sonia had not been interested in her input about the wedding planning and there had been multiple incidents in the past where she had made decisions which involved her and her family without checking it out with her. Sonia respectfully listened to each one of the reported incidents and apologized for upsetting her. Sonia recommended that they try and improve their relationship by talking on the phone once a week and have lunch together every few weeks to help improve their relationship. Stella agreed to do this but requested that she would appreciate if Sonia took the lead in initiating the calls and planning the lunches with her. In the past, Stella had felt that she was stuck having to do this and wanted things to be different. Sonia agreed to honor Stella's wishes. I pointed out to both of them that I was glad that they agreed to meet with one another and make plans for the future to improve things and I predicted that because their communications difficulties had been so longstanding that it may be a bumpy road for a while with trying to strengthen their relationship because this was new territory for them and to expect that they may run into some potholes and slip into their old habits and patterns with one another. Sonia thanked me for having her come and trying to help them to resolve their communications difficulties. I recommended to both women that we meet again in two weeks to see what further progress they were making. One week later, Stella came in complaining about Sonia's failing to call her over the week to check in to see how she had felt about the meeting and how she was doing in general. Additionally, she found out after the fact that Ron had made some future family holiday plans with his mother without involving her in the decision-making process. It was like a powerful rubber band that had been stretched out as far as it could go and snapping back at us after what had appeared to be a productive session with Stella and Sonia and it felt like we were back to square one. Although I had predicted change would be a "bumpy road" for Stella and Sonia, this did not seem to matter as a normalization of what had transpired after my seemingly good meeting with the two women. Next, Stella launched into an angry verbal assault at Ron for not wanting to change, that his mother was not changing either, and that she was considering divorcing him. I calmed Stella down and validated her feelings of frustration and anger. Although Ron apologized to Stella, she did not believe he was sincere and shared something along the lines of, "You are more married to your mother than me" and recommended that he go and live with his parents. Stella walked out of the session and Ron chased after her and they both left. I had done phone outreach to both partners but Stella claimed she was done with couple therapy and Ron. Ron wanted me to keep the door open if he could get Stella to come back. I tried to outreach to Stella but she refused to respond to my texts, phone calls, and emails. The couple ended up dropping out of therapy.

In reflecting on this case and what I could have done differently if I had had another shot at working with the couple, I think it might have been useful to make room for storytelling with Stella by creating a safe space for her to talk about some of her past negative traumatic experiences with her father and having been bullied in high school and at her last job with her "controlling" boss. Although I am speculating but it could be these experiences are like constraints for Stella and they contribute to her high level of emotional reactivity when triggered by Ron's drinking and Sonia's controlling and intrusive behaviors. It could be that I put the wagon before the horse with pushing for reconciliation sessions with Stella and Sonia before she was truly ready for it. Having worked with many couples in the past where one or both partners had diffuse boundaries with their parents and had a tendency to go underground and have private complaint conversations about their partners with them and have had a great deal of success with firming up the partners' marital relationship boundaries, using unbalancing to rebalance the power and control dynamics in their relationships, and have successfully gotten them to directly resolve their conflicts without involving their parents. I also have found it to be productive to conduct conflict-resolution sessions with the partners and their in-laws without the other partners' presence as a buffer or mediator. Based on my past experiences having seen this couple presentation before, I relied too heavily on pattern recognition and the matching therapeutic action steps presented above and my overconfidence that what I chose to do therapeutically would work was really putting all of my eggs in one basket, which in looking back was risky and the timing of this intervention was too premature. It might have been helpful to give it more time with the couple in terms of helping them to bring back more warmth and positivity into their relationship first before introducing the conflict-resolution session idea with Sonia. In looking back, I fell prey to a number of the mental traps and biases discussed earlier, such as: predictive bias with believing that I had the recipe for future success with this couple since I had been successful in the past working with similar couple situations; the halo effect and anchoring had compelled me to be too simplistic with my clinical formulations, in that I thought that by resolving Stella's conflicts with Sonia it would improve the couple relationship and I had failed to take the time to have Stella elaborate more on the current impact that her past traumatic life experiences were having on her relationships with Ron and Sonia; and the salient analogies, confirmation bias, and availability biases also misled me to keep things simple, become to wedded to my clinical thinking and strategies, and stop gathering more information to make better sense of the couple's problem situation. Finally, it may have been helpful to have a colleague sit in on one of our sessions to observe and reflect on things we may be missing that would have been worthwhile for us to learn about and address.

In conclusion, I have presented in this chapter both the advantages and disadvantages of relying on practice evidence-based wisdom and experience to aid us with our clinical formulations and therapeutic decision-making as a resource. Much of the research presented earlier in this chapter can be of great benefit in informing our clinical practices. Two cases were presented that illustrate both how practice evidence-based wisdom and experiences can in some cases serve as a roadmap for change with a family and with a challenging couple situation, pave the way for a premature client drop-out situation due to our mental traps and biases that we need to be mindful about in our clinical work and critically evaluate throughout the course of treatment if they are influencing our thinking and therapeutic actions.

Key Takeaways

- Keep growing your mental storehouse of patterns by exposing yourself to couples and families presenting with a wide range of problems and who come from different cultural backgrounds.
- Ask yourself when prematurely locking down on one problem explanation or intervention choice, "What are a second, third, or fourth possible explanations for the couple or family's presenting problem situation? What are two or three other possible interventions that may have a better shot at working?"
- When faced with complex client problem cases, step back and reflect, incubate, play with different problem explanations and ways to intervene in your mind, and have a colleague or two serve as a consultation team and share what their thoughts are about your difficult cases to learn about how we may be getting stuck and to offer us some fresh ideas.
- Use reflection-on-action to help you to critically evaluate your clinical formulations, therapeutic decision-making, keep an open mind, and stay therapeutically flexible.

The Therapist's Use of Self Toolkit

The Therapist's Use of Self Toolkit

In this chapter, I present eleven different ways therapists can use themselves in the therapeutic process as the catalyst for deepening therapeutic alliances, empowering their clients to achieve their goals, and optimizing for therapeutic breakthroughs with our most challenging couples and families' difficulties. It's all about taking risks outside of our comfort zones and operating out on the edges with our clients where change happens, not within the confines of a particular therapy model. Case examples are provided to help illustrate each one of the use-of-self tools and strategies in action.

Strive for Extraordinary Presence

Through keen observation, generous listening, and emotional responsiveness, our clients will *feel felt* by us. When this occurs, clients often respond with something like, "Yes, you get it … that's how I feel." They feel validated and understood by us, which helps strengthen our alliances with them. We should strive for with all of our clients' *extraordinary presence*, which consists of being highly focused on what is being said by the clients and how they are responding nonverbally to us in our in-session interactions with them and at the same time, keenly aware of what we are thinking and feeling in response to our clients without being distracted and losing focus of what is being discussed in the moment (Hayes & Vinca, 2017). Emotional resonance is a key element at work with extraordinary presence for both clients and therapists alike. We need to be able to feel and tolerate our clients' pain and suffering and make it emotionally safe for them to take risks with us, their partners, and family members. The case example below not only demonstrates how our clients can move us emotionally and be inspiring with how they had overcome adversity but also can pave the way for crafting intriguing questions to pose to them.

In the context of workshop, I provided a family therapy consultation to a Caucasian family consisting of a single-parent mother and her three daughters ages

DOI: 10.4324/9781003334460-4

17, 14, and 12. All three daughters had been sexually abused by their father, as well as their 18-year-old brother who was in long-term residential treatment for sexually abusing a younger boy. The mother and the daughters shared how much they missed their brother. Cindy, the mother, had shared with me that she was an adult survivor of child sexual abuse and had spent years in therapy as an adolescent and young adult learning how to better cope with this traumatic experience. I also had learned earlier in the session that the father somehow had a great lawyer and was able to get off the hook with the child protection organization involved and with the local police department. The 17-year-old daughter Sandra had courageously written a scathing complaint letter to the governor of their state to let him know how both the child protective system and the police department had let her family down and how her father was never held accountable for victimizing her and her siblings. While sharing her courageous act with me, Sandra was crying and voiced how each sibling had been negatively affected emotionally by her father's sexual abuse. I could feel Sandra's emotional pain and provided empathy and support. The horrible mishandling of their family case situation by the child protective and police departments had compelled the mother to apply to law schools to earn a law degree with a special emphasis on family law, so that she could help other families not go through what her family had gone through. After hearing this, I found the mother to be not only resilient but quite inspiring. It emotionally resonated with me and it sparked a question in my mind to ask the daughters, "In what ways has your mother inspired each of you as young women to be all that you can possibly become with your futures?" Each daughter took turns sharing how their mother had inspired them to "not give up," "follow your dreams and they can be whatever you want them to be," and "someday work with her" in her law practice. They also praised the mother for being both a mother and father to them and that they loved her for that. The mother cried and was touched by all of the beautiful things the daughters had said about her. I shared my vision in my mind with the family picturing all these strong women working together in a law practice someday making a difference in society. According to the therapist and the family, this was the first session they had had together where each family member respectfully listened to one another and the daughters had held up their mother and acknowledged all that she had done for them to help them to have hope and heal.

Seizing Anomalies and Sparkling Moments

Buddhists have long believed that change is in a constant state of evolutionary flux and all afflictions or problems are transitory (Hanh, 1998). There are always spaces in between when problems are not occurring in couple and family relationships. Our job like good super sleuth detectives is to carefully listen and observe for our clients' anomalies and those sparkling moments when they are using their self-generated coping and problem-solving strategies to successfully prevent difficulties from occurring, and how they have surprised or impressed themselves and us with their courage, resilience, creativity, and resourcefulness when faced with challenging relationship and other adverse life situations. We need to go into our couple and family sessions expecting the unexpected or you won't learn about or observe for it. The case example below illustrates how resilient and resourceful clients can be even after experiencing multiple traumatic experiences. By seizing, amplifying, and consolidating our clients' anomalies and sparkling moments, we are inviting them to compliment themselves on their resourcefulness.

Forty-one-year-old Adela, a Latina woman, was involved in a highly toxic relationship with a man named Hector who was not only unfaithful to her but emotionally abusive towards her. He refused to join her for our consultation session in spite of efforts to get him to come with her. Apparently, this pattern of hooking up with men that mistreated her had haunted her throughout her adulthood. When asked what her best hopes that she wanted to get out of our conversation were, Adela had shared that she wanted help with trying to stop the suicidal thoughts that she had been having since age 10. I explored with her if there had been any triggering events that had occurred prior to age 10. She disclosed that she had been sexually abused by her older brothers and her maternal uncle. Adela further added that she had been cutting herself since adolescence and had made two suicide attempts in the past. After hearing her past painful story and chronic difficulties with having suicidal thoughts, the light bulb lit up in my mind to ask her what her secret was about how she had stayed alive over all of these years. This was a major client anomaly worth seizing and inquiring about. My question opened up space for Adela to share important details about her "anchors" that have kept her alive, such as the following: her loving and caring maternal grandparents who were "better parents" then her biological parents that she no longer communicated with; her cousin Fernanda who was a "big support"" to her, "caring and loving," and "always there" for her; and her 11 cats that loved her unconditionally, who were "soft and furry," comforted her, and made her feel good. By deconstructing Adela's anomaly, I discovered important building blocks for solution construction that could be both amplified and prescribed to empower her to not cave into cutting or to her fleeting suicidal thoughts. Adela also shared that the most powerful anchor for her when pushed around by her suicidal thoughts was to "think about" her maternal grandparents and how much they loved her and she could not do this to them. Additionally, she had discovered that by rapidly contacting Fernanda and snuggling up with her cats when having suicidal thoughts those anchors would take her out of harm's way as well. I also learned from Adela that she had had a recent epiphany about finding a different type of man than Hector who would "accept me for who I am as a person, loyal, caring, and treat me in a respectful and affectionate way." Adela had decided to leave Hector and "try and find a better man." In an effort to find meaning and purpose in her life other than her stressful business job, Adela had started a journal of her "positive thoughts" that gave her hope to carry on with her life, to return back to writing her "fantasy book about cats and mythology," and get back into "opera singing," which she used to love. Adela left our consultation session smiling and more hopeful about the future then at the beginning of our meeting armed with a roadmap for change, which consisted of using her anchors more, getting out of her toxic relationship with Hector, adding daily entries to her "positive thoughts" journal, finishing her fantasy book, and taking opera singing lessons.

In addition to illustrating how resourceful and resilient our clients can be, Adela also decided to get out of her toxic relationship with Hector and had an epiphany that she can do better with choosing more healthy and respectful intimate partners in the future. Adela's case situation also demonstrates that it is not necessary to have both partners present in couple therapy in order to change the relationship. One partner can serve as the agent of change. Adela ended up breaking up with Hector and had decided to take a long hiatus from being in a serious relationship for awhile.

Sparkling moments can take the form of our clients displaying courage, grit, quickly bouncing back from adverse life situations, doing something dramatically different than how they typically manage or act in certain situations that benefited him or her, being successful at mastering a task or life challenge, and so forth. When hearing about or observing in our sessions sparkling moments, we need to punctuate and celebrate them with the client. Like client anomalies, we need to deconstruct the sparkling moments of our clients by soliciting from them the thinking behind their positive actions and the specific steps they took to pull off what they had accomplished.

Respectful Curiosity

Curiosity requires openness and humility. As therapists, we really can't gain a good grasp of our clients' stories and lives when we are actively trying to move or sway our conversations in a particular therapeutic direction and/or working with them within the confines of our choice therapy models. Goolishian and Anderson (1988) contend that there is always more to know about our clients' stories, particularly those clients that have been oppressed by their difficulties for a long time and have had extensive treatment histories. They have long stories to tell which we should honor and respect. According to Guzman (2022b), "people are wonderful mysteries." She contends that a good question is one that fills the gap between what you don't know and what you want to know with new knowledge (Guzman, 2022a). When there are still gaps in our understanding of the client's problem story, we need to ask another question and another one after that until we have enough information to have a good grasp of all of the unique meanings to the client's story. We need to provide a therapeutic context ripe for inquiry, a mutual search for new meanings, and the co-creation of novel solutions. Respectful curiosity also involves generously listening to in awe and inquiring about with deep interest our clients' storylines of resilience and courage and about their self-generated creative coping and problem-solving strategies, which underscores their resourcefulness and engenders hope and optimism that they can have a better future. Goldenberg (2022) contends that radical curiosity is built upon an optimism that the extraordinary is possible. The case example below illustrates a nice balance of using respectful curiosity to come to know the client's problem story and concerns, as well as seizing her creative self-generated coping and problem-solving strategies that were already making a difference for the client in her life.

Twenty-one-year-old Alejandra, a Latina young adult, was brought for a consultation by her mother Raquel for her concerns that she was having problems with anxiety, depression, and for difficulties staying on top of her university schoolwork. She majored in both psychology and business. Alejandra had her own apartment. Raquel was a psychologist and owned a boutique. Alejandra disclosed that she was experiencing at times dissociation and de-realization episodes, which she had suspected by being traumatized and betrayed in the past by family members and friends. She also had been cutting herself, has had suicidal thoughts, and used to abuse a variety of drugs. Prior to our consultation, she had seen six other therapists since her early teens but felt that these treatment experiences failed to offer her any relief from or coping tools or strategies to resolve her difficulties. I asked if it would be helpful to her to learn a few coping tools that she could use when experiencing emotional distress and she voiced a desire to learning these strategies. I recommended counting all of the objects in her bedroom, six deep breaths slowly, and mindful walking, since she loved being out in nature. Alejandra shared that she felt that her parents often invalidated her and that they did not understand her. They often would tell her to smile and be emotionally strong. Apparently, the parents seemed to be much more interested in her getting good grades than her emotional state and struggles. Alejandra had had enough of her parents emotionally invalidating her and decided to move out and share an apartment with a good friend. Throughout our consultation, the mother was quiet and appeared emotionally detached from Alejandra, even when she would shed some tears and disclose painful life experiences that had occurred in her life. It was as if her mother was a spectator in the stands watching us talk. I have encountered this before when I have worked with other parents who were psychotherapists. At one point in the session, Alejandra had shared that there were times where she did "feel normal." I was curious to learn about what she told herself and did during those times that helped her to "feel normal." Alejandra reported that she worked out, did karate, draws, hangs out with family and friends, and she wrote about "theories about herself and people." This really perked my interest and I voiced my desire to learn more about her "theories." Alejandra had discovered that "it is important to self-reflect, keep an open mind, look for patterns in one's thinking and behavior and in the behaviors of others, and remind oneself that during the darkest times when one is really being pushed around by negative thoughts and feelings that everything will pass, don't worry." I discovered that this was a self-talk strategy she had used to prevent herself from caving into cutting herself, abusing drugs, and to help her to calm down. I shared with her that the Buddhists had discovered centuries ago that thoughts and feelings are temporary visitors in our minds and will exit on their own, so that there was no need to be scared or flee from them and that by detaching from them, they cannot own or control us. I pointed out how she had already arrived at this discovery by going a whole month without cutting herself or doing drugs by telling herself after being triggered: "Everything will pass, don't worry." I circled back to her "theories" eager to learn more about what further she had discovered about herself and other people. We talked about how she had applied her theoretical ideas to her relationships with her parents. She pointed out that she has had to be a "human chameleon" with them in order to get along with them. With her mother, she has to take an interest in what is meaningful to her, such as make-up, fashion, and health. When she is with her father, she has to "act like a son," which meant "talking about soccer" and having to "act confident and be strong." By doing so with both parents, they would get along and would reduce negative interactions. In wrapping up our consultation, I complimented Alejandra on her tremendous insight into herself and on what works in her relationships with her parents, and how useful self-reflecting, having an open mind, and being flexible has worked for her. I pointed out how all of her deep work on herself has helped generate post-traumatic growth for her. I shared that maybe someday she will publish her theories in a book that may become a text used in university psychology courses. She smiled. By the end of our session, Alejandra declared that she planned to continue to work on "leaving behind all that is hurting me." She left the session smiling, more confident, and hopeful about her future.

Navigating Through Ambiguity, Uncertainty, and Complexity

Goldenberg (2022) contends that when faced with an ambiguous situation it is not something we have to avoid or struggle to figure out how to manage it but rather, it can be viewed as an opportunity for new possibilities. The same is true with uncertainty or not knowing, the sky is the limits in terms of the possibilities. However, our brains do not handle ambiguity and uncertainty well (Schwartz & Gladding, 2011). We like to know, be in control, and have grave difficulty being in No Man's Land with not knowing what our clients consider to be the *right problem* to work on changing first and not having well-defined goals, which can lead us to feeling anxious and stuck. In some cases, the goal posts may be shifting all over the therapy playing field or we do not know from the clients how they will know when their presenting problems are really solved. What is being described here are what are called *wicked problems* (Camillus, 2015; Rittel & Webber, 1973). Wicked problems have the following characteristics:

1 The perceived "problem" is difficult to define.
2 There are multiple causes to the perceived problem which are intertwined and cannot be separated.
3 Wicked problems are always described as a symptom of other problems.
4 They do not have a "stopping rule." They lack an inherent logic that indicates when they are solved.
5 There is no end to the number of solutions or approaches to a wicked problem.

The greater our ability as therapists to embrace ambiguity and uncertainty through both acting and adapting, the greater are confidence in navigating in, with, and through the unknown will be. Acting requires that we make choices, take risks, and not allow ourselves to get paralyzed by fear (Small & Schmutte, 2022; Wucker, 2021; Labalme, 2021). At times we may want to rapidly experiment trying different change strategies out (acting) and at other times, step back and reflect or incubate about the big picture, what we might be missing, and explore other therapeutic options that may have a better shot at working (adapting). Furr and Furr (2022) contend that there is always a phase of uncertainty behind every brilliant insight, choice, action, and innovation. Research indicates when faced with uncertain environments it is important to take small steps, switching between different demands that the problem situation requires rather than trying to change everything all at once (Ott & Eisenhardt, 2020). When applying this research finding to families presenting with multiple problems and symptom-bearers, it makes the most sense to work with individuals and subsystems and establish separate goals and work projects until the situation becomes more stabilized and then bring family members back together for conjoint work. The complex case below with multiple symptom-bearers illustrates the challenges of working with wicked problem client situations and winging it session-by-session not knowing what might work or happen next in the therapeutic process.

George, a Caucasian 45-year-old, came to therapy with his wife Beth, and their 12-year-old-son William. According to Beth, George had an extensive treatment history for alcohol and pain pill abuse, depression, a suicide attempt, and back surgeries. He had been unemployed for a year since the family had moved here from New England so that Beth could take a "dream job" as an administrator for a company. George had been a highly successful engineer but his alcohol and abuse of the pain medication Vicodin for his chronic back problems had begun to impact on his job by missing days of work and making costly mistakes on work projects. His inability to find a similar position locally pummeled him into a deep depression, leading to his heavy abuse of hard liquor and abusing more Vicodin. George had pointed out to me when he would attempt to abstain from alcohol or Vicodin, he would get highly depressed, anxious, and experience tremendous back pain. Prior to seeing me, he had been to several outpatient therapists and he had been in three inpatient chemical dependency programs. The couple argued all the time about his drinking and Beth was threatening to divorce him unless he goes for treatment. Unfortunately, William had often observed his parents' arguing and would come home from school and find his father passed out on the couch or on the floor after a heavy drinking episode. All of the stress that William had to endure resulted in his developing stomachaches and headaches. Beth reported that she was crying all of the time and had to be placed on anti-depressants. What was an interesting feature of this complex case was that George would come fifteen minutes early via a taxi to our family sessions intoxicated on alcohol. I found this encouraging in that I believed that although he was physiologically dependent on alcohol and Vicodin there was a healthy part of him that wanted relief from all of his problems and that he was taking responsibility by showing up. What was most challenging about working with George and his family was the following: there were multiple symptom-bearers and that a change in one family member did not result in changes with the other members; changes that did occur were short-lived and were not perceived as noteworthy by the family members; working with individuals and subsystems of the family made no difference, in spite of negotiating tiny and realistic goals and coming up with together separate work projects; the clients' goals were constantly shifting from resolving the couple's arguing problem, to helping George stop drinking and abusing Vicodin, helping Beth be less depressed and stabilizing William's symptoms. Attempts to negotiate smaller more realistic goals went absolutely nowhere with the family. Although all of their difficulties were interconnected, each family member's individual difficulties disconnected them from one another, almost like they were on their own individual islands in the same family. William was very quiet in our sessions and I had decided to have him do the imaginary feelings X-ray machine exercise with me so we can learn about his emotions being expressed somatically through his stomachaches and headaches. He was to lay down on a long sheet of paper and with a crayon his mother drew an outline of his body. Next, he was to show us where his feelings lived in his body and scenes from his life that captured those feelings. William drew a sad face over his stomach, which according to him represented his fear and sadness that his father might die from his drinking. Inside his head area, he drew a big red bell ringing, which represented how the family problems are loud and painful to experience. Over his heart, he drew chains and locks around it to not let his father in because of all of the "forgotten promises" of letting him down with not stopping his drinking and forgetting about plans they had made to do some high-quality activities together. When the parents' had seen and heard from William the meanings of the drawings in his X-ray, Beth began to cry and even George had shed some tears. Both parents got up and hugged William and apologized for how bad family life had become for him. Observing this reminded me how children are like shaman and they can reach their parents' hearts and minds and heal them in ways that therapists cannot come close to in impact. Much to my pleasant surprise, the family came to our next session together and George did not come intoxicated. He was holding a large maple leaf in his hand that he gave to me. I asked him what the leaf meant to him and he shared, "I am turning over a new leaf today and please take me to a rehab." When asked about how he came to this decision, he shared that William's drawing had had a profound impact on him in terms of his guilt and shame about his drinking and how it has devastated his family relationships. I complimented him on taking this courageous step and made arrangements with an excellent psychiatrist and colleague who specialized in addiction medicine at an area hospital-based chemical dependency program. Once in the program, George had had the most severe and longest withdrawal process the psychiatrist had ever experienced in his career, which included delirium tremens. After getting out of harm's way, George actively participated in all of his therapy sessions and was working really hard to change. While George was in the hospital, I had met two times with Beth and William. In our second meeting, Beth shared that she had decided to divorce George and move back to her former northeastern state with William. My efforts to try and convince Beth to postpone pursuing the divorce until we see how George is doing after getting out of the hospital proved to be futile. Beth contended that she could no longer take the emotional roller-coaster ride with George anymore. Thank goodness George was still in the hospital where he could get a lot of support around the impending divorce situation. I had done some joint sessions with his therapist at the hospital to offer additional support. George appeared to be handling this painful situation well, knowing that he could still have telephone and social media contact with William. Once George got out of the hospital, he daily attended Alcoholics' Anonymous (AA) meetings, got a veteran AA sponsor, and moved into a men's sober living residence. I saw George weekly for relapse prevention training and to consolidate his gains. He also had regular contact with his AA sponsor for added support. After achieving nine months of sobriety, George decided to move back to his parents' farm and helped his father manage his successful produce business. He also had eventually had the opportunity to have William visit him at the family farm over some holidays and summers.

In reflecting back on this complex case situation, it reminded me of the qualitative research findings of Bohart and Tallman (2022, 1999) and Greaves (2022) that indicates that it is the client who makes the therapy work, not the therapeutic tools and strategies of the therapist and that clients can actively self-heal and have epiphanies that can transform their situations. Yes, one can argue that by providing a safe and comfortable therapeutic climate that embraced George unconditionally and that William's imaginary feelings X-ray drawing had greatly impacted on him, ultimately, he had decided the time was now for change. When working with complex and wicked problem cases like George's family situation, we need to be able to thrive in ambiguity, uncertainty, complexity, and allow ourselves to be surprised by our clients' responses to our risk-taking in sessions with them and our rapid experimentation with having them implement proposed therapeutic tools and strategies that we think could benefit them. Finally, we have to be patient with the change process because it may take time to find strategies that work. It was an unexpected and pleasant surprise in our last family session that George had moved into the action stage of readiness for change (Prochaska, Norcross, & DiClemente, 1994) on his own, which successfully got him on the road to recovery.

The Use of Metaphorical Questions

Often, our clients' presenting problems are a metaphor for a relationship conflict or difficulty. For example, I once consulted with a family where the adolescent daughter had a four-year history of bulimia, including two psychiatric admissions. I asked her "Was there anything that happened to you in the past or recently that has been difficult for you to stomach or digest?" She replied with, "Yes, my issues with my father." The client further added, "His drinking, swearing, and not listening to what people are saying to him." I responded with, "That is a lot to stomach." I had another client who was cutting herself for the past six months daily. When asked, "Now that I know that you are cutting, what does it mean to you and how does it fit into your life story?" She shared with me that she felt "cut in two." I asked what she meant by this and she went on to say that six months before we started working together, she had discovered that her father was having an extra-marital affair after reading a text exchange on his phone with his lover. The client was simultaneously upset with her father and felt badly for her mother, feeling "cut in two." In an effort to protect both parents and numb out her anxiety and depressed moods by harboring this secret, she turned to cutting herself, which she had felt was the best solution for managing the situation. The case below illustrates the power in the use of metaphorical questions to both get at the "not yet said" or the unexpressed, gain a better understanding of the unique meanings of a client's presenting problem and how it is connected to the family drama, and for identifying what specifically needs to change and potential solutions.

> Sebastian, a Latino 12-year-old was brought to therapy for his explosive and aggressive behaviors, regularly getting into fights with his peers both at school and at home. According to the mother, she would receive calls from Sebastian's school anywhere from 3–4 times per week regarding his fighting and disruptive classroom behavior. The parents Carlos and Juanita had marital problems and had separated for a few months due to their arguing all of the time. Both parents were hard working and stressed out by Sebastian's behavioral difficulties. Earlier in the year, Juanita became suicidal after giving birth to their second child and saw a therapist for post-partum depression. While discussing the parents'

arguing problem and their disagreements about how to manage Sebastian's behavior, Sebastian started to tear up. I also had learned that when the parents had
big arguments typically the next day in school Sebastian would get into trouble
for fighting and the parents would have to come in for a meeting with the school
principal. This made me think that maybe Sebastian's fighting behavior was a
metaphor for fighting to keep the parents together and there was an element of
noble intent behind it. I circled back to asking Sebastian the following question,
"If your tears could talk to us, what would they say?" He responded with, "I just
need their support." I asked him what he needed their "support" with. Sebastian
confirmed my hunch: "I want them to stay together with me?" I asked him if
that was his catastrophic fear that they would divorce and he agreed that this
was a worry of his. The father was alarmed by this and Juanita started to tear
up. I then turned to the father and asked him to speculate, "If Sebastian's tears
could talk, what would they say?" The father shared that he is a perfectionist and
puts a lot of pressure on Sebastian to work hard in school and stay on top of his
chores. He admitted that at times he yells a lot at him and once hit him after
getting suspended from school for fighting. Carlos also shared that he thinks he
may be too strict with him. I explored with Sebastian did he think his father put
too much pressure on him and was too strict. Sebastian agreed and admitted
that this was hard for him and it stressed him out. I could tell that the father
was taking this to heart by his generously listening to him. Next, I turned to the
mother and asked her to speculate, "If Sebastian's tears could talk, what would
they say?" Juanita shared that she yelled too much at him and Carlos. I added,
"So, if his tears could talk, they would say, 'Stop yelling so much!!!!'" Both the
parents and Sebastian laughed. I checked in with Sebastian, who visibly was
smiling and looking happier, and asked him, "If your father was less strict and
did not put so much pressure on you and your mother cut back on her yelling,
would that make a big difference to you?" Sebastian responded with, "Yes, that
would help." During my individual session time with Sebastian, I praised him
for courageously opening up about what was worrying and stressing him out. I
also told him that he did his job of getting his parents into counseling and that
I could now take over and help them to improve their marriage. He agreed to
let me takeover with his parents. The parents during our private time together
agreed to do couple therapy.

As can be seen with this case example, metaphorical questions can provide valuable
information about the story behind the client's presenting problem. By seizing the
opportunity in the therapeutic process to learn about the meaning of Sebastian's
tears, we gained a wealth of information about family stressors that were fueling his
fighting and school disruptive behaviors. The use of metaphors with clients in general is a helpful way to have them picture images in their minds that we would like
them to think about how it relates to their presenting difficulties or can offer them
alternative ways of viewing their current dilemmas that can be transformative for

them. The great hypnotist Milton H. Erickson often used metaphors and storytelling to alter clients' rigid beliefs and to trigger new interactions in their couple and family relationships (Short, 2020; Battino, 2002; Havens, 1996).

Improvisation, Humor, Absurdity, and Playfulness

To help lighten up the atmosphere in sessions and take the sting out of our clients' difficulties, the use of improvisational moves, humor, absurdity, and playfulness is the perfect antidote. Humor helps us to relax and feel good and can provide a mini vacation for our clients from their problems and stressful lives. I always know I have gotten off to a great start with kids when they say at the end of the session, "That was fun!" In my sessions, anything and everything can happen, there are always surprises, such as: telling jokes and sharing funny stories; singing; dancing; playing my djembe drum loudly and fast when things are getting out of hand in the session or jam with my clients who brought in their instruments; fall out of my chair out of amazement when people share their sparkling moments and big steps they had taken between sessions; and sometimes spontaneously getting up and leaving my office, and the clients have no idea if I am coming back or not. Like a TV series where at the end of the show they want the viewers to be on the edge of their seats for the next episode, I want my clients to be eager to come back for our next session in anticipation of what surprises await them when we get together again. The case example below illustrates how by being playful, using humor, and tapping the inventiveness and artistic talents of a child with eating-distressed behavioral difficulties rapidly created a therapeutic context ripe for change.

Luis, a Latino 10-year-old was brought in for a live family consultation for what was being described by his parents as *avoidant/restrictive food intake* difficulties. The parents Gabriela and Pedro had been separated for a year due to their marital problems. Luis's 15-year-old sister Sandra came with the family and shared she was an "A" student in school, had lots of friends, and liked art. Luis looked depressed, had his head down, and he was frail-looking. This problem had developed six months prior to our consultation. According to the mother, when Luis had discovered that there were two obese male students, he had become quite anxious and fearful that if he was not careful and watched what he was eating he could turn out like them and "get fat." For months, Luis had been ruminating and worrying about falling prey to obesity. This resulted in his only eating certain foods he liked such as quesadillas and sushi and he would refuse to eat other foods, which led to power struggles around eating, tempers flaring up with one another, and the parents worrying about his weight loss. I had discovered earlier in the consultation that Luis loved *Marvel* superheroes and drawing cartoon characters. He also wanted to learn how to cook and work in the kitchen with his mother. Knowing that Luis was into Marvel superheroes, I offered him the opportunity to do the art activity *my superhero comic strip* (Selekman, 2017).

I asked him if he could be a new Marvel superhero what would he call himself, what would he look like, and what super powers would he have. On my legal pad, I had him draw in the first box of the comic strip his new superhero that he would become if worrying about getting fat started to push him around. He called his new superhero *Ninja Hombre* (Man). Luis drew an incredibly detailed ninja warrior, with the robe, bandana wrapped around his head, and carrying in his belt a large and razor-sharp Samurai Katana Sword. In the second comic strip box, he was to introduce what an objectified version of "worrying about getting fat" would look like as the super villain. He was to give him a name and let us know what superpowers he had. Luis called him "Owner of the Land," and drew this large roundish character with arms and legs. When asked about the name he came up with for worrying, Luis shared that he had been ruling over his life for some time, controlling his thinking, and he could use materials from the land to create dangerous cement weapons to either use to defend himself or conquer superheroes like Ninja Hombre. In the subsequent comic strip boxes, he was to draw action scenes of how he will outsmart and conquer the Owner of the Land super villain. He used Karate chops and drop kicks and the Owner of the Land tried to hit him with his large spiked cement ball. Finally, in the last comic strip box, Ninja Hombre slayed and sliced up into pieces Owner of the Land with his Katana Sword. I had this outrageous idea that had suddenly popped into my mind after I saw how nicely Ninja Hombre had filleted the Owner of the Land, which was presenting the idea of creating a new type of sushi roll out of him. Luis and his family laughed. I recommended that Gabriela buy a sushi roll maker, sushi rice, and Luis could pick out the ingredients he would like to have in the new, first of its kind Owner of the Land sushi roll. Luis perked up and got super excited about working in the kitchen with his mother and creating this new type of sushi roll. I recommended that if he really liked the taste of it that they market it to Japanese restaurants in his city. Again, the family laughed. At this point in the consultation, Luis shared with us that if he could produce a series of comic books with his superhero Ninja Hombre, maybe some day the Marvel Studios will ask him to make a movie with Ninja Hombre starring in it. Luis shared with me that he promises to put my name in the film credits. We all laughed and I said, "That would be real-cool!" We laughed. Suddenly, Luis declared with his head cocked back sporting a big smile on his face, "Worrying is gone!" In wrapping up our consultation, I shared with Luis and his family a great quote from the jazz virtuoso and Buddhist the late Wayne Shorter that nicely captured his conquest of the Owner of the Land super villain and how to manage any future worries that may strike, "Remember to be a warrior, not a worrier" (Jackson & Shorter, 2023, p. 30). Luis and his family really liked the quote and found it to be quite inspiring. I wrote the quote right underneath Luis's superhero comic strip so that he could always remember Shorter's wonderful words of wisdom. The family left smiling and much more hopeful about their future.

And now, an improvisational move on my part – a recipe for my readers! One of my house specialties that I make for my family and friends is a lasagna made with roasted wild mushrooms and vegetables in a pumpkin sauce (see the recipe below).

Roasted mushrooms and vegetables ingredients:

- Two pints of wild mushrooms (combination of porcini, cremini, portobello, and chanterelles), chopped
- Two zucchinis, chopped into small squares
- One eggplant, chopped into small squares
- Two red peppers, chopped into small squares
- One green pepper, chopped into small squares
- One fennel bulb, chopped into small pieces
- One butternut squash, chopped into small cubes
- One sprig of fresh rosemary, finely chopped
- One sprig of fresh oregano, finely chopped
- Salt
- Freshly ground mixed peppercorn berries
- Three or four tablespoons of olive oil

Toss all of the ingredients together in a large bowl, pour them into a large casserole dish, and roast them at 350 degrees for 45 minutes or until the butternut squash cubes and the fennel are soft.

Pumpkin sauce ingredients:

- Three or four shallots, finely chopped
- Four cloves of garlic, finely chopped
- Five or six basil leaves, chopped
- One 32 oz can of pumpkin puree
- 24 oz crushed San Marzano tomatoes
- One 16 oz can of coconut cream (healthy alternative to regular cream)
- One 16 oz can of coconut milk
- Half a cup of white wine
- One drop of white truffle oil
- Salt
- Freshly ground mixed peppercorn berries
- Sprinkle of dried chili flakes
- Two tablespoons of olive oil

Sautee in a large pot the shallots and garlic and add salt and pepper. Add the pumpkin puree, coconut crème, and half of the coconut milk. Add the crushed tomatoes and basil, sprinkle in the chili flakes, and a drop of white truffle oil. Stir together at a low heat and add additional salt and pepper for taste. Simmer at a low heat for 45 minutes to an hour.

Lasagna pasta and cheese ingredients:

- One box of Granoro lasagna pasta (gluten-free and no need to boil)
- Two packs of part-skimmed milk shredded mozzarella cheese

In a large casserole dish, pour some of the sauce into the dish coating it. Next, put down 3-4 rows of the lasagna pasta and place on top some of the mushroom and vegetable mixture. Pour some of the sauce over it and add cheese on top of it. Pour a little bit of the sauce over it and lay down on top of it another 3-4 rows of lasagna pasta and add sauce on top of that with the rest of the mushroom and vegetable mixture. Sprinkle the remaining cheese on top of it. If you have enough sauce and cheese left you could add another layer. Bake at 425 degrees for close to 45 minutes to an hour, or until the lasagna noodles are soft and the top is nice and brown. I recommend you garnish this dish with Italian flat-leaf parsley, serve a side of asparagus or green beans, a tossed salad in a balsamic vinaigrette, a baked crusty and chewy baguette, and a nice Italian red wine. Bon appetit!

Being Transparent and Sharing Your Gut Hunches

There are times that we hear or see something that occurs in the session that touches us or we have a visceral reaction to, or a hunch, therapeutic experiment ideas, great quotes that captures our clients' problem situations enter our minds that are worth sharing. Sharing our gut hunches with clients often comes from practice evidence-based wisdom where we had successfully matched up effective change strategies with particular couple and family problem-maintaining patterns and presenting difficulties in the past which had disrupted those patterns and stabilized there presenting problems. We need to give ourselves permission to share our thoughts and feelings with our clients and even the playing field with them. Most importantly, what we choose to share with our clients should be done in purposeful way and believe it can benefit them. The family case example below of a 14-year-old bulimic and self-injuring lesbian female illustrates how taking risks with being transparent and sharing one's gut hunches can help pave the way for an in-session breakthrough.

Fourteen-year-old Olivia, a Latina adolescent, was grappling with depressed and anxiety moods, fleeting suicidal thoughts, and cutting herself for the past two years daily. She also recently came out to her parents that she was lesbian, which had been difficult for her parents to accept. Olivia had two older siblings: Pedro (19 years old) and Tanya (24 years old). The parents reported that Olivia refuses to open up to and isolates herself from them. Olivia disclosed that her parents don't understand her and do things that upset her like yelling at her after cutting herself, for not opening up to them, and don't understand her lesbian sexual orientation. In fact, the mother's attempted solution to try and make her more feminine-looking was to buy her "girly-looking dresses," which greatly angered

Olivia. Olivia and I made a strong empathic connection and she freely opened up about how she felt all alone in the family. I could feel her emotional pain and profound sense of aloneness. I shared with her that it sounded like she was all alone on an island in the family. Olivia agreed and further added that she could not count on her parents for support. I learned that what kept her at a distance from her parents was fear of being mistreated. Apparently, when Pedro was a teenager, he had major behavioral problems. The mother chimed in and shared that she and her husband badly mishandled Pedro's behavioral problems, such as yelling at him a lot and sometimes hitting him. Both parents expressed their guilt and shame about this and voiced their desire to do a better parenting job with Olivia. Olivia began to cry and shared that it was so awful how they treated her brother and that she was afraid to go to them out of fear that they would treat her the same way. The mother got out of her seat and hugged Olivia and shared that she and her father loved her and they want to be there to support her. Since the parents were eager to learn a parenting strategy that they could regularly use with Olivia when she would experience emotional distress, to help prevent cutting episodes, I taught the family a strategy that I had found to be quite helpful with self-injuring clients and their parents. Whenever Olivia would experience emotional distress and/or be triggered to cut herself, she was to approach her parents and they were to do the following: listen, validate, and sooth her with a hug and comforting words. I had Olivia and her mother practice this in the session. Although Olivia was pleased that her parents were willing to change their ways with her, she voiced her concerns that they may not stick with the strategy and resort back to former invalidating interactions with her. I stressed that the more they practiced this new strategy it would become the go-to response. I also pointed out that there should be no reason why in her own family Olivia should feel all alone, isolated on her own little island. The parents agreed and expressed to Olivia that they want to be there to comfort her. Since the parents came from religious conservative homes, they were new to LGBTQ sexual orientations and shared their desire to have them gain a better understanding from Olivia about her lesbian sexual orientation. The mother also said that she would stop buying her "girly-looking dresses." Another parenting idea I had that popped into my mind was for Olivia at the end of every week to offer her parents feedback on how well they were doing in the parenting department, both positive and negative constructive criticism. Based on Olivia's feedback, the parents would do more of what works and make the necessary adjustments she was recommending to them to improve the quality of their relationship with her. Olivia and her parents thought this could be helpful. At the end of the session when I solicited feedback from family members about what the meeting was like for them, the mother shared that she felt like a "miracle" had happened. I explored what she meant by this and she shared that Olivia had not been this open with them about her thoughts and feelings for the past two years! The father got out of our session the importance of "listening to your daughter, not being emotionally reactive to her." Olivia shared that she thought our meeting was good and she was more hopeful that things could get better between her and her parents. Suddenly, Olivia started to cry and she disclosed that she had been bullied and teased at school about "dressing like a boy and being fat," which led her to developing a problem with bulimia. The parents were troubled by Olivia's keeping this from them and the mother went over to her to hug and comfort her. We also learned that for the past two years Olivia would go to her older sister Tanya for support because she understood her better than the parents did. In fact, there had been times when Olivia wanted to die and Tanya was there to support her. The parents did not know this. I shared with Olivia that it was my hope that she would give her parents a chance to practice being there for her by taking risks and going to them when she was not in a good emotional state and that this needed to be a team effort. I stressed that it will be hard work and not always go smoothly but that the only way to get good at communicating better and responding constructively to one another was through regular practice and Olivia's giving her parents weekly feedback on how well they were doing with her in the parenting department. The family left smiling and more hopeful about the future.

Having worked with self-injuring adolescents and their families for over 30 years, I have observed some common problem-maintaining family interactions, such as: emotional disconnection and invalidation, conflict-avoidance, and difficulties with affective expression in the family. These dynamics serve as the problem-life-support-system for self-destructive behaviors like self-injury and eating-distressed behaviors, which Olivia was engaging in because she had to take matters literally into her own hands to sooth herself when experiencing emotional distress due to her parents not being able to provide this function for her. I taught Olivia's parents new ways of responding to her, such as listening, validating, and soothing her when she would experience emotional distress and as a way to prevent her from caving into cutting or bingeing and purging episodes. By doing so, my hope was that eventually the parents would become more empathically attuned with Olivia and takeover with soothing her so that she would no longer have to rely on her self-destructive habits for emotional relief.

Using Time in Therapy

The exciting thing about the future is that it has not happened yet. The sky is the limit in terms of the possibilities the future can bring us. Exploring with clients the *what can be* possibilities of the future is a great therapeutic direction to pursue when it feels like we are at a standstill in the treatment process, the therapy sessions are feeling too humdrum, or the clients are feeling paralyzed by and like prisoners trapped in their problem-saturated dominant stories. We also can have our clients go back into their pasts to relive positive and meaningful relationship events and times together, which triggers positive emotions for them while they reminisce and can engender hope about the possibilities for having a brighter future together. Next, we can have them identify which aspects or elements of their past positive experiences they would like to put back into their relationships today.

James and La Tisha, an African-American couple, sought therapy for James' infidelity. The couple had been struggling with communications, conflict-resolution, and sexual intimacy issues since their son Terence had been born a year ago. La Tisha had pursued couple therapy after she had discovered that James had been having an affair with a former girlfriend from high school. Whenever La Tisha would bring up the unresolved infidelity issue, James would get defensive and say, "How many more times do I need to apologize to you. Why can't we move on." La Tisha felt that this was not a sincere apology and she was not ready to move on, trust him, and let alone being sexually intimate with him. James was not keen on the idea of going for couple therapy but he begrudgingly came in with La Tisha. Picking up on the skeptical look on James' face and his leaning away from us in his chair, I strived to make him feel as comfortable as possible by connecting with him on our mutual passion for watching both college and NFL football. Apparently, he was a star fullback on his high school football team and had been recruited by several colleges, however, he had sustained a bad knee injury, which crushed his promising future football career. I empathized with how painful this must have been for him. I explored with the couple how they had met one another and decided to marry. I discovered that they were not only high school sweethearts but that Tammy the woman James had an affair with was still quite upset with La Tisha for stealing him away from her and eventually marrying him. I was curious to learn about James' story about what led him to re-connecting with Tammy at this time. James shared that Tammy had contacted him because she had heard from mutual friends that he and La Tisha were having marital problems. She communicated with him via text, on Snapchat, and on Instagram daily until he agreed to meet with her at a hotel. He shared that he was in a vulnerable place and was wrong to fool around with Tammy. I asked if it had stopped after this one encounter and they ended up at the same hotel three more times until he ended it. La Tisha was crying and quite upset with James for being unfaithful and being unwilling to solve this problem in a mature adult way. I explored with La Tisha what steps James would have to take to rebuild trust and help relieve her emotional pain. La Tisha was able to spell out concrete steps James could take in the short-run to help rebuild trust with her, they were: give her all of his social media account passwords, check in with her during the work day each day via text to see how she and their one-year-old were doing, block Tammy on all social media sites, no responding to Tammy's texts, phone calls, or emails, and when out with his male friends let her know who he is with, where they are going, and let her know when he will be home. James agreed to take these steps to win back her trust and help heal their relationship. I praised James for his willingness to take these steps to show his wife that he loved her and was committed to improving their relationship. At this point in the session and in an effort to move our conversation in a more positive direction, I decided to have each partner hop into my imaginary time machine and take it back to the early stages of their relationship where there was a lot of passion and desire for one another. The partners went back to their senior prom in high school. Next, I had them both use all of their senses, including color and motion to relive this special time together. While describing each of their experiences they were smiling and looking at one another as they described this magical evening. James remembered them slow dancing by a large ballroom window and seeing a bright full moon above them and how he loved the feeling of La Tisha's head cheek-to-cheek with him. La Tisha smiled and shared how happy she was with James. She said he was the most handsome man at the prom. It was quite obvious that their reminiscing about this romantic experience was triggering a lot of positive emotions for each partner. After the prom dance was over, they had gone to a party and made love for the first time at a friend's house, which they both indicated was very special. When asked about other things they used to enjoy doing together both as high school seniors and during their college years, James and La Tisha reported they liked going to dance clubs, concerts, going out for dinner, snuggling up together on the couch and watch movies, and socializing with friends. I asked each partner what pieces of these positive past experiences they think would be great to put back into their relationship now that could help improve it. Both partners agreed that they needed to bring back more physical closeness into their relationship and do more fun things together like go out dancing, go out for dinner, pick a concert to go to, and snuggling up on the couch and watching movies together. I had discovered from La Tisha that her mother had offered to babysit if they ever wanted to go out. I encouraged them to take advantage of this kind offer. Next, I had the couple respond to the following question, "Let's say, you both hop back into my imaginary time machine and take it four months into the future, long after we successfully completed counseling together. Once you step out and grab a seat in my office, what changes will each of you be eager to share with me?" La Tisha shared that James was being faithful to her, they were no longer arguing, and they were going out on dates again. James agreed with everything that La Tisha shared and added that they were much more intimate with one another and grew closer together. Another change that happened in this session was that James got up out of his chair and joined La Tisha on the couch holding her hand while they both described all of the changes they planned to make happen in the future. I encouraged the couple to pretend over the next week that the future was already here and experiment with their great ideas about how to further improve their relationship.

Storytelling

Everyone likes a good engaging story that touches on their emotions and has themes of the protagonist's courage, perseverance, and overcoming adversity. Stories can offer wisdom and inspire our clients to muster up the courage to step out of their comfort zones and venture into new territory in their lives. In a purposeful way, we can share our own stories of how we conquered difficulties individually or as a couple or family to help normalize for and engender hope with our clients struggling with similar difficulties. Another way we can normalize our clients' struggles and engender hope with them is to share what creative steps former clients took to resolve similar difficulties, which is illustrated in the case example below.

Ramesh and Indira, an Indian couple, sought marital therapy for communications and conflict-resolution difficulties. The couple had been married for 18 years and had two children aged 10 and 12 years old. Although Indira reported that Ramesh was great with the kids when he was at home, but she was upset about how he would "come and go as he pleased getting together with friends and doing his own thing" without consulting with her." Whenever she would confront him about this, he would get defensive and at times, they would argue about it. Ramesh felt that he was justified to do his "own thing" because he had a stressful job as a doctor and he was the breadwinner. According to both partners, before the children were born, they used to go on exciting trips, loved hiking and biking together, and there was a lot of passion in the relationship and a longing to be together sexually. I shared with the couple that I had worked with another Indian couple whose presenting complaints and dynamics mirrored their situation and that they were able to quickly improve their communications and resolve their conflict difficulties by instituting into their daily regime two mindfulness practices. I asked Ramesh and Indira if they were interested in hearing about what mindfulness practices my former clients had implemented that worked for them. They were all eyes and ears. I described to them the first ritual I had given to the other couple that was developed by the late and great Vietnamese Buddhist monk Thich Nhat Hanh, which is called the *Two Garden* mindfulness practice (Hanh, 2011). I shared with them that it is a wonderful mindfulness practice that can help bring back the warmth, passion, and love that couple partners are both longing to have back in their relationship again. I began by sharing with them that with every marital relationship, there are two gardens that equally need to be watered and taken care of daily. Each partner has his or her own garden to tend to daily, which could consist of the following: exercising, having individual time be alone to relax or engaged in a meaningful hobby, and communicating with or hanging out with a friend. By taking care of our individual garden, we can be fully present with and emotionally available to our partners. We also have to devote an equal amount of time and care to watering our couple garden daily. This can consist of the following: daily being affectionate with our partners, daily let each other know how much you love and appreciate him or her, and doing nice things for one another that each partner will notice and really appreciate, such as bringing home flowers or cooking a favorite meal for the other, and so forth. If we don't carefully take care of our gardens daily, particularly our couple garden, the weeds will grow rapidly and squeeze the life out of the beautiful tall flowers and plants, which will turn into anger, hurt, resentment, and despair. Both Ramesh and Indira were onboard with experimenting with the Two Garden mindfulness practice. We discussed what each them could do to take better care of both their individual and couple gardens. For example, Ramesh had stopped regularly working out, which he openly admitted led to his coming home from work "stressed out and on edge with Indira." Indira shared that she too felt "out of shape" and "depressed about not working out anymore." We explored what each of them could do to better water and attend to their couple garden. They both agreed that "doing little somethings" and expressing daily appreciation to one another about all that each partner contributes to their relationship and the family would be helpful. Having remembered from earlier in the session that the couple used to do a lot outdoor adventure activities with one another, I introduced them to a second mindfulness practice that my former couple clients found helpful to do, which is called *mindful walking, biking, or hiking*. I shared with them while doing this mindfulness practice they are to pay close attention to everything they see, hear, and smell. To provide them with a nice example of my own special mindful hiking experience, I shared with them my hiking up a mountain adventure a few hours inland from Anchorage, Alaska. I had been in Anchorage giving a two-day workshop and my host asked me what I wanted to do on Saturday and I shared with him my desire to hike up a mountain. My host gave me a heavy coat, bottled water, and granola bars to be able to handle the challenging mountain climb. While traversing the big boulders and rugged mountain terrain, I slipped quite bit because there had been an overnight frost that had covered the rocks. Three hours later, I had come to a large ledge and pulled myself up on it. Suddenly out of the blue, a giant and beautiful golden eagle with a huge wingspan had landed about twelve feet from me. It looked at me and then I looked at it, and all I could think about was that the Creator (First Nation people believe that the eagle represents God) was wishing me good luck to make it to the summit of the mountain. For me, this was a spiritual experience and inspired me to continue the challenging mountain climb. Both Ramesh and Indira appeared to be entranced by my story. About four hours later, I finally made it to the summit. On top of the summit was a circular pond of water that was mirroring the sky up above. You could see the clouds and blue sky being reflected on the surface of the pond. I shared with Ramesh and Indira that I truly felt like I was in God's country. After sharing my story, I encouraged the couple to experiment with mindful walking daily at their local forest preserve paying very close attention to all that they see, hear, and smell. With much enthusiasm, they were eager to institute both of the daily mindfulness practices. I shared with the couple that by doing the daily mindfulness practices they will discover that they will become much more present and much better listeners with one another, their relationship bond will grow much stronger day-by-day, and they also will discover the healing powers of being out in nature together.

After three weeks of religiously doing the two mindfulness practices, the couple's communications and conflict difficulties greatly improved and they had felt that they brought back the warmth and love they used have in their relationship again.

Strategic Use of Confusion and Incompetence

Throughout our professional careers, we have all had those couple and family cases where the following has occurred: when pushing for specificity with having the clients identify what they perceive as the *right* problem they wish to work on changing first; they demand that we help them to change all of their presenting difficulties all at once or when attempting to negotiate small and realistic treatment goals they respond with vague or highly unrealistic goals; the couple or family's goals keep changing every week; both couple partners or the family members are pre-contemplators and it is unclear who the customer for change is in client eco-system; the couple or family's presenting problems appear intractable and impervious to well-timed and agreed upon implemented change strategies; the treatment process initially got off to a great start and all of a sudden, it feels like you had run into a brick wall with the clients, without any identified reasons for it happening, almost like an unsolved detective mystery; and couple and family therapy veteran clients that are like master chess players, are gamey and provocative, and while on the treatment circuit, had frustrated and defeated many therapists along the way.

When faced with the clinical dilemmas described above, they can make us wish Scottie, the engineer on the *Starship Enterprise* from the TV series *Star Trek* would beam us up to escape from feeling confused, frustrated, and incompetent. In the TV show, Scottie would beam his crew up from planets they were investigating or when they were in danger of being attacked or captured by alien beings. Rather than trying to rid ourselves of feeling confused or incompetent, I have found it to be most advantageous to let it shine through with the challenging couples and families we are struggling with. It is quite inviting for clients to want help the confused and bungling therapist out because they will feel sorry for him or her. There are several ways we can make strategic use of our confusion and incompetence they are as follows:

1 We can share with the clients that we feel like we are really blowing it with them and offer to talk to our supervisor about getting them a new therapist.
2 We can share with the clients that our supervisor will not be happy to hear when we meet with her later in the day that not only that their (the client's) situation is not improving but has become much worse! Next, we can share with the clients that you are worried that you will be taken off their case and more than likely they will be given a new therapist, which means having to tell their story all over again.

3   We can ask, "Is there something I am missing or we have failed to address with your situation that may be contributing to my confusion and why I am feeling so stuck right now with making sense of your situation?"

4   We can ask, "It seemed like we got off to a good start and all of a sudden, we have run into a brick wall. Is there something we have not talked about yet that may need to be talked about now?"

5   We can ask, "If the four of you (the family) were serving as my family therapy consultation team and I were to work with another family just like you, what advice would you have for me in terms of what questions I should ask them, what I should be working on changing with them, and what I should avoid doing with them at all costs?"

With the five therapeutic strategies presented above, clients often respond by sharing with us the following,

- "You're not so bad. We are not ready to give up on you."
- "Oh, we don't want to tell our story again."
- "Would you like us to talk to your supervisor for you?"
- "We have not talked about X (the painful undiscussable or secret)."
- "This is really uncomfortable to talk about but _____ happened six months ago ..."

Not only do some clients become more forthcoming about what they really want help with in an effort to not lose their therapists but they might start to talk about secrets or critical life events that that they think might be contributing to the maintenance their difficulties. With the last therapeutic strategy, it empowers a family or couple to be expert consultants to us about how best to foster a cooperative relationship with them, helpful questions to ask them, specifics about where in their client system change strategies need to be targeted and what might work, and what specifically to steer clear from doing with them so as to avoid alliance ruptures or a premature drop-out situation from occurring with them.

The case below is of a 12-year-old explosive African-American boy named Donny who had an extensive treatment history with both outpatient therapists and had had six psychiatric admissions after becoming aggressive and violent both at home with his siblings and at school with his fellow students. Donny also was diagnosed with ADHD and had not responded well to many of the medications used to treat this condition. Cynthia, the mother, was constantly receiving calls from his teachers and the school principal about his aggressive and disruptive behaviors. Donny had no friends and struggled to adjust with the three major moves the family had to make due to his father Harold's being transferred to different military bases.

Donny was the only male and the oldest of five children. The youngest child was 2. When upset at home, Donny would tease and torment his younger siblings.

His father Harold was away a lot due to being in the army and having to go on deployments and to out-of-state trainings. When Harold was around, the frequency of Donny's aggressive and disruptive behaviors would decrease. They had a great relationship and would play sports together when he was at home. Harold also was much stricter and consistent with limit-setting than Cynthia. Cynthia was often feeling overwhelmed and stressed out by having to manage all of the kids most of the time by herself. Her parents and adult siblings lived across the country and they typically visited with one another around holiday times. Although I was able to connect with Donny around our mutual love for playing and watching NFL football games on TV, he could not share any specific triggers for his explosive and aggressive behaviors and made it clear to me that he did not want to talk about his difficulties. Cynthia, however, went on a long monolog about how bad Donny's behavior was and his lack of motivation to change. In collaborating with Donny's teachers and school psychologist the consensus was that they felt like Cynthia and Harold were not stepping up enough as parents in setting limits and disciplining Donny. In our family meetings, which Harold infrequently attended, I tried to stress to the parents that they must be consistent with enforcing their rules and consequences with Donny to help him to make better choices with his behavior and be less impulsive. However, this went absolutely nowhere because Cynthia was either too tired to deal with Donny and would resort to yelling at him and eventually would acquiesce with no consequence given to him for his misbehavior. After collaborating with his teachers, the psychologist, and principal, we came up with a plan to unify their efforts with the parents to better manage Donny's behaviors and as an attempt to foster a cooperative partnership between the school and the parents. The plan was to institute *The Three Ss* with Donny both at school and at home (Selekman, 2017). The Three Ss are: self-awareness (When I am triggered what am I thinking, feeling, and what is happening physiologically inside of me?), self-monitoring (What can I do to regain control? Which coping tools and strategies can I use to regain self-control? Have I lost self-control?), and self-advocacy (Who can I turn to for support? (my teacher, the psychologist, or my mother at home and can talk about what is upsetting me). I taught Donny a variety of mindfulness practices (take four deep breaths slowly, the sound meditation), counting all the objects in the room, and some visualizations he could use in the self-monitoring stage to help him to center himself and disrupt negative thought patterns that would compel him to lose physical control. The teachers came up with cue cards to remind Donny about using The Three Ss when he appeared triggered, made themselves available with support, and would allow him to go see his psychologist when necessary. Additionally, when he would come to school all wound up or had a lot of nervous energy, we worked it out with one of the gym teachers that he could go shoot baskets with him. After four weeks of trying out The Three Ss at school, Donny's behavior had greatly improved in the classroom and he had not gotten into one fight with other students. At home, he had stopped tormenting his younger siblings and he had been more cooperative with following his parents' rules. However, two weeks later, after Harold was deployed for an indefinite amount of time and Cynthia was left all alone with the kids again, she resorted back to yelling at Donny, not making herself available to him with support when he attempted to self-advocate for himself with her, and she stopped using the Three Ss strategy with him at home. Donny had a major behavioral regression where he had hit both his mother and one of his siblings, which resulted in his being psychiatrically hospitalized for three days. After hearing about Donny's being hospitalized, I was quite upset with myself for not predicting for the family after Harold left that there might be some slipping back into old behavioral patterns with the increase in stress and with not knowing how long the father would be gone. I apologized to Cynthia for not forecasting their slipping backwards and doing fire drill training with them so that they knew concrete steps they could take if a crisis should occur. Cynthia was not upset with me about failing to predict their setback and shared with me to not feel bad about it because it was going to happening sooner or later. I also was totally confused by Cynthia's giving up on the Three Ss strategy that had been working so well for Donny. I took a risk and asked her the following question, "Is there something else going on that you and I had not talked about yet that may be contributing to your decision to jump ship on The Three Ss strategy with Donny?" For the first time Cynthia shared with me that she thought she was "depressed" and "feeling trapped" and all alone with having to manage the children, which was zapping her of all of her emotional and physical energy. After learning about the "depression" piece, I offered to hook her up with the psychiatrist I use to have her evaluated for depression. Once she had been assessed by my psychiatrist, he ended up putting her on an anti-depressant. The school staff were incredibly supportive with Donny and warmly welcomed him back after being discharged from the hospital. They were committed to keeping The Three Ss strategy in place there since it was working so well and regularly sharing with Cynthia Donny's progress with her. Once Cynthia was less depressed, she re-instituted The Three Ss strategy with Donny, which helped get him back on track behaviorally at home. Through the local recreational park district, we were able to get Donny signed up for a football team, which he was really excited about. During some of our sessions together, we would throw the football around and I was very impressed how fast a runner Donny was and what great hands he had when catching my passes to him. Donny eventually opened up to me about how hard it is having his dad away so much and being the only other male in the family. I validated his thoughts and feelings about this and encouraged him to work on making some friends on his new football team. He did share with me that he had become friendly with one boy in his class who he really liked.

Having worked with many children and adolescents who have one or both parents in the Armed Forces, it is particularly rough on their families to have to uproot every 3–5 years, give up close friendships, make new friends, adapt to new locations and schools, and so forth. When one of the parents is deployed, it is confidential where they are being sent to and how long they will be gone for. This can be quite disruptive for family life and anxiety-provoking for the children and remaining parent not knowing if they will return. With Cynthia and Donny, Harold's absence had a major impact on both of them emotionally and with high stress levels in the family. Once we got Donny's explosive and aggressive behaviors under control, he was better able to open up about his sadness and anger about his father's constantly having to go away and better manage his negative thoughts and feelings.

Being Provocative

With couples and families deeply entrenched in their rigid problem-maintaining patterns of interaction, presenting with longstanding chronic and intractable mental health and addiction difficulties, and have had long, unsuccessful treatment histories, being provocative in direct and indirect ways may help pry them out of or liberate them from their problem-saturated situations. Minuchin and Whitaker were masters at being highly provocative in direct ways through the use of metaphors and sharing their absurd and crazy thoughts as they are sparked in sessions with their clients. For example, with a tyrannical and defiant 12-year-old boy who was wielding all of the power and in charge of the emotional climate in his family, Minuchin might ask, "How did Johnny get so tall in this family? Next, he would have Johnny and his father stand back-to-back and would ask the father, "How can Johnny be both shorter and taller than you at the same time? That's amazing! Johnny, how do you do that!" The family members would laugh because it was quite obvious that the father towered over Johnny in height. In this family, the father had become too peripheral and disengaged from Johnny and supporting his wife as a co-parent, thus she became the heavy and had to contend with trying to manage alone Johnny's challenging behaviors. Minuchin's next moves would be to reel the father back in as a co-parent, unify the parents as a team, and build more closeness into the father-son relationship that had been lacking for some time, which was what Johnny was the most angry and sad about.

If Whitaker were working with a couple where the husband had had an affair and was not taking any steps to repair this serious rupture in their marital relationship, he would turn to the husband and say, "This is really outrageous to me. You have this beautiful, intelligent, and wonderful wife sitting right next to you and you [the husband] are so laissez-faire about the affair situation. Most men would die for a woman like your wife. In fact, if I were not married I would find your wife to be a great catch!" Although Whitaker's comments about how his client looks and being a "great catch" for men is sexist, and other words could have been used to support and compliment her, he was trying to provoke her husband to step up and take responsibility for his poor choice-making with the affair and fight for his marriage. Once the husband would get upset with Whitaker's provocative words, it will be tempting to prove him wrong by trying to repair his relationship with his wife and show him by being more active in the session.

Another way we can use provocative and counter-illogical with our clients is to be indirect with them, such as the following: being curious about the negative consequences of clients giving up their problems and speculating about what some of the costs might be for them (an increase in arguing or another family member becomes symptomatic); for couples that argue a lot, coming up with a weekly schedule at different times each day to have time-limited arguments and that a ritual rule was they must refrain from arguing during non-scheduled times; or for the child or adolescent who has temper tantrums when frustrated or not getting his or her way, to pick a few times over the next week to pretend to have a temper tantrum and not tell the parents whether it is the real deal or he or she is pretending. The parents have to guess. We can have clients practice in session giving these therapeutic experiments a test-run before they implement them at home.

Being provocative also can be helpful to our clients by helping them gain a meta-position to themselves to see how absurd their situations have become. When clients can see how their problematic behaviors are really costing them in their important relationships, psychologically, and in some cases physically, and spending an inordinate amount of time in therapy sessions or in treatment programs, where instead they could have used all of this time to further themselves by pursuing their life goals and dreams, the door to change can suddenly swing open and transformation can occur.

Camilla, a 17-year-old Latina, was referred to me for her five-year history of bulimia. Her parents were divorced because they were allegedly arguing with one another daily for years and her father had had multiple affairs as well. Camilla's mother Juanita had given up one of her two jobs to be at home with her more and to try and prevent binge/purge and self-injuring episodes from occurring. Prior to making this change, Juanita was working all of the time and they rarely did fun things together anymore. Additionally, Juanita had given up her socializing with friends and her hobbies to attend to Camilla. Camilla also was not going to school on a regular basis. She had seen four different psychologists and a psychiatrist over the past five years but was inconsistent with attending her scheduled appointments and deemed noncompliant with using the dialectical (DBT) and cognitive-behavioral therapy (CBT) tools that had been taught to her and with regularly taking her Zoloft as prescribed. According to Juanita, the psychologists were frustrated with Camilla's noncompliance and lack of motivation to change. To learn more from Camilla about how her bulimia has benefited her, I asked Camilla a provocative and counter-illogical question, which was, "What would be the disadvantages of you giving up throwing up?" Camilla responded with, "For my mom to pay attention to me. Not just my mother but everyone." I responded with, "That would be a lot to give up. Do you think you would become an invisible person?" With the help of my questions, I learned about the secondary gain Camilla was getting from having a serious problem. Her bulimia served an intimacy function in that it demanded her mother's attention and increased involvement with her. Not only was her bulimia demanding her mother's attention, but Camilla's close friends were regularly texting her to see how she was doing and the psychologists that she had been working with were also regularly outreaching to her as well. Juanita shared that Camilla had always been extremely dramatic, even as a young child. I asked her what she meant by this and Juanita added that "Camilla always loved to be in the spotlight." I followed up with Juanita by asking her if she ever had gotten Camilla involved in children's theater before, so that she could take center stage as an actress. Apparently, Juanita had signed her up for a children's theater program but Camilla eventually lost interest and dropped out. I turned to Camilla and shared with her that her performance over the last five years should have earned her an Academy Award. They both laughed. Camilla had shared that there had been times that she had thought about getting back into acting again. The mother shared that Camilla's high school has a great theater program. We discussed the steps Camilla could take to get involved in her school theater program and who to contact. However, Camilla agreed that she first needed to get caught up in school, pick up her grades, and use her coping tools and take her medication as prescribed in order to be able to be considered for her school theater program. While meeting alone with Juanita, I offered her an experiment to do to help empower her and to support her strong need to have a life outside of taking care of Camilla. Whenever Juanita wanted to go out shopping or socialize with her friends, she was to leave the home without telling Camilla where she was going or when she was returning. Upon returning and when Camilla would question her, she was to respond with an arbitrary comment like, "Oh, I just felt like going out." She was not to provide any details about where she went and who she was with. After a week of doing this experiment, Camilla started attending school regularly and meeting with her teachers to see how she could get caught up in their classes. She also started using her DBT and CBT coping tools and strategies and over time, greatly reduced her binge/purge episodes. The best news of all was that Camilla landed a part in a school play, so that she could shine on stage and get a lot of attention in a positive way. Another important change was that Camilla and Juanita were spending more high-quality time together on the weekends. Eventually, Camilla's bulimia completely stopped because it became irrelevant in that she was getting more time and attention from her mother and friends in positive ways. Juanita also found the balance in her life by socializing with her friends and getting back into her artwork and gardening hobbies.

In this chapter, I have presented eleven different ways we can use ourselves in the therapeutic process to strengthen our alliances and spark transformative breakthroughs with challenging couples and families. In a circular manner, based on how our clients respond to what we say and do will determine which of or what combination of the eleven therapeutic tools or strategies we choose to use next. However, what is most important is that whatever we choose to say or do is done in a purposeful manner with the intent of liberating our clients from the shackles of their difficulties and have the kind of future realities they wish to have.

Therapeutic Brick Walls

Trouble-Shooting Guidelines for Getting Unstuck

In this chapter, I present trouble-shooting guidelines for when we run into *therapeutic brick wall* situations that may occur with our clients in the therapeutic process and how to get unstuck. By therapeutic brick walls, I am referring to those times with our clients where the treatment process can come to a sudden standstill, we feel like we are trapped in a maze with our clients' problem situations, and at a loss for what to do. Therapeutic brick wall situations can occur in three different ways: *therapist-generated*, *client-generated*, and *therapist–client–ecosystemic-generated*. Under each of these categories that lead to therapeutic brick walls occurring, there are specific contributing factors that occur in the therapist–client relationship and therapist–client–ecosystemic interactions with involved helping professionals and concerned resource people from our clients' social networks that are critical to assess for and address. If we fail to quickly attend to and successfully ameliorate each of the contributing factors as they occur, this can lead to clients feeling like they have a weak emotional connection with us, feeling unsafe in sessions, becoming demoralized, and losing their faith in our ability to help them to resolve their difficulties, which can eventually lead to their prematurely dropping out of therapy. Psychotherapy research has indicated that the stronger our therapeutic alliances are with our clients greatly optimizes for the likelihood of client retention in treatment and positive treatment outcomes (Duncan, 2019; Schucklard, Miller, & Hubble, 2017; Maeschalck & Barfnecht, 2017; Diamond, Diamond, & Levy, 2014; Friedlander, Escudero, Heatherington, & Diamond, 2011) Below, I discuss the three major types of therapeutic brick wall situations, describe how they can occur, and practical steps therapists can take to remedy each one of the contributing factors.

Therapist-Generated Contributions

When we begin with new clients, it is important for us to provide a safe therapeutic climate so that they can build a strong emotional connection with us, take risks with us and their couple partners or family members about their needs and concerns, be listened to and respected, and gain clarity about what their theories of change, expectations, preferences, and goals are. Also, we need to demonstrate to our clients that

DOI: 10.4324/9781003334460-5

we are culturally sensitive, gender-sensitive, and gay-affirmative with our LGBTQ clients. When we successfully provide this climate ripe for change, we can rapidly build strong alliances with each couple partner and family member. By regularly soliciting session-by-session feedback from our clients on the quality of our therapeutic relationships with them and their perceptions of the change process, we can make the necessary adjustments to strengthen our alliances with them and determine what we need to do differently in the therapeutic process to co-produce with them the changes they desire. Below, I describe eleven contributing factors to therapist-generated therapeutic brick walls and practical steps we can take to remedy them:

1   The therapist has failed to provide a therapeutic climate that is safe for couple partners and family members to take risks with one another.
2   Failure to explore how clients of color feel about working with a Caucasian therapist and demonstrate awareness, cultural-humility, and sensitivity to the inherent power imbalance in the therapeutic relationship.
3   Failure to either tailor-fit your choice therapeutic approach to the unique characteristics of clients from different cultural backgrounds or use a different therapeutic approach that is known to be a better fit with clients from a particular cultural background.
4   The therapist failed to ask their LGBTQ clients' what their desired pronouns are, use them in their conversations, and is perceived as not being gay-affirmative.
5   The therapist has failed to elicit from the couple partners and family members their theories of change, treatment preferences, and expectations.
6   The treatment goals are still too big, unrealistic, or vague.
7   Mismatch between clients' stages of readiness for change and trying to implement particular therapeutic experiments with couple partners or family members who are not in the action stage of readiness for change.
8   Weak therapeutic alliances exist with the male partner in a heterosexual marital relationship or the one couple partner in a same-sex relationship who wields the most power in the couple relationship, and with parents or the adolescents in family therapy.
9   The therapist talks too much, has an interrogative interviewing style, or is too central in the therapeutic process.
10 A couple partner, the parents, or the adolescent perceive that the therapist is taking the side of one couple partner or family member against the other(s).
11 A therapeutic alliance rupture occurs with a couple partner or family member and the therapist failed to rapidly repair it.

Client Emotional Safety and Strong Emotional Bonds with the Therapist

Couple and family therapy outcome research has indicated that emotional safety and having strong emotional connections with their therapists are highly rated by clients (Duncan, 2019). Additionally, therapist *structuring skills*, that is actively taking charge in sessions when destructive interactions occur and displaying good timing with breaking up the couple or family and meeting alone with individual partners, family members, or subsystems (Alexander, Waldron, Robbins, & Neeb, 2013). Therapists must strive to in their very first couple or family therapy sessions to make it clear to the couple partners and family members that everyone's voice will be heard and respected and being attacked or threatened will not be tolerated. Clients need to know that our sessions are going to be like a sanctuary for taking risks and freely sharing their needs and concerns with one another, which can provide a therapeutic climate ripe for healing and change. If the therapist fails to make it safe and take charge in sessions when destructive interactions occur, a couple partner or family members may decide to drop-out of therapy due to losing their faith and hope in his or her ability to change their situation and it may feel like to them no different than what happens in their home. Some clients may decide to give the therapy a little bit more time to see if things change but are more cautious about what they might be willing to bring up in sessions or what change strategies they are willing to implement out of fear of negative repercussions occurring. In this clinical scenario, the therapeutic process may begin to drift or eventually come to a complete standstill.

Cultural Humility and Sensitivity to Inherent Power Imbalances in Therapeutic Relationships with Clients of Color

It is important to explore at the very beginning of couple or family therapy how clients of color feel about working with a Caucasian therapist due to the inherent power imbalance that exists in the relationship. Often, clients of color respond with, "Thank you for asking" or "It isn't a problem." Although they may say this, the underlying concern of sharing how they may truly think and feel has to do with trust and emotional safety concerns, particularly of taking the risk of not being believed or understood due to historical trauma, oppression, systemic inequality, feeling devalued, having experienced racist therapists or institutional racism, and social injustice in our society. In addition to exploring with clients about their feelings about working with a Caucasian therapist, it can be quite beneficial to explore with them from a position of respectful curiosity what past negative experiences with racist therapists and other individuals they have had, as well as where they experienced institutional racism, felt devalued, disrespected and/or mistreated due to the color of their skin. If we fail to do so, and their underlying thoughts may be, "How do I know that you're no different than all of the other white professionals we have had to deal with over the years" or "He can't possibly understand me and what my people have been through," this will greatly impact on our ability to build strong alliances with them because of our failure to convey sensitivity to their experiences of racial trauma and injustice. Hardy (2019) would argue that these true unexpressed feelings and concerns are due to the clients of color feelings of being "silenced and learned voicelessness" and an "assaulted sense of self," which is a "culmination of chronic and persistent experiences of being defined and silenced" (pp. 144–145). Unless we provide our clients of color with a safe space to share their past negative experiences with racist Caucasian therapists and other professionals and being disrespected and mistreated in general, this will lead to discomfort with implementing their therapists proposed therapeutic change strategies in their couple and family relationships. Hardy (2019) contends that therapists need to have "a thorough understanding of the dynamics of socio-cultural oppression, as a precursor to oppression trauma, which is necessary to work across cultural boundaries, especially with marginalized populations" (p. 134). Greene-Morton and Minkler (2020) and Tervalon and Murray-Garcia (1998) propose that therapists and the professional licensing boards and associations they are affiliated with move away from the old cultural competence model, in that it is too top-down and an expert-driven approach about what skills culturally competent therapists are supposed to have and instead, adopt a "cultural humility" mindset and approach. According to Tervalon and Murray-Garcia:

> Cultural humility is a life-long commitment of critiquing and increasing our self-awareness in order to identify and examine our own patterns of unintentional and intentional racism, classism, and homophobia. It also involves conveying to our clients' recognition and respect for their cultural priorities and practices.
> (Tervalon & Murray-Garcia, 1998, p. 120)

To help increase our self-awareness and be more present and effective healers with our clients of color, we can do a deep dive into critically examining our own racist biases and prejudicial ideologies or beliefs that we may still carry and had learned in our families of origin, primary social groups, or communities, and make a commitment to identifying and eliminating them (Hardy & Laszloffy, 2005). Finally, we need to both serve as racial justice allies and leverage our white privileged status we have to elevate and empower our clients of color.

Tailor-Fitting Our Treatment Approach to the Unique Needs of Clients of Color and Different Ethnic Backgrounds

When working with clients of color or of different ethnic backgrounds then us, we need to be flexible therapists and tailor-fit our choice therapeutic approaches to the unique characteristics, customs, values, and beliefs of the couple or family's cultural background or use a particular couple or family therapy approach that has been found to be a good fit and clinically effective with a particular cultural group. For example, brief strategic family therapy is an empirically supported approach that has consistently shown good clinical results with Latino substance-abusing and delinquent adolescents and their families (Szapocznik & Hervis, 2020). No matter what therapeutic approach we use, we need to be able to see past our own assumptions about how we think things should be in a marital relationship or family in order to better understand the experiences and values of others (McGoldrick, Giordano, &

Garcia-Preto, 2005a). What may look problematic to us can be a norm and expectation in a family of a different cultural background than our own. For instance, the eldest daughter in a Latino family may be expected to stay home and help out with their younger siblings, cook, and have other household responsibilities until she gets married. A Caucasian middle-class therapist may view the daughter as being trapped in this role as a parentified child, which will squelch her independence, not allow her to successfully launch, and become a self-sufficient adult. The belief here is that once one turns 18 years old they should either go away to college or move out because this is what young adults should do. Another way therapists can inadvertently offend couples or families of different cultural backgrounds, is by using certain therapeutic interventions that impinge on and counter their traditional beliefs and values. For example, when working with Asian and Arabic families and turning to a teenage son or daughter and asking, "Do you have any advice for your parents about how they could argue less?" Although the parents may have shared with the therapist that they do argue a lot and their kids have repeatedly witnessed this happening in front of them, this is not only a private adult matter but a son or daughter is expected to honor and respect his or her authority figures and not criticize or critique how they operate as a couple or parents. So, such a therapeutic move could not only offend the parents but for the son or daughter, make him or her feel very uncomfortable and balk at answering the question. If we want to be effective therapists when working with clients of color or from different ethnic backgrounds then our own, it behooves us to use respectful curiosity and ask questions as one way to learn more about certain customs, values, rituals, and role behaviors and demonstrate to your clients your desire to learn from them about their cultural realities. Another thing we can do is search for resources in the literature and in the community that can provide us with valuable information for working with clients of color and different ethnic backgrounds than our own. Two wonderful family therapy books that offer a wealth of information on this subject are: *Ethnicity and Family Therapy*, 3rd edition (McGoldrick, Giordano, & Garcia-Preto, 2005b) and *Re-Visioning Family Therapy: Addressing Diversity in Clinical Practice*, 3rd edition (McGoldrick & Hardy, 2019).

Being Gay-Affirmative with LGBTQ Couples and Families

Similar to asking clients of color how they feel about working with a Caucasian therapist, it is important if you are a straight therapist to ask how LGBTQ clients feel about working with you or if they would prefer being referred to a therapist who specializes in working with LGBTQ couples or families. If they choose to stay with us, it is important to ask what their preferred pronouns are, use them consistently in your conversations with them, and avoid at all costs projecting onto a lesbian, gay, or transgendered couple your own heterosexual biases and beliefs about how an intimate couple should function. As Kort (2008) has pointed out, "the erroneous belief" that a "couple is a couple" does not apply with LGTBQ couples. He contends that the "doubling factor" comes into play, that is "it intensifies the traditional gender role conditioning of both partners" (p. 26). Male partners are often more detached, struggle with emotional expression, are competitive, and may be conflicted about sexual expression in the relationship. He has observed in his clinical practice with female couples a strong tendency to be too emotionally engaged and struggling with boundary and sexual expression issues in their relationship (Kort, 2008).

As a straight therapist, we need to be in touch with our own covert homophobia and stereotypes we may have about LGBTQ individuals that can get in the way of our being truly present and being effective clinicians. We also need to be sensitive to the impact of the traumatizing effects of covert cultural sexual abuse on our LGTBQ clients, such as: having experienced gay-bashing and/or physical assault, hearing about on the news hate crimes regarding LGBTQ individuals being shot and/or killed, being rejected by one's family after "coming out," always feeling like they have to put up a "straight façade" at the workplace or in other settings, and recent fears of the Supreme Court overturning the right to have same-sex marriages (Kort, 2008).

As a helpful thought exercise for straight therapists to enhance their empathy and compassion and as a way to prepare clients for drumming up the courage to "come out" and/or transition and the aftermath of "coming out" and beginning the transitioning process, Nealy (2019) asks us and the clients to respond to the following:

Imagine realizing that you identify as a gender different from the sex you are assigned at birth and that you plan to begin using a new name and new pronouns:

- How would you feel?
- What concerns would you have?
- Imagine sharing this information with your family?
- Imagine telling your friends?
- Imagine telling your colleagues or classmates
- How might these various people respond to your news?

(Nealy, 2019, p. 375)

Not only is this thought exercise helpful for straight therapists putting themselves in the minds, hearts, and in the shoes of their LGBTQ clients contemplating "coming out" or transitioning but it can be helpful for the clients to prepare themselves for the process, the benefits, the bumpy road ahead, and potential costs of being true to themselves.

When working with LGBTQ adults and adolescents and their families, there are a wide range of negative family responses that may occur once your client attempts to "come out," they are as follows:

- The parents and/or siblings think that it is just a "phase" he or she is going through or a popular fad among young people today perpetuated by social media.
- The parents blame their son or daughter's intimate partner as corrupting or "seducing" him or her into becoming gay, lesbian, or transgendered.
- The parents and/or siblings may view him or her as "sinning" and violating their religious beliefs and cultural values.

- The LGBTQ son or daughter "comes out" to his or her mother and she protects him/her/them by not telling the father.
- With transgendered adolescents wishing to begin the transitioning process, the parents put up roadblocks to supporting them with this until they are adults.
- One or both parents respond to their son or daughter's "coming out" as a way of hurting them or making them feel like failures as parents.
- The parents may blame themselves for causing their kid's LGBTQ sexual orientation due to their intense marital discord or divorce, rigid or poor parenting practices, past traumas, or due to their mental health, alcohol or substance abuse difficulties.
- Parental disconfirmation—"You don't exist to us anymore." This reaction can lead to being kicked out of the home or a longstanding or permanent emotional cut-off from the family.

Needless to say, as an LGBTQ individual experiencing these painful negative family reactions described above, it is no surprise that this population has high rates of depression, anxiety, suicide attempts, and engaging in self-destructive behaviors like self-injury, substance abuse, and in unsafe unprotected sex (Nealy, 2019; Kort, 2008; Selekman, 2009; Selekman & Beyebach, 2013; Whitlock, Muehlenkamp, & Eckenrode, 2008; Garofalo, Wolf, Wissow, Woods, & Goodman, 1999).

Nealy (2019) contends that in order to be effective family therapists with LGBTQ individuals and their families, the therapist needs to be highly active and provide a therapeutic climate that is emotionally safe. The family therapist needs to validate the LGBTQ client's and family members' feelings and concerns. He recommends that parental rejection can be reframed into "fear for the child's safety, their deep love for" him or her, and his or her "well-being" (p. 379). He also recommends using a narrative therapy approach to empower families to break free from their oppressive problem-saturated stories of "being a disappointment, unloved and unlovable, or even sinning" (p. 380).

Honoring Couples and Families Theories of Change, Preferences, and Expectations of the Therapist

There are three client extra-therapeutic areas therapists must attend to, they are: clients' *theories of change*, *their preferences*, and *expectations of the therapist*. First, in order to best satisfy our clients' needs we need to know from them what specifically has to be addressed in our work together and has to be solved in order to have a positive treatment outcome. We can ask our clients the following to secure this important information:

- "You have seen many therapists before me. What did they miss or failed to address with you as a couple/family that we need to resolve in our work together, so that you will leave completely satisfied?"

- "How will you know that this problem is really solved?
- "What has to be addressed first in order to put us on the road to change?"
- "How will you know you are really succeeding in counseling"

By securing answers to these important questions, we will know what is most pressing to the clients that needs to be addressed, learn what the signposts are from them about how we will know we are on the road to change, and ultimately, when we have arrived at the clients' ideal outcome destinations.

Second, we need to honor our clients' preferences. For example, seeing an adolescent and her parents separately at the beginning of family treatment because the young person had already had three negative family therapy experiences in the past, which left a bad taste in her mouth regarding having to be in the same room with her parents and with having to do family therapy again. We can still maintain a systemic relational focus working this way and as the adolescent begins to see the parents changing and she views the therapist as being competent and making a difference in her relationship with her parents, she may be open to the idea of bringing everyone together. The parents also may want help with their parenting skills or concurrently with family therapy working on their marital relationship.

Third, clients enter couple or family therapy with certain expectations about what the therapist needs to work on with them and how they would like the therapist to be, such as being active and conversational and not passive, to give advice and offer them lots of tools and strategies and things to work on between sessions, and so forth. This can help us to determine with each couple and family member what the best *relationship-of-fit* would be for them (Norcross & Lambert, 2013, 2011). Additionally, when working with couples in particular it is important that the therapist accurately assesses where each partner is at the beginning of treatment with what their expectations are for the couple therapy work together and the therapist's role, that is does he or she want to work on improving and saving the marriage, are one or both partners ambivalent about whether they want to continue the marriage, or do they want to work on constructively dissolving the marital relationship (Trembley et al., 2008). Once the couple therapist knows what each partner wants, he or she can tailor-fit his or her treatment approach to each partner's or the couple's needs and best hopes. To learn what their expectations are, we can ask them the following:

- "Before coming in here today, did any of you have any pictures or expectations in your minds about how you wanted me to be as a therapist with you?"
- "Are you looking for a therapist who is interactive versus more laid back and non-directive?"
- "With your past therapists, was there anything they said or did that made you upset or really turned you off so that I don't make the same mistakes?"
- "With your most favorite past therapist, what did you like the most about him or her as a person, his or her style, and what he or she had offered you in your work together that really helped?"

- "Just to help me better understand where each of you (the couple partners) are at in terms of the work we will be doing together and what your best hopes are with your outcome goals, are one or both you hoping to improve and save your marriage, are one or both of you feeling stuck or ambivalent about what to do about your marital relationship, or are one or both of you looking to work on constructively dissolving your relationship?"

The answers to these questions can guide us in how best to tailor-fit our relationship styles and ways of using ourselves in the therapeutic process in order to best meet the unique needs and wishes of each couple partner or family member.

Couples and Families Take the Lead in Determining Their Treatment Goals

Clients should take the lead in defining what their goals are for couple and family therapy. Research indicates that when there is consensus between therapists and clients about what the treatment goals are and how they will be achieved often leads to positive treatment outcomes (Duncan, 2019; Owen, Duncan, Anker, & Sparks, 2012; Tryon & Winograd, 2011; Friedlander, Escudero, Heatherington, & Diamond, 2011; Horvath, Del Re, Fluckiger, & Symonds, 2011). Our job is to negotiate with them small, realistic, and solvable behavioral goals. It is important to remember that goals are the start of something new, not the end of something. Therefore, it is important to let our clients know that establishing small goals and setting in motion small changes can cascade into bigger changes. As part of the goal formulation process, we need to break down into bite-size pieces whatever problem the clients wish to change first. For example, the couple shares, "We would like to improve our communications." It is too vague and too big of a goal to accept that as is. However, we can ask the following questions:

- "Over the next week when the two of you are communicating better, what will that look like?"
- "What will be the first sign or indicator that will tell you that you are communicating better?"
- "What else, will you be doing differently that will convince you that you are communicating better?"
- "Which sign or indicator of better communications do you want to work on changing first, 'not interrupting your partner when he or she is talking,' 'being a better listener,' or 'staying on the topic at hand until there is a mutually agreed upon end point?'"

After determining what piece of the couple's presenting problem they wish to work on changing first to serve as our initial treatment goal, we can use *scaling questions* to gain a sense of where the couple was at on the scale a month before therapy, two weeks ago, and currently, which will serve as our baseline (de Shazer, 1991; Selekman & Beyebach, 2013). Let us say the couple chooses as their initial treatment goal "not interrupting your partner when he or she is talking," on a scale from one to ten, with ten being listening intently to your partner without interrupting him or her and one being not listening to and frequently interrupting him or her, we can secure ratings from each partner where things were a month ago, two weeks ago, and where they would rate this difficulty today. Like good detectives, we need to secure details from each partner of any improvements with this difficulty, albeit small that occurred between a month and two weeks ago and to the present time. We want have them increase their self-generated problem solving and coping strategies and anything else they are doing that works. It is okay if each partner has different ratings for their presenting difficulty and with his or her next action steps are to further improve their situation. Once we secure this important information and learn what each partner's current rating of the difficulty is, we can ask each of them, "What are you going to do to get one step higher on the scale over the next week?" We want to secure from each partner in great detail the *what, when, where,* and *how* of what goal-attainment will look like. Often, I will pull out my trusty imaginary crystal ball and have the couple partners and family members gaze into it over the next week seeing themselves taking the necessary steps to achieve their goals, which helps co-create a positive self-prophecy for them. If either partner identifies any potential obstacles or roadblocks that may occur while pursuing their goals, we need to take the time to problem solve with them about how we can remove or work around them to optimize for their achieving their goals (Oettingen, 2014). If we fail to cover the back door and have in place a solid plan for constructively working around or managing the client identified obstacles, the clients can get stuck or fall short of achieving their goals, which can have a demoralizing effect, and lead to their feeling like they are back to square one.

When the clients' goals remain vague, too big, we have failed to remove barriers to goal-attainment, we don't know what the clients' goals are, or we have not moved the clients beyond complaining about their multitude of problems, the therapeutic process will drift and eventually reach a complete standstill. At this point, the clients may become demoralized since their situation is not improving but getting much worse and possibly dropout. One way we can prevent this negative outcome from occurring is to ask the *miracle question* (de Shazer, 1988; de Shazer et al., 2007). Not only does this project the clients rapidly into a future reality where all of their problems are solved (their ideal outcome) but it can help us learn what the signposts of what change will look like individually, in all of their significant relationships, and in the major contexts they regularly interface with. Once we have expanded the possibilities with each couple partner or family member regarding what they will be the most surprised with and pleased about what changed for them individually, in their key relationships, friendship groups, at work or at school, and the positive effects of these changes on them, we can ask the *miracle scale question* (de Shazer et al., 2007). The miracle scale is as follows:

- "So, on a scale from 0 to 10—where 0 means when you decided to seek help and 10 means the day after the miracle—where would you say you're at today?"

The advantage of using the miracle scale is that all of the changes the clients had reported in the miracle inquiry have already happened, therefore their situation has already improved and is much better. When asked, let us say the couple partners rate the situation post-miracle happened at a 6 and 7 respectively. Next, to help secure our well-articulated initial treatment goal, we can ask the partners, "What are you going to do over the next week to get one step higher on the scale to a 7 and 8?" Not only have we succeeded with this couple moving from vagueness, a litany of complaints about one another, or no clue what their goal is, to having a clearly negotiated goal to further improve their situation in miracle land. Finally, if clients have grave difficulty entertaining the prospect of miracles happening in their life due to their high level of pessimism and chronicity of their difficulties, we can use the following coping and pessimistic questions (Selekman, 2017; de Shazer et al., 2007) to better cooperate with their pessimism and try to establish a very small behavioral goal:

- "It sounds like Johnny's behavior can really stress you out, tell me what steps have you (the mother) taken to prevent the situation from getting much worse?"
- "So, you discovered by not reminding him about doing his homework he actually started to do it on his own. Are you aware of how you arrived at the idea of deciding not to 'remind' him?"
- "What else are you doing to prevent the situation from getting much worse?"
- "So, cutting back on your 'nagging' has helped as well. Which of your creative parenting strategies would you like to further increase doing, reducing or eliminating the 'reminding' or the 'nagging,' or is there something else you would like to work on changing?"
- "Some couples in your situation would have given up on counseling a long time ago and I'm the eighth therapist you have been to! What keeps you hanging in there and not throwing in the towel with the relationship?"
- "What would be the tiniest of changes or baby steps the two of you would need to make happen over the next week that would give each of you a glimmer of hope that your situation has improved at least a little bit?"

Questions like these not only help to foster better cooperative partnerships with pessimistic clients but they offer us alternative pathways for goal-setting and setting in motion small changes that can cascade into bigger changes.

Accurately Assessing the Stages of Readiness for Change of Each Couple Partner and Family Member

Another important area that therapists need to accurately assess for is determining at what stage of readiness for change each couple partner and family member are currently in and matching what he or she does therapeutically with what stage he or she is in. According to Prochaska and Prochaska (2016) and Norcross, Krebs, and Prochaska (2011), only 20% of the clients we see are in the *action stage* of readiness for change across a wide range of presenting problems at the beginning of therapy. However, many therapists and treatment program teams make the errone-ous assumptions that just because their clients showed up and appeared cooperative that they are in the action stage armed with goals and ready to do the hard work, when in reality, they are either *pre-contemplators* (don't think they have a problem) or they are *contemplators* (are stuck or ambivalent about changing). When clients have difficulty with identifying any specific problems they wish to change, can't identify their goals, and/or do not comply with implementing proposed change strategies, they are often labeled "resistant," "in denial," "defensive," and "noncom-pliant," and blamed for the privileged expert professionals' inaccurate assessments and mismatching their therapeutic approaches with the stages the clients were pres-ently in. If this mismatching process continues to occur, eventually the therapeutic process will come to a crashing halt, the therapist or treatment program team and the clients will become frustrated with one another, and the clients will drop-out of therapy or the program.

Collaboratively Determining with Couple Partners and Family Members the Best Relationship-of-Fit for Them to Help Build Strong Alliances

When engaging in alliance-building with each couple partner or family member, we need to strive to establish the *relationship-of-fit* with each individual, which by doing so, will help us to develop strong working partnerships with them (Norcross & Lambert, 2013a, 2011b). For example, a couple partner may voice a strong desire to work with a couple therapist who is much more interactive than the previous therapists she and her partner had seen in the past that were too passive. A mother may voice a strong desire to work with a family therapist that is action-oriented and gives her and her family lots of tools and strategies to practice and use both in and out of family therapy sessions. The best way we can determine with our clients that our therapy alliances are strong or weak is through soliciting session-by-session feedback from them on both the quality of our relationships with them and their perceptions of the change process or lack of (Duncan, 2019; Schucklard, Miller, & Hubble, 2017; Maeschalck & Barfnecht, 2017; Miller, Mee-Lee, Plum, & Hubble, 2005). Duncan and his colleagues found in their couple therapy research that solic-iting session-by-session feedback on both the quality of the therapeutic relationship and the clients' perception of the change process not only increased the clients' confidence in their therapists and prevented premature drop-out from occurring, but couples that had the opportunity to give regular feedback to their therapists also had much better treatment outcomes at follow-up then couples that received treatment-as-usual and had no opportunity to give feedback to their therapists (Duncan & Miller, 2000; Duncan, 2019). They also found that when the male partner had a strong alliance with the therapist throughout the couple treatment process the couples had better treatment outcomes. In my own couples therapy practice with gay and lesbian clients and through the use of soliciting regular feedback from them, I have found that when I had been able to establish and maintain strong alliances with the partners that wielded the most power and control in their relationships, I not only gained the necessary leverage to balance out this dynamic in their relationship but had better treatment outcomes with them as well.

When working with adolescents and their parents, it is like walking a tightrope in that we have to build strong alliances with both parties and session-by-session attend to both sides of the generational fence. We need to find out what both the parents' and the adolescents' expectations and goals are that will come out of our work together. Research indicates that when therapists establish strong alliances early in family therapy it is predictive of positive treatment outcomes (Diamond, Diamond, & Levy, 2014; Robbins, Turner, Dakof, & Alexander, 2006). One of the major challenges in family therapy work with adolescents and their parents is that both parties don't see eye-to-eye nor agree upon what the treatment goals are or the parents have identified a problem they want changed with their adolescent but he or she is not even a window-shopper for counseling he or she does not think they have a problem. The remedy for this stalemate is to establish separate goals and work projects with the parents and the adolescent and with the latter, go with whatever he or she wishes, be it getting social control agents off of his or her back, reducing a particular annoying behavior of the parents', and so forth. This is how to break the stalemate and foster cooperative relationships with adolescents. The parents may still want to work on changing one of the adolescent's behaviors even if the latter is not onboard to work with them on eliminating it. Once we can get the parents to abandon their unproductive attempted solutions, which are inadvertently maintaining the very behavior they want changed, we can offer pattern interruption strategies like the do-something-different experiment to try and stabilize the adolescent's behavior. Sometimes parents may want to contract to change their yelling, nagging, lecturing, pleading, and criticizing behaviors as their target goal area and work project with the therapist. Prior to ending each couple or family therapy session, we can ask them the following questions:

- "What ideas did you find most helpful in our meeting today?"
- "Are there any adjustments you would like me to make that can better improve the quality of our relationships?"
- "Is there anything we have not yet talked about in our meetings that you think we need to address the next time we get together?"

- "Has there been anything that I have said or did that was upsetting to any of you that you would like me to stop doing?"
- "In what areas of your lives are you experiencing the most changes?"
- "Are there still some areas in your relationship or life that you feel we need to do further work together?"
- "Which one of those areas do you feel we should address first?"

Another reliable option we have for soliciting client feedback is to use both the *Session Rating Scale* (SRS), which rates the quality of the therapeutic relationship or alliance and the *Outcome Rating Scale* (ORS), which measures change occurring in major areas of the clients' lives (Miller, Mee-Lee, Plum, & Hubble, 2005; Duncan, 2019). These instruments can be used across the course of couple and family therapy process to gain accurate measurements of how strong alliances are, where change is happening or not, and make the necessary therapeutic adjustments along the way, to help prevent premature client drop-out from occurring, and to optimize for clients having successful treatment outcomes. Since the therapeutic process can be so ambiguous, like a wicked, unpredictable, emotionally charged environment at times, and we never know where we truly stand with our clients, soliciting session-by-session client feedback from them by asking the above questions or regularly using the SSR or ORS can help optimize for better delivering what our clients need from us and desire as their outcome goals.

Avoid Talking too Much, Using an Interrogative Interviewing Style, and Being too Central

When conducting couple and family therapy sessions therapists need to be careful not to talk too much, adopting an interrogative interviewing style, and avoid being too central in terms of being the switchboard operator in sessions and robbing clients the opportunity to talk to one another and practice in-session skills together. Beyebach and Carranza (1997) found that therapists who talked too much and had an interrogative interviewing style lead to their clients dropping out prematurely from solution-focused brief therapy. By an interrogative interviewing style, the researchers had observed that the therapists in their study would ask questions and either not give their clients enough time to respond to them or think about the questions they were being asked and/or bombard them with too many questions, like being interrogated by police officers at the station. Nylund and Corsiglia (1994) refer to this therapist behavior as "solution-focused forced therapy." Goolishian and Anderson (1988) and Minuchin, Colapinto, and Minuchin (1998) have also weighed in on the dangers of becoming too solution-focused forced as a therapist. Goolishian and Anderson contend that one of the dangers of therapists being too sharply focused on the positives or one part of clients' realities is that we can become narrative editors and block them from sharing their concerns and problem stories. This also can become a constraint for alliance-building with a couple partner or family member who may indicate on the session rating scale at the end of the session that he or she did not feel heard, understood, and respected by his or her therapist who was too wedded to the solution-focused model, where one is supposed to avoid engaging in *problem talk* with his or her clients (de Shazer et al., 2007; Nylund & Corsiglia, 1994; Gingerich, de Shazer, & Weiner-Davis, 1988). Minuchin and his colleagues (1998) contend that solution-focused and other brief therapy approaches provide little space for resolving longstanding conflicts that left untouched could continue to maintain a couple or family's presenting problems. They also believe that solution-focused and other brief therapists are too central in that they are directing the session interview by asking questions, responding to the couple partners' or family members' responses by asking more questions, and so on. Fishman (2022), a master structural family therapist and trainer, has had similar criticism for therapists using a narrative therapy approach. It is their contention that therapists need to get couple partners and family members talking to one another and through the use of *enactments* in sessions as a way to learn new and more adaptive ways of communicating and resolving relationship conflicts (Fishman 2022; Minuchin, 1986; Minuchin & Fishman, 1981).

Finally, therapists need to use self-disclosure sparingly and it has to be used in a purposeful manner. Therapists who self-disclose too much not only turn off their clients but leave them feeling like who is supposed to be the client here! We need to learn how to observe and listen more and talk less in our sessions. The wise Hindu elephant god Ganesha who has large ears and a very small mouth serves as a great metaphor for us to become better listeners and talk less, and as a result, we will discover when others feel listened to in a generous way, positive things will happen in our relationships.

Be Sensitive to Couple Partners' and Family Members' Perceptions of Our Side-Taking in Sessions

When couple partners or family members perceive that the therapist is taking the side of one of the couple partners, the parents, or the adolescent against them, this could not only lead to an alliance rupture, make it unsafe to take risks with one another in sessions, and premature dropouts occurring. I once worked with a bi-racial adolescent named Candace who had had 16 therapy experiences in every type of treatment setting and had been court-ordered for 9 months to a long-term juvenile detention center. Candace, 16-years-old, had been running away from state to state, polydrug abusing, prostituting, had gang-involvement, and had been criminally charged for theft and assault and battery charges multiple times. Her mother was a recovering heroin addict and alcoholic and married five times to abusive men. The mother brought to our first family therapy session a massive fork-lifted file folder of all of her daughter's past treatment records. In leafing through the file folder paperwork, there were pervasive themes of mother-blaming and labeling Candace with the worst DSM-V diagnoses in the book. Since Candace wielded all of the power in the family and controlled the family mood, I decided to meet alone with her and asked her the following question: "You've seen a lot of therapists before me. What kinds of thing did they do that was a real drag for you or you didn't like so that I don't make the same mistakes?" Candace quickly responded with, "Siding up with my mom against me … and that makes me real mad!" When this would happen, Candace would exit out of family therapy. She went on to share that her past therapists regularly violated her confidentiality and were not interested in what she wanted out of counseling. We made an agreement that I would set aside each family meeting 20–30 minutes for her own private time with me to address her concerns, needs, and the parental behaviors she wished for me to work on changing so it would be more comfortable for her to hang around rather than run away again. Candace smiled and agreed that we had a good plan. This set in motion the beginning of a strong working alliance throughout the course of family therapy resulting in Candace's stopping her drug use and not running away anymore. The family interactions greatly improved as well.

With some families where the parents have highly conflicted relationships with their adolescents, having strong alliances with their adolescents can be perceived as a threat by them and they may feel like they are in competitive relationships with the therapists for their adolescents' affection and better connection with them, which can alienate the parents and weaken our alliances with them. In extreme situations, the parents may terminate the therapy altogether (Muñiz de la Pena, Friedlander, Escudero, & Heatherington, 2012; Selekman, 2017). This is why it is so important for family therapists to find that balance between meeting the needs, expectations, and goals of the parents top down and the adolescent's needs, expectations, and goals bottom up. We have to be intergenerational negotiators and keep parents abreast of what we are trying to do with their son or daughter to both stabilize his or her difficulties and improve their family relationships.

When working with couples, we also have to strive to deliver equally with each partner in terms of honoring their preferences, expectations, needs, and goals. If we fail to do so it can lead to alliance ruptures and premature drop-out occurring. One of the challenges of using the structural family therapy technique of *unbalancing* to rebalance the power and control dynamic in their relationship is that if we have a weak alliance with the partner who wields the most power, he or she can become defensive, feel slighted by us, and worse yet, storm out of the session and not come back. Not only does the timing for when we use unbalancing with a couple but we must have a strong alliance with the partner who has the most power in the relationship.

Rapidly Identify and Repair Alliance Ruptures in Couple and Family Therapy

The last therapist-generating contributing factor for therapeutic brick walls occurring that requires our immediate attention is the repairing of alliance ruptures with couple partners and family members. According to Sander (2002), mis-attunement, which can contribute to an alliance rupture is inevitable and can occur with our clients up to 70% of the time. Attunement, on the other hand, is when we have a good grasp of our clients' subjective realities and we are keenly aware of what is happening between us in our interactions with them. Muran, Eubanks, and Samstag (2023) and Muran and Eubanks (2020) contend that alliance ruptures can occur when the following happens:

- There is a disagreement in how the couple and family should work together (the therapeutic approach, main focus of treatment) and to achieve what outcome.
- A deterioration in the emotional bond with the therapist where distrust and disrespect occur between him or her and their clients.
- The therapist and clients have grave difficulty negotiating their respective goals, needs, or desires.

Muran, Eubanks, and Samstag (2023) and Friedlander and Escudero (2023) have identified three *interpersonal markers* for therapists to regularly assess for that can contribute to alliance ruptures occurring, they are:

1 withdrawal markers;
2 confrontation markers; and
3 intrapersonal markers.

With withdrawal markers, therapists should be looking for how either they or a couple partner or family members are becoming more distant and detached from one another or silent. Other withdrawal markers to look for are the couple partners or family members changing topics or are being overly compliant with us just to avoid conflicts.

Confrontation markers are movements against one another, such as tension in the air, aggression, and vying for who is going to be in control of the treatment process. A couple partner or family member may test the integrity of the therapist by being critical of the therapy or his or her competency as a therapist, triggering his or her anger and defensiveness, or one of the couple partners or family members become highly manipulative with him or her. Both parties equally contribute to the alliance rupture.

Intrapersonal markers take the form of emotional invalidation or empathic failures on the therapist's behalf. The therapeutic climate becomes unsafe for one or both couple partners or a family member. This could be a repetition of what a couple partner or family member is currently experiencing or experienced in their families of origin. By using ourselves as an emotional barometer to better understand what the clients are experiencing with us, and sharing what we are feeling with them, can be a teachable moment, an opportunity for client growth, and a way to repair the alliance rupture.

When alliance ruptures occur, we must rapidly repair them with our clients. We need to be emotionally responsive. Otherwise, the likelihood of the clients prematurely exiting from therapy greatly increases as the rupture and the distrust of the therapist festers. Both clients and therapists contribute to alliance ruptures either deliberately or completely out of their awareness. Ideally, alliance repair needs to be a collaborative effort. Some constructive steps the therapist can take to begin the repair process is by first acknowledging with the client what the rupture was, exploring with the clients how they think it occurred (both parties' contributions) and sharing our thoughts through the use of respectful curiosity, and exploring with the clients what he or she could do differently as a therapist to better meet their needs and strengthen their working relationship. Conveying to clients' *therapist humility* regarding the limitations of our knowledge base, the limits of what we can attend to in a given session, how we too have blind spots, sometimes we too prematurely try things out before clients are ready to hear or experience them, how therapy is not an exact science, and that we are just as fallible as they are, can be helpful to share. Additionally, we can revisit with our clients if our treatment approach suits them or whether we need to use a different approach, revisit their theories of change, expectations of us, and their treatment goals if they need to be smaller or renegotiated (Eubanks, Samstag, & Muran, 2023; Muran, Eubanks, & Samstag, 2023; Muran & Eubanks, 2020).

Client-Generated Contributions

Client-generated therapeutic brick walls can occur when couple partners or family members report that they had had past painful and traumatic life experiences or iatrogenic injuries sustained from negative treatment experiences with their couple partners, family members, and/or past therapists and treatment program staff. In some cases, we don't learn about their past painful and traumatic life or iatrogenic injuries until a few sessions into the therapeutic process when the therapeutic brick wall suddenly pops up and we are at a standstill. At this point, one of the couple partners or a family member may come late for sessions, miss appointments, or prematurely drop-out. In Rachel Aviv's haunting and provocative book, *Strangers to Ourselves: Unsettled Minds and the Stories That Make Us*, shares the stories of individuals, including her own story of experiencing iatrogenic injuries by privileged expert psychiatrists, therapists, inpatient treatment program staff, which had a profound impact on their identities and the course of their lives (Aviv, 2022). These clients also may be a secret-keeper, a trauma survivor, or for undisclosed reasons, may not feel safe with the intimacy of the therapeutic encounter or opening up with his or her partner or other family members. Their past traumas or iatrogenic injuries may be contributing to the maintenance of their presenting problems and serve as constraints for the change process. Below, I describe five contributions to client-generated therapeutic brick walls and practical steps we can take to remedy them:

1 A couple partner or family member is responding to the therapist with a high level of psychological reactance to the therapeutic encounter or in response to proposed or mutually agreed upon therapeutic tools and strategies to implement.

2 Clients' hostility, rage, and cynicism is due to a long history of being mishandled by past treatment providers, multiple treatment failures, and their problem situations had gotten much worse.

3 The couple or family are therapy veterans and have amassed while on the treatment circuit many therapists who had become their casualty victims.

4 One of the couple partners or parents is a practicing therapist and has assumed a spectator role watching us do the work.

5 One of the couple partners or family members is harboring a secret, which is serving as a constraint with the change process.

Be Sensitive to and Cooperate with Couple Partners' or Family Members' Psychological Reactance

There are a couple of treatment populations that tend to have high levels of psychological reactance to the intimate nature of the therapeutic encounter and being brought to or forced to see us by a social control agent who has the power to enforce response and action, they are: victims of child physical and sexual abuse, the adult victim of domestic battery and the perpetrator, male or female adolescents and adults that had experienced sexual assault outside of their homes, court-ordered parents and juvenile offenders, and oppositional defiant adolescents that are coming to us under duress. Some clients have experienced iatrogenic psychological injuries as a result of being mismanaged by past treatment providers and other psychologically negative aspects of the treatments they had received. Client psychological reactance is a normal and natural response to protecting oneself from being harmed, violated, controlled by others, and protecting one's personal agency (Norcross & Wampold, 2013; Beutler, Harwood, Michelson, Song, & Holman, 2011). When working with clients with high psychological reactance levels, we need to put them in the driver's seat of control with deciding what is the *right* problem to work on changing first, goal-setting, setting session agendas, with treatment planning, and have plenty of choices among options of therapeutic tools and strategies to experiment with. They are the experts on their situations and know what is most comfortable and best for them to try out. If therapists privilege their treatment agendas as if they know what is best for their highly reactant clients, more than likely a therapeutic brick wall will occur, and the clients will either start missing appointments, or possibly dropout of therapy. This is not client resistance or noncompliance but it's about self-protection. They are not going to allow any therapist to try and control them or put them in a vulnerable position.

With victims of child physical or sexual abuse, sexual assault outside their homes, or domestic battery, the intimacy of the therapeutic relationship can be threatening and make it difficult to build trust and establish a strong alliance with them in the early going of couple or family therapy. Additionally, their past traumatic experiences can contribute to sexual intimacy, communications, and conflict resolution difficulties in the couple relationship, as well as self-destructive behaviors and other emotional difficulties occurring with the victimized partner. We need to honor and respect their *protective shields* used to cope with their past and present traumatic experiences, such as eating-distressed behaviors, self-injury, or substance abuse. These protective shields are often used to ward off flashback activity and negative thoughts and emotions they are struggling to cope with. If the therapist too prematurely tries to remove their protective shields, this can lead to the client possibly having suicidal thoughts and dropping out of treatment. Once a strong and emotionally safe alliance has been built, they will be more receptive to learning alternative coping tools and strategies. Additionally, with trauma survivors they need to decide what the focus of treatment should be. The effects of their past traumatic experiences may be fueling their current presenting difficulties and we can explore with them which one of the effects they would like to work on changing first. My clinical experience has been that once one of the effects are stabilized it can trigger a ripple effect and the other reported effects can begin to lessen in intensity and become ripe for change. Sometimes we will work together in systematically stabilizing each effect in the order of priority for the clients. Throughout my career, I have worked with a number of trauma survivors who experienced iatrogenic psychological injuries because their therapists' agendas dictated the focus of treatment, which was to take them back into the past to their traumatic life experiences in order to work them through. I have had a number of former clients who had become suicidal as a result of their past therapists' mismanagement and had to be psychiatrically hospitalized.

When working with court-ordered, highly oppositional defiant, and powerful tyrannical adolescents who rule the household, we need to be like the bullfighter with how he makes masterful use of his cape with the charging bull by utilizing adolescents' high level of psychological reactance in a constructive way, by putting them in the expert position. We can ask them the following questions:

- "If you were the clinical director of our treatment program, how would you change things?
- "What type of activities or groups would you offer that kids like you would really like?"
- "If you were to hire the most perfect staff, how would they be as people that kids like you might really warm up to?"
- "If you were my family therapy consultant and I was working with a family just like yours, what would you recommend I change first with the family that the teen would be most happy about?"
- "What else would have to change with this family that would help make the teen less stressed out and happier?"
- "What's your parents' most annoying behavior that you would like me to work on changing?"

Adolescents enjoy being leaders and having the power to make a difference in their families, schools, and communities. In the same way that parents get stuck, if we take highly reactant adolescents head on in the attempt to take away their power and control, put the parents in charge, not only will we needlessly antagonize them but they will win the battle for control and decide to boycott attending future family therapy sessions.

Maintain Your Cool with Hostile, Enraged, and Cynical Couple Partners and Family Members

When taken off guard by hostile, enraged, and highly cynical clients coming at us with a verbal assault, it is quite easy to get lead-footed and defensive. However, we need to remind ourselves that there is always a back story to how these clients got to this place of anger and frustration and we need to greet them with loving-kindness and compassion (Hanh, 2001, 1991). Additionally, we need to give them plenty of space to share their long problem-saturated stories of being mismanaged by, disrespected, and in some cases blamed for their child or adolescent's or couple relationship difficulties by past treatment providers. They may feel demoralized by the fact that no past treatment experiences had successfully stabilized their difficulties and their situations had gotten much worse. Using respectful curiosity, we need to find out from these couple and families what their past providers had missed with their situations and what to avoid saying or doing with them at all costs. Once these clients have had ample opportunity to vent and share all of the details about their past negative treatment experiences, they often settle down and we can begin to build therapeutic alliances with them. We can inquire with them what their theories of change are, their expectations of us, their current goals or best hopes are, and how they will know that they really succeeded in couple or family therapy.

When working with angry and frustrated parents, we need to learn how they get stuck trying to manage their child or adolescent's most challenging behaviors and help them to abandon their unproductive problem-maintaining attempted solutions. These parents often are desperate to learn strategies to change their kids' behaviors and can make good use of such pattern interruption experiments as: *do-something-different* (de Shazer, 1988) or *benevolent sabotage* (Watzlawick, Weakland, & Fisch, 1974) described in Chapter 1. Another therapeutic option that we can pursue with these parents is *externalizing* the "anger" that may be intergenerational and is getting the best of the parents, the child or adolescent identified client, other family members, their peer relationships, and wreaking havoc for him or her at school. We then can set up a *habit control ritual* (Durrant & Coles, 1991; Selekman, 2017) to help empower the family to conquer the "anger" that has been getting the best of their relationships and lives for a long time.

Honor and Respect Therapy-Veteran Clients or You Will be the Next Therapist Casualty Victim

We all have worked with clients who appear gamey, are masters at "Yes ... butting," and will surprise us by pointing out which of the therapy books on our bookshelves they have read and easily recite passages from them. Not only are these clients' scholars on their DSM diagnoses and recommended empirically supported treatments for them but they will not hesitate to let us know when we are off the mark with what we are trying to do with them therapeutically. For these therapy-veteran clients, the map is the territory in terms of their diagnoses, how they view their problem situations, and they will balk at any therapeutic attempts to sway them from their problem views such as using reframing or presenting alternative constructions of their difficulties (Selekman, 1996). I once worked with a couple where the husband was diagnosed with Psychotic Disorder, NOS. He used to heavily abuse hallucinogens and it was unclear if all of the drugs had produced his paranoia, fleeting delusions, and sometimes hearing voices. Sean had been to twenty therapists before me either having seen them individually or with his wife and he had been psychiatrically hospitalized six times. His wife Cindy pointed out to me how bad their past couple therapists had been in that they would take her side, blame Sean for their problems, and he would get angry and drop out of couple therapy. In our first session, Sean tested me by asking me lots of questions about my credentials and experience in the field and if I had the knowledge and skills to work with him and his wife. He further shared with me that he had read many of the couple, family, and psychotherapy books on my bookshelf and he could tell me specific interventions that had not worked with him individually or with his marital relationship. I asked him to give me a grand tour of his most memorable therapeutically botched treatment experiences. He reeled off about six that he could vividly remember. I asked him and his wife if they had a wall in their home of Ts, all of the therapists they had defeated over the years, names, and dates. They both laughed. Sean had a great sense of humor and shared with me his most recent exchange with his worst psychiatrist ever:

> I went to see Dr. Smith to see if we needed to increase my Risperdal dosage. He responded in 15 seconds with his head down, "Here is your script for 50 milligrams, see you in three months!" There was no eye contact or further conversation. I could have told him I killed and ate three people and probably he would have been totally oblivious to what I just said.

After I took ample time to find out how not be a therapist with him and his wife, I was able to begin to build therapeutic alliances with them. At the end of the session, Sean shared with me what he appreciated most about me was my humility, strong desire to learn from him about what doesn't work with clients like him and his wife, and not presenting myself as the expert. One of the major benefits of working with therapy-veteran clients is their high level of knowledge and wisdom they can impart on us regarding our future work we do with clients carrying particular types of diagnoses and presenting problems and what to avoid doing with them at all costs.

The Art and Challenges of Working with Therapists
Who are Your Clients

One of the biggest challenges as a therapist is working with couples or families where one of the couple partners or parents is a practicing therapist. In some cases, the therapist client will adopt an observing position up in the stands of a stadium watching you work with his or her couple partner or family and not initially include himself or herself as part of the solution construction process. Even after spending an adequate amount of time trying to build good rapport with him or her, he or she may continue to not budge from his or her spectator position. When this occurs, I may ask him or her up in the stands the following questions:

- "How am I doing with your wife?"
- "Are there any missing pieces to your wife's description of what the issues are in your relationship or did she leave out anything more I need to know about?"
- "Have I established a good enough connection with your son?"
- "Should I use more humor with him or are there other techniques you think I should try?"
- "If you were to work with a couple in your office that was just like you and your wife, what therapy approach do you think you would use, and what set of techniques and strategies do you think would have the best shot of working with that couple?"

Often, this way of trying to engage the therapist couple partner or parent sparks laughter from him or her and/or the couple partner, other parent, or even the kids putting pressure on him or her to join our conversations and be part of the solution construction process. In many cases, the therapist couple partner or parent had done research on us in terms of our alleged expertise on their presenting problems and initially may want to see if we have lived up to the positive publicity press on us and whether or not we are a good enough fit for resolving his or her couple relationship or family difficulties. Sometimes therapist clients worry about their confidentiality being violated or get hung up on the erroneous belief that therapists should not have personal problems, which may keep them from initially including themselves as part of the solution construction process. If the therapist couple partner or parent is worried about these concerns, we should let them know that their confidentiality will be protected and that we are fallible just like our clients and this is nothing to be ashamed about. I let them know that the stressful nature of our work can take its toll on our own marital and family relationships and sometimes we need an objective third party to support us through tough and stressful times in our lives. Finally, purposeful use of self-disclosure of our own experiences seeking a therapist for individual, couple, or family difficulties also can help normalize therapist clients' concerns.

A Couple Partner or Family Member's Secret May be a Constraint and Keeping the Change Process at a Standstill

With some couple and family case situations, a couple partner's or a family member's secret is serving as a constraint and keeping the change process at a standstill. In couple relationship difficulties, the secret can take many forms: one partner is having an extra-marital affair with a porn star in a chatroom, on a cheating dating site, or with an off-line lover; one of the partners has a behind-the-scenes gambling, substance abuse, or over-spending difficulty; or a couple partner had been sexually abused in the past, never talked about with his or her partner, and it is contributing to the couple's sexual intimacy difficulties. Secret-keeping children in the family may be covering up their accidental discovery that one of their parents is having an affair, has a gambling, alcohol, or substance abuse problem or that they had been sexually abused by one of the parents or a close relative. Children are benevolent by nature and are protective of their parents. Unfortunately, for adults and children who are the secret-keepers it can take its toll emotionally and lead to the development of anxiety and depression difficulties, and acting in by engaging in self-destructive behaviors like self-injury, eating-distressed behaviors, and possible substance use to cope and keep a lid on the secret.

When we are picking up on innuendos of secrets, change is not happening after a few sessions, or it appeared that we got off to a great start and all of sudden we have run into a therapeutic brick wall, from a position of respectful curiosity we need to inquire about what's not being talked about. We can ask the following questions:

- "It seemed like we were moving along in a positive direction and all of sudden, we have run into a brick wall. What's not being talked about here that we need to talk about?"
- "For any of you, was there something unpleasant or painful to talk about that you told yourselves you were not going to bring up in our sessions?"
- "Sometimes couple partners or family members discover things about their partners or other family members that could be upsetting to them but out of love and a desire to protect them, they keep a lid on their discoveries. Have any of you ever had these experiences?"

One exercise I like to use with couples and families where I am picking up on innuendos of secrets is called *question-storming* (Selekman, 2018, 2017). I give each couple partner or family member a pen and pad of paper and respond to the following central question, "What has not yet been asked about our couple/family situation?" Each partner or family member is to come up with 5-6 questions beginning with qualifiers like: "What?" "What if …?" "How?" or "Why?" I like to give them 20–25 minutes to come up with their questions. The couple partners and family members are to take turns sharing their questions and allowing plenty of space for the others to reflect and respond to each other's questions. This can not only lead to the revelation of secrets but the couple partners and family members learning about certain life events that troubled them, concerns and wishes, why family emotional cutoffs have occurred with certain family members and relatives, and so forth. I make it clear to the couple and family that I want everyone to feel comfortable and safe with the questions they choose to share. I usually do this exercise once I have built alliances with the couple partners and family members and trust and safety has been established. When it comes to families, I only do this exercise with young adults and adolescents. Often, couples and families engage in highly meaningful, albeit emotional dialogues in response to each other's questions and this can carry over into multiple future session conversations. When secrets are revealed, it is important that we make it safe for the disclosing couple partner or family member and honor his or her preference to meet alone privately if he or she would feel more comfortable processing the secret situation and how best to cope with or manage the possible fallout of his or her disclosure. Occasionally, as a result of this exercise, I have had to make reports to child protection or contact the police with domestic violence situations. Finally, I would not do this exercise with young children. Because of adolescents' cognitive development and curiosity, they tend to make good use of this exercise, coming up with bold and intriguing questions to ask their parents and siblings.

Another therapeutic option when picking up on innuendos of secrets or feeling stuck with a couple or family, is to invite two or three of your colleagues to serve as a reflecting team (Andersen, 1995, 1991; Lax, 1995). About 40 minutes into the hour the therapist and the couple or family will have the opportunity to observe and listen to our colleagues' sharing their thoughts with one another about what is not being talked about, offer alternative perspectives on the presenting problem situation, and their thoughts about how we and the couple or family have gotten stuck. Additionally, they are free to take risks and be provocative with what they share with the family and us. The consultation team's reflections typically lasts for 6–7 minutes and then the couple or family are invited to respond to the teams' reflections. In some cases, the teams' reflections can open up space for the secret-keeper to courageously take the risk of disclosing his or her secret. The couple or family are also asked what particular team ideas really resonating with them or triggered epiphanies and new ways of looking at their situation. Sometimes the reflecting team conversation triggers for couple partners or family members an *afterglow effect*, where they continue to think and dialogue about what the team had shared with them long after the session is over (Erlich, Erlich, & Pepper, 1994).

Therapist–Client–Ecosystemic Contributions

With these therapeutic brick wall situations, there are involved helping professionals and concerned members from the clients' social networks that are entrenched in longstanding problem-maintaining interactions, which can keep the change process at a standstill. Once we enter conversations with our clients and these involved and powerful individuals, we need to be mindful of the fact that we become part of the problem system, treat all parties with respect, keep an open mind, and be therapeutically flexible. Below, I describe four major contributions to therapist–client–ecosystemic-generated therapeutic brick walls, followed by practical steps we can take to work with and remedy them:

1   The referring person is the customer for change, not the clients.
2   A couple/family-helping system knot exists, which is further exacerbating the clients' presenting difficulties and keeping the change process at a standstill.
3   There are over-involved in-laws or extended family members that have coalitions with one of the couple partners or with the identified child or adolescent client, which are contributing to the maintenance of the clients' presenting problems.
4   The adolescent's *second family* has dethroned his/her parents.

Keys to Fostering Cooperative Partnerships with Concerned and Highly Involved Referring Professionals

There are many different theoretical perspectives on how therapists view the referring person, how to work with him or her, and make sense of the referring process (Selekman, 2017; Selekman & Beyebach, 2013; Goolishian & Anderson, 1988; Anderson, Goolishian, & Winderman, 1986; Imber-Black, 1988; Boscolo, Cecchin, Hoffman, & Penn, 1987; Bergman, 1985). Some of the theorists cited above view the referring person in a negative light, that is he or she is a Dr. Homeostat contributing to the maintenance of the couple or family's difficulties by clinging to narrow fixed views of the clients' problem situation and/or engaging in unproductive attempted solutions, being too pessimistic, pathology-minded, or intrusively over-involved with the identified client, couple, or family (Boscolo, Cecchin, Hoffman, & Penn, 1987; Bergman, 1985; Selvini-Palazzoli, Boscolo, Cecchin, & Prata, 1980). My mantra is that with the referring person and other involved helping professionals with my clients I adopt the mindset of: *there are no villains or Dr. Homeostats, only allies.* I like to view the referring person and the other involved helping professionals as potential allies that can offer the clients and I novel perspectives, creative ideas, wisdom from working with similar clients in the past, and advocacy in their respective larger systems. They also are part of the new solution evolving, solution construction system along with the couple or family, other involved professionals, and the therapist. We also can't lose sight of the fact that these professionals have certain mandates and policies related to liability issues in their respective larger systems or organizations they represent that they must uphold. Additionally, the work contexts they represent can have a profound impact on how they view and approach client problems. For example, if a high school student is either caught in the act or has fresh cut marks on her arms, the school administrative officials will more than likely contact the parents and possibly recommend that she be evaluated by the district psychiatric consultant or be taken by the parents to nearest emergency room of a hospital with the concern that she may be suicidal.

Once I receive a referral of a new couple or family, I may get verbal consent initially from my new clients to let the referring person know that we made contact and set up appointment. In my first sessions with couples and families, I secure signed consent forms from the clients to be able to continue collaborating with the referring person and the other involved helping professionals to keep them abreast of clients' progress but be able to address any concerns they may have across the treatment process. With referring professionals in the community that I often work with, they have expressed appreciation that I let them know that the clients made contact with me, that we have appointments, and they like that I give them regular progress reports. I also let clients know that sometimes it is quite helpful to have the referring person or other involved helpers come to our sessions so they can bear witness to the changes they are making and for them to share with the helpers' certain needs or requests they have so they can advocate for them.

With some couple and family case situations, the referring person somehow became intrusively over-involved or over-stepped their boundaries playing the role of therapist to a couple partner or family member and alliances had been built, making it quite difficult for the new therapist to establish an alliance with their referred clients (Imber-Black, 1988). Rather than getting into a power struggle with the referring person over turf issues or putting them on the defensive, it is more productive to use respectful curiosity to come to better understand from him or her what is driving his or her *commitments*, that is his or her problem views, concerns, and compelling him or her to be overly involved (Kegan & Lahey, 2001). Just like with over-protective parents, there is often a backstory fueling their concerns and over-involvement. For example, I once received a referral from a school social worker of a 17-year-old self-injuring and bulimic adolescent female named Jackie. The social worker had been seeing Jackie 3–4 times per week, taking her out of classes that she liked. Jackie complained to her mother about missing class time and feeling like it was an over-kill on the social worker's behalf to see her so often. The mother complained to her daughter's high school dean and the principal about the social worker. I had seen the family three times and Jackie had completely stopped her self-injuring and bulimia. She had even told her social worker this great news but since the latter saw her still being at-risk to returning to these behaviors and insisted that they still have multiple times per week. The mother called for a school staffing to get to the bottom of why the social worker was making her daughter's school experience such an ordeal for her. In the meeting with the daughter's academic advisor, social worker, dean, principal, and two of her teachers, I posed the following question to the school social worker, "Is there something you think the mother and I might be missing with Jackie's situation that is making you worry and driving your strong desire to make sure that she is safe?" The social worker started to tear up and shared with all of us that in her last school social worker job she had lost a student to suicide who had been cutting herself. After learning about this terrible tragedy and every therapist's' worst nightmare of losing a client from the social worker, we finally learned what was driving her commitments. Once this important information came out, not only did all of the participants around the meeting table rally around the social worker with their support, including Jackie and her mother, but she felt much more at ease with my completely taking over the counseling process on my own and giving her regular progress reports.

Sometimes we get referred to us *no-problem problem* couples and families (Selekman, 2005; Eastwood, Sweeney, & Piercy, 1987). This can be a couple or family that would not have pursued counseling with us if it were not for the referring person who has the power to enforce quick response and action from the clients to go for counseling. For the majority of these couples and families, they are functioning quite well in most areas of their lives and had no past involvement with child protection, the police, been on court supervision before, or with kids, school administration involvement. Whether the referring person is a child protective worker, a probation officer, a school dean or principal, a couple partner's boss we need to build a cooperative relationship with them, engage the couple or family for counseling, and ask him or her the following questions:

- "What was Charles doing or had done that made you decide to refer him and his partner/family to me for counseling?"
- "What is your theory about why this behavior is occurring?"
- "What specifically do you think has to change with Charles so that this behavior will stop?"
- "How will you know when Charles has truly succeeded in counseling?"
- "What else will be major indicators of change for you?"
- "Anything else that you would need to see or hear about Charles behavior-wise that would indicate to you that he can stop counseling?"

The work with the no-problem problem couple or family is present and future-oriented. We discuss steps they need to take presently, and in the future to work their way out of the child protection, juvenile or adult justice systems, get off work probation, and as a way to get the referring person/social control agent off their backs. We can ask them the following questions:

- "What do you think Mr. Johnson would need to see changed first that would make him less concerned about you?"
- "What steps are you going to take over the next week to make that happen?"
- "Once that happens, what else would Mr. Johnson need to see changed that you think he would be pleased with?"
- "How else will he know that you are really succeeding in counseling?"

By regularly communicating with the referring person about our clients' progress, occasionally inviting him or her to join our sessions, he or she will be less alarmed and may be willing to relinquish not only the counseling mandate but close out the clients' child protection opened cases or get off court supervision or probation sooner. Finally, we need to consolidate the clients' gains and have them steer clear from what had originally led them to their being mandated for treatment to begin with, such as staying away from certain people and places and making better choices with avoiding drug use and anger management.

Keys to Untangling Couple/Family-Helping System Knot Situations

The more extreme and dramatic a couple partner's or family member's presenting problems are, the more likely they will attract an army of helping professionals around him or her like a magnet. When this happens, a couple/family-helping system knot situation can occur, which can become a therapeutic brick wall blocking the client change process. Often, the concerned professionals representing major larger systems and involved relatives from the couple or family's social network have different problem views, don't see eye-to-eye about how to resolve the clients' difficulties, are not regularly meeting or communicating about what they are doing to try and solve the clients' problems, which knots up the couple/family-helping system. Once we can start meeting as a group and the clients can have the lead voice in articulating their concerns, needs, and goals, the involved helpers and concerned relatives can learn how they can help the couple partners or family members in the best way possible. When hosting these meetings, we need to provide a safe climate for everyone's voice to be heard and respected, avoid privileging our own views or solution ideas and instead, use multi-partiality and model the use of "Yes and …" with piggy-backing meeting members' ideas and proposed solution strategies, and use respectful curiosity when exploring meeting members' concerns, expectations, and best hopes for the clients. By using all of these collaborative tools and strategies, it should help untangle the couple/family helping system knot and lead to productive meeting dialogues and teamwork and help the couple or family to stabilize their difficulties and achieve their goals.

Constructive Management of Over-Involved In-Laws and Relatives in Coalition with One Couple Partner or a Family Member

With couples, it is not uncommon during stressful times in their relationships it will be very tempting for one or both partners to breech the relationship boundary and complain to their parents about their problems. Naturally, the parents are going to protect their adult son or daughter, offer constructive or in some cases bad advice about how to manage the difficulty, or in worst case scenarios, verbally attack or blame the alleged couple partner for making their son or daughter unhappy or scared. Unless addressed, this will fuel more anger and conflict between the couple partners and can create emotional distance in the relationship and spending more time apart from one another. One therapeutic option we can pursue with this clinical situation are to use in-session enactments of whatever the hot conflict is between the partners to show you what the conversation about this conflict issue looks like in action. Once we see how each partner contributes to an escalation where the conversation becomes quite negative, we can then intervene directly and help them learn more constructive ways of communicating and solving conflicts. We also need agreement from each partner that they will keep up firm boundaries between their relationship and their parents when it comes to personal matters. Another option we have when it has been a chronic in-law boundary issue problem possibly dating back to the planning of the marriage is to bring the complaining partner together with his or her in-law parent for a session to directly try and resolve this difficulty. If the angry and frustrated partner would be willing to courageously meet with the boundary violating in-law, we can attempt to address this problem head-on, once and for all, to see if it can be resolved. Before having such a meeting, we need to do some coaching sessions with the brave partner to strategize a plan A, B, or C if a straightforward approach does not work. We can create a nice and non-threatening script that will be shared with the in-law. I always let partners know that in spite of their most respectful Herculean efforts to improve their relationships with their in-laws it does not always work for the better.

Another type of clinical dilemma is when one of the partner's parents or adult siblings of one of the parents is in a coalition with identified child or adolescent client and undermines their parents' authority with him or her. The grandparent or aunt or uncle are critical of their sibling's parenting abilities and go out of their way to sabotage parental rules and consequence enforcement. Sometimes they directly tell the child or adolescent not to listen to his or her parents. They also have a tendency to spoil the child or adolescent with money and gifts that are given behind the scenes. There may be long-standing sibling rivalry between one of the parents and the offending adult sister or brother and they getting even by undermining their parenting and using their son or daughter as a tag team wrestling partner. What both the grandparent and adult sibling are missing is that the mixed messages the child or adolescent are receiving is fueling his or her symptoms or acting out behaviors. With this clinical dilemma, I ask the frustrated parent if they would be willing to meet with one or both of their parents or the adult sibling and try and resolve their conflicts directly so that we can disrupt the destructive problem-maintaining patterns of interaction. Like with the couple partner confronting an intrusive in-law, I will do coaching sessions with the parent and come up with a solid script to use as a guide for how best to gain his or her parent's or sibling's cooperation and support.

Constructive Management of the Adolescent's Second Family's Powerful Grip on Him or Her

When there are poor communications, a high level of conflict, and emotional disconnection between adolescents and their parents, they will often gravitate to the *second family*, which is often a peer group of other adolescents who are angry, frustrated, and are disconnected from their parents (Selekman, 2017, 2005; Taffel & Blau, 2001). In the second family, they may feel a strong sense of connection, feel valued, respected, feel powerful, and have people watching their backs. These adolescents spend little time with their families and would rather be with their second family friends that they can count on. Often, the parents have not met their adolescent's second family members. As a result of this challenging situation, the parents' power and control is completely neutralized and they are dethroned. While with their second families, adolescents may be exposed to a lot of self-destructive and delinquent behaviors, which may be fun and exciting initially but can come back to haunt them in some big-time ways down the road. Family therapy will remain at a standstill unless we directly address the second family issue.

There are two therapeutic options worth trying with this therapeutic brick wall situation. One is to have them invite two or three of their closest second family friends to meet or bring in some former adolescent alumni who also were adopted by a second family, but the consequences of being affiliated with groups of unsavory peers led to juvenile detention time, being admitted into a psychiatric hospital, and residential treatment. The first option is to have them bring in their closest second family friends to meet. Once they show up, I go over the rules of confidentiality, I have my client have their friends and their friends' parents sign off on my significant other permission consent form, and I collect it from him or her. I treat the friends like royalty and we discuss how we can help my client re-connect with at least one of his or her parents or siblings so he or she could have some kind of connection with his or her family. Often, at least one of the second family friends had a need to re-connect with his or her family and was glad that they put forth the effort to do so. Also, I enlist the support and creativity of the friends in coming up with some strategies or solutions for my client to help him not get in to further trouble at home and at school. The friends often come up with some great ideas that the client can experiment with. When we wrap up our first meeting with the friends, I thank them for being a big help and coming and ask if they would be willing to come again. When it has been a productive meeting with lots of conversation, the friends often agree to come in again.

Another therapeutic option is to bring in adolescent alumni who discovered that joining a second family was a huge mistake and cost them big-time. Using my significant other permission consent form, I get parental, alumni, and client written consent to participate in a session together. In this meeting, I have the two or three adolescent alumni share their horrific stories of being part of some very negative second families that led to severe consequences for them. After they share their stories and our clients have had room to ask questions, we can have the alumni share how they reconciled with their real families and turned their lives around. Often, alumni have a lot of wisdom and great ideas about finding one's path in life to share with our clients. If this meeting proves to be helpful to the client, I will explore with both parties if they would like to meet again in the future.

In this chapter, I have presented 20 contributing factors that therapists, their clients, and the complex interactions between them, their clients, and involved larger systems professionals and concerned resource people from their social networks can play a role in therapeutic brick walls occurring. For each of the contributing factors presented, I have offered trouble-shooting guidelines for getting unstuck, dismantling the therapeutic brick walls, and liberating our clients from their difficulties.

Improvisational Theater on the Screen

The Therapist's Use of Self in a Virtual Tele-Health Therapy Context

The COVID-19 pandemic and all of the ensuing restrictions this nightmarish situation had imposed on all of us worldwide had turned our lives upside down. Many of us for the first time had to rely heavily on Zoom and other streaming services to conduct our therapy sessions virtually with our clients, which could feel stifling and unnatural in that as humans we much prefer building in-person relationships with them. The same is true for us trainers and consultants that love working hands-on with groups and enjoy making connections with people in-person rather than on Zoom where we may be able to see some of the participants in boxes but there are many participants that cannot be seen and we don't know where we stand with them. These life and professional challenges can be approached with a doom and gloom mindset or we can adopt a radical acceptance position of "It is what is," which can be quite liberating (Brach, 2004; Selekman, 2021). Once I embraced this true Buddhist position, I could begin to see all of the possibilities and opportunities these constraints provided for our clients and therapists alike.

In this chapter, I discuss some of the major advantages of doing couple and family tele-health therapy for both our clients and us. This will be followed by a brief discussion on the use of improvisational skills, creative ways we can use our clients' strengths and resources, life passions, top skills, cherished mementos, children's favorite toys, pets, and hobby items to aid us in crafting intriguing and bold questions and with co-designing therapeutic experiments. Finally, in an effort to further make our clients tele-health sessions more fun and engaging, I present eight idea-generating skill-building exercises and seven couple and family games that they can do together in tapping their inventiveness to co-construct their own creative high-quality solutions for their difficulties.

Experiencing Couples and Families in their Natural Habitats: The Therapeutic Advantages of Virtual Tele-Health Couple and Family Therapy

In the late sixties and early seventies, Kantor and Lehr (1975) conducted a groundbreaking naturalistic study with nineteen families from Boston and surrounding suburbs. As an important component of the study, university students spent time as

DOI: 10.4324/9781003334460-6

participant observers living with these families in their homes to learn about the following family processes as: how family members solved conflicts, problems, and crises; affective expression in family relationships; learn about their rituals; values; identifying individual member and family strengths in action; what family members were passionate about and found meaningful doing; children's responsibilities; how well parents worked together as a team; how well the parents disciplined and comforted their kids when they experienced emotional distress; closeness and distance in family relationships; the fostering of dependence versus independence, was family member privacy valued and upheld; were family ties strong with extended family members, how strong the family's connections were with neighbors and friends; how open and strong were their communications with the outside world. Not only did Kantor and Lehr's research provide a fascinating insider's perspective of family life and functioning but it led to the creation of a new theoretical framework for family assessment and treatment.

When conducting virtual tele-health couple and family therapy sessions, it affords us with a unique insider's perspective, similar to the research of Kantor and Lehr (1975) of couple and family life, we can learn about the same aforementioned couple and family processes, certain undiscussables, critical life events, painful traumas or losses, or even secrets that we may not have gained access to in our offices. By working with couples and families in the safety and comfort of their homes, they tend to be less guarded, more relaxed, and more likely to lower their drawbridges and welcome us in to their lives past and present. There is a *distanced intimacy* that occurs online in our conversations with our clients that may feel much more comfortable and safer for them than in-person in a therapist's office (Zeavin, 2021).

Other advantages for working virtually with couples and families is it provides us ample opportunities to further hone our observation and listening skills. With observation skills I am not just referring to observing for both repetitive problem-maintaining and positive solution-building interactions but paying closer attention to the nonverbal communications of couple partners' and family members.' We are forced to listen more deeply and generously with our clients, almost like having a third ear. Another advantage of working virtually is that we can tap into the inventiveness of our clients to craft intriguing and bold questions to ask themselves about their situations and co-design high-quality therapeutic experiments together. Finally, in an effort to keep our tele-health sessions more upbeat and engaging for our clients, we can use fun idea-generating skill-building exercises, couple and family games, our improvisational skills, humor, and playfulness to help strengthen our alliances with them and have them on the edge of their seats eager to come back and experience what surprises await them in their next sessions.

Improvisation and All that Jazz: Playing Out on the Edges with Couples and Families

One of the best examples of playing out on the edges can be heard in what is touted as the greatest jazz concert ever at Massey Hall in Toronto, Canada 1953 with the all-star line-up of Charlie Parker, Dizzy Gillespie, Bud Powell, Charlie Mingus, and Max Roach (Parker, 2006). On all of the tunes on this recording one can hear improvisation at its best on popular jazz standards, like "Salt Peanuts" and "A Night in Tunisia." Like great jazz performances, change happens in our sessions out on the edges, seizing opportunities as they present themselves in the moment, and improvising off of what our clients present to us by introducing something novel and surprising. Most couples and families come to us feeling stuck and limited in their ways of viewing and doing with one another. By bringing to couples and families lively up-tempo energy, giving ourselves permission to take risks, using ample amounts of humor, playfulness, and novelty in our sessions, such as sharing quotes, telling jokes, engaging stories that mirror their situations, and absurd ideas that pop into our minds in response to something that a couple partner or family member had shared, can not only create a context ripe for change but can help liberate them from the clutches of their difficulties.

Creative Uses of Clients' Life Passions and Interests

In addition to coming to know our clients by their strengths and resources, life passions, interests, and top skills, when working virtually with them we will gain access to their pets, good luck charms, meaningful mementos, children's favorite toys, and hobby items, which we can use for crafting intriguing and bold questions and co-designing therapeutic experiments. Some examples of the type of questions we can ask couples and families in our tele-health sessions with them are as follows:

- "If Ralph (the family dog) could talk and offer you and your mother advice about how the two of you could argue less, what would he say?"
- "How might that help?"
- "What else would he (Ralph) recommend the two of you do differently that could help the two of you get along better?"
- "Let's say the spirit warriors woven into your Navajo rug (highly cherished rug bought on a trip to New Mexico) on the wall could step down and help you to not cave into using alcohol, what would they say to you (a couple partner) and recommend you do to stay on track and stave off a slip?"
- "If Spider-Man and Iron Man dropped by to meet with you and your family, what would they recommend that you should work on changing first?"
- "What creative ideas would they have for you that would help you put an end to your clashes?"
- "If your most favorite Alebrije (Mexican wooden folk-art sculpture) of an owl (most valuable memento) could suddenly talk and offer you (a couple partner) valuable words of wisdom to avoid saying or doing the next time you get upset with your partner, what would it say to you?"
- "Let's say your Star Wars Lego spacecraft could magically beam outside into your backyard and was now human-size. What planet would you take it to?"
- "What would the two of you (father and son) come to know about one another over the light years you are traveling together in the spacecraft?"

- "When you come back to the planet Earth, what will the two of you be the happiest about that changed in your relationship?"
- "Let's say your turquoise and silver pendant (a good luck charm) suddenly had magical powers. How would you use its powers to transform your relationship with your husband?"
- "How will he be different with you?"
- "What affect would his changes have on you?"

Some examples of how we could co-design therapeutic experiments with couples and families based on their responses to the questions asked above, are as follows:

- Based on Ralph's recommendations, family members can practice new ways of interacting with one another that they think he would be happy about and help him to bark less due to family members' not arguing as much.
- The spirit warriors would recommend that the couple partner (abstinent alcohol-abuser) practice on a daily basis as an experiment *Walking in Beauty* and engaging in *hozho*, which consists of choosing healthy alternatives to rapidly pursue when triggered to drink, such as: exercising, engaging in a meaningful hobby, playing an instrument, eating healthy foods, get together with non-using friends, spend high-quality time with family and extended family members, take breaks from technology usage, and get more sleep (Alvord & Cohen-Van Pelt, 2000).
- Based on Spider-Man's and Iron Man's advice, the family would practice enacting what they would recommend for them to change first such as working on being better listeners or when conflicts occur, take turns hearing each other's positions on what they are upset about without interrupting, think before talking, or be less emotionally reactive with one another. When practicing listening skills with one another, they could pretend that Spider-Man fired webbing at their mouths so they could not talk when another family member is speaking. Iron Man might fire a stun beam at family members that are engaging in destructive interactions with another member, so that they can try and catch themselves from blaming and criticizing to avoid having a stun beam fired at them.
- Once we learned from the father and son what changed in their relationship while in outer space together, we can have them practice their new ways of interacting with one another and engaging in other meaningful and high-quality activities together as their therapeutic experiments.
- With the couple partner utilizing the words of wisdom of the wooden owl she could experiment with avoiding using certain words or ways of interacting with her partner that have blown up for her in the past when upset with her and see how she responds differently to her. Once the partner discovers what works, she should do more of it with her partner whenever disagreements occur.

- With the couple partner who possesses the turquoise and silver pendant with magical powers, we can not only have her wear it when attempting to settle disagreements with her partner but experiment with new ways of approaching him, that is changing her vocal tone and posture, being more relaxed, and notice how he responds differently to her. Before approaching him, she is to visualize in her mind what the transformed partner will look like and what affect those changes will have on her.

The following case example below illustrates how to make use of a child's favorite and trusty stuffed animals as a consultation team:

> Lisa, a precocious Caucasian 10-year-old, had experienced multiple traumatic experiences while living with her biological mother after her parents had divorced. Her mother abused drugs and had sex in front of Lisa with multiple partners, who she also witnessed battering her mother. There were a few nights where the mother would not come home until the next day. These experiences triggered anxiety, depressed mood, and bed-wetting difficulties for Lisa. Once the child protection department had completed their investigation abuse and neglect allegations were determined, she lost custody of her daughter, and Lisa went to live out of state with her biological father and his new wife. After I built an alliance with Lisa, I had her bring into our online sessions her four favorite stuffed animals: Daffy (duck), Porky (pig), Wilbur (lion), and Henrietta (rooster). It had been six months since her mother had contacted her and Lisa was quite angry and depressed about her neglecting her. I asked Lisa to consult with Daffy, Porky, Wilbur, and Henrietta about what they thought she should do about the lack of communication with her mother. I had her pretend to be their voices and have them respond to the following questions:
>
> - "Should Lisa try and contact her mother to help open up the lines of communication again with her?"
> - "Do you think her mother is going through a tough time right now and it could be a good thing for Lisa to reach out to her?"
> - "Do you think Lisa should let her mother know that she is upset with her about not communicating with her and get this off her chest?"
> - "Is it possible that her mother feels badly about losing custody to Lisa and she might feel too ashamed to talk to her, and that's why she cut off the communications with her?"

Lisa did a great job of pretending to be the voices of her stuffed animals and having them dialogue about what she should do about her situation with her mother. The stuffed animal team came to the conclusion that Lisa should call her mother, let her know that she was upset with her about cutting off the communications with her, and explore with her if she was interested in resolving the situation with her. With the support of her parents and I in the next session, Lisa drummed up the courage to call her mother to find out what had contributed to the communications breakdown, express that she missed not talking to her, and to catch up on what was going on her life. The mother had apologized to Lisa and shared with her that she had to go into a drug treatment program for over a month and is trying to turn her life around. She started to cry and made a commitment to Lisa that she would not allow this to happen again. Lisa and her mother picked a day and time that they could speak weekly. The father and stepmother supported this plan and thought it was a good idea. We praised Lisa for her tremendous courage and doing such a great job with how she spoke with her mother. As the weeks past, Lisa and her mother were regularly communicating again, her bed-wetting stopped, and her anxious and depressed moods dramatically decreased.

As mentioned earlier, couples and families tend to be much more relaxed and upbeat in their home environments, they are less guarded, and may be experiencing a wide range of positive emotions, which provides the perfect climate for effective and creative problem-solving (Fredrickson, 2009). Our clients bring to the virtual tele-health therapy context a treasure trove of strengths and resources, skills, life passions, varied interests, and meaningful possessions that we can utilize to craft intriguing questions and co-design therapeutic experiments derived from their responses to the questions we had posed to them.

Broadway Theater on the Big Screen: Therapist as Director and Choreographer of New Couple and Family Dramas

Another way we can liven up our virtual tele-health therapy sessions is to be like a *Broadway* director and choreographer of a new couple and family theatrical production of both their presenting problems and preferred future solution-determined realities. The couple partners or family members are free to wear costumes, use props, and provide a soundtrack for their choreographed works. Below, I describe how to use *couple choreography* and *solution-oriented family choreography* (Papp, 1983; Selekman, 2017).

Couple Choreography

One way we can co-produce with couples a more preferred future relationship outcome is to use couple choreography (Papp, 1983). Each partner will take turns closing his or her eyes and have a dream or fantasy about their partners and visualize what symbolic form he or she would take in the dream or fantasy, such as: an animal or other physical objects out in the world, a historic figure, a character from a movie or popular book, a cartoon, and so forth. Next, each partner will visualize what form he or she will take in relationship to whatever form they came up with for their partners. They are then to imagine what movement or dance would take place between these two forms, given the presenting problems they described to you. As the director of their theatrical production, you have them enact each of their dreams or fantasies one at a time physically with one another. They are invited to discuss while in motion in their dramatizations to provide details about time, setting, mood, and the movements they are engaging in. After each partner enacts his or her dream or fantasy, we can have them reflect on their thoughts about what they came up with, central themes, how the patterns of interactions and their reciprocal roles have become redundant and rigidified, and have them be curious about what the possible negative consequences of changing their ways of interacting with one another would be. With the help of each couple partner, we can revisit each of their dramatizations of their dreamt or fantasized depictions of their current relationship situation and have them co-choreograph with us more preferred and adaptive ways of interacting with one another that they think would make a difference in helping them have a more satisfactory relationship. Once they come up with the new dance steps or ways of being with one another in each of their dramatizations, we can have them enact it in motion, and have them take it off the stage and practice at home to help consolidate their new ways of interacting and role behaviors in their relationship.

I once worked with a Latino couple where the partners had drifted apart emotionally from one another, they rarely went on dates or spent time together, and there was no sexual intimacy. I used couple choreography with them. Rosalita, the wife, visualized the image of her husband Alberto as a giant loving gorilla and her image for herself was that she was a female tapir in the jungle. I had them stand up and enact Rosalita's scene in the jungle with motion. I asked her ideally what she wanted the gorilla to do with her as the tapir. She invited the gorilla to give her warm, loving hug. Rosalita started to cry and express how she misses the closeness and intimacy in their marriage that they used to have. I had Rosalita and Alberto discuss how they thought they could bring back the intimacy in their relationship and what steps they could take over the next week to begin to make that happen. Alberto had a visualization in his mind that Rosalita was a tall pyramid and he was a court jester dancing around her, making funny faces and jumping around in an effort to get her attention and interact with him. Alberto shared that his pyramid image was capturing her rigidity, keeping her distance from him, and balking at his attempts to spend time with him and have fun together. We discussed how both partners had the same goal and various ways they could build in daily intimacy time doing something high-quality together and institute a weekend date night. Both partners took responsibility for allowing them to drift apart from one another and committed to turning the situation around. They both shared that it was helpful to do the couple choreography exercise because it helped them to step outside of their stuck relationship drama and see from a metaphorical perspective how bad things had gotten in their relationship and were now fired up to remedy their situation.

Solution-Oriented Family Choreography

Solution-oriented family choreography can be used with children and adolescents and their parents as a way to co-choreograph with them a compelling family drama of their ideal future outcome of endless possibilities (Selekman, 2017). To begin with, I have the parents and kids identify any positive pretreatment or between session interactions that are occurring that are helping them get along better and the originally reported problems are absent. One of these solution-building patterns of interaction that the child, adolescent, or parents have found to be most meaningful or helpful can be enacted in motion in the form of a choreographed dramatization of it. The family members can wear costumes, use props, choose their favorite tunes that they would like to play in the background, decide how family members will interact or dance with him, her, or them, and what the nonverbals will look like, such as facial expressions, and so forth. Not only do family members laugh and enjoy playing with one another doing this exercise but it can be transformative in helping them to co-choreograph a more preferred solution-determined drama with them. They can decide as a group which of the family members' choreographies they would like to practice implementing over the next week. Another valuable resource for accessing family members' compelling future realities is to ask the following questions:

- "Let's say our work together proves to be helpful to all of you beyond your wildest dreams and your problems are now solved, what changed with your situation?"
- "What difference will that change make for you?"
- "How will that help the two of you get along better?"
- "How else will you be able to tell that your wildest dreams were really happening in your family?"
- "I'm curious, sometimes people's wildest dreams started to happen a little bit before they came here. Have any of you noticed your wildest dreams happening a little bit already?"

Once we know what each family members' wildest dreams changed family interactions would look like, we can have members take turns enacting their ideal scenarios in motion in the session. Using the same processing format as described above, family members can take turns presenting their choreographed wildest dream ideal interactions to one another. Together, they can decide which of the wildest dreams patterns of interaction they would like to practice over the next week.

The Use of Couple and Family Idea-Generating Skill-Building Exercises and Games to Co-generate their Own Unique Solutions

In this section of the chapter, I present couple and family idea-generating skill-building exercises and games that tap our clients' inventiveness and help strengthen their communications and problem-solving skills. Not only are these exercises fun, engaging to do, trigger positive emotions, and help liven up our tele-health sessions for couples and families but they invite the clients to co-generate their own unique solutions for their presenting difficulties. Brown and Vaughn (2016) contend that "The times we feel most alive, those that make up our best memories, are moments of play" (p. 6). The idea-generating skill-building exercises and games can be used in in-person office sessions as well. Below, I present seven games and eight idea-generating skill-building exercises for helping couples and families co-generate their own unique solutions.

The Family Strengths Game

DeFrain and his colleagues (DeFrain 2007; Stinnett & O'Donnell, 1996; DeFrain & Stinnett 1992) over the past three decades in their research on *strong families*, have identified six characteristics of strong families, they are as follows:

- appreciation and affection for each other;
- commitment;
- positive communications;
- spend enjoyable time together;
- the ability to manage stress and crisis effectively; and
- spiritual well-being.

They have found all six characteristics in culturally diverse families from all socioeconomic levels and struggling with a wide range of difficulties. Some families are stronger in one or more of these family strengths areas than other families. As part of my family assessment process, and after presenting the six characteristics of strong families to the clients, I inquire with them about how high they would rate on a scale from one to ten each of the six family strengths with their family. Some families voice a desire to work on strengthening their weaker family strengths in family therapy. When a family shares their top family strength that they think their family shines in, I ask for members to give me concrete examples of their family strengths in action and how they have used them to resolve difficulties, conflicts, and manage crises successfully. The *family strengths game* consists of having the family first writing down on slips of paper the six family strengths which will be placed into a small box or shoebox. Next, each family member will blindly pick a family strength written on one of the slips of paper that they will commit to trying to implement in their relationships with one another over the next week. However, whatever family strength they select, they are not allowed to share with other family members which family strength they chose to put into action over the next week. They are simply to enact their selected family strength in their relationships with other family members and not tell them what they are doing. This is repeated until all family members have taken turns selecting their family strengths. While enacting their chosen family strengths, they are to pay close attention to how family members respond to them in positive ways. When the family and I meet the following week, they compare notes and see if family members can accurately guess who enacted what family strength and what positive differences did their actions have on their relationships. As part of this discussion, family members may voice a strong desire to strengthen their weaker family strengths or increase using their selected family strengths due to their improving their relationships and helping them to resolve their presenting difficulties.

Back from the Future

The nice thing about the future is that it has not happened yet, so why not co-invent it with our clients. This exercise can be used with both couples and families to help propel the treatment system into a future reality of client liberation from their presenting difficulties and change. The exercise is particularly helpful when clients are feeling stuck and frustrated with their current state of affairs or we have run into a therapeutic brick wall in the treatment process. Once we know what our clients' ideal outcome pictures will look like, we can have them walk back from their positive future reality spelling out the steps they took to arrive at their ideal destinations. I have the couple partners or family members pretend to hop into my imaginary time machine, which I had transported over to a location in their family or living room. Clients are to hop into the imaginary time machine and travel into the future one year from their travelling date and while on their journey all of their problems are completely solved. They are told that they will not notice all of their positive changes until they exit the machine. I than ask them to respond to the following questions:

- "What will you be the most surprised with that changed in your relationship with Linda?"
- "What affect has that change had on you (the husband)?"
- "Linda (the wife) how has Steve changed and what difference has that made for you in your relationship with him?"
- "How else will things be better in your relationship?"
- "If each of you were to walk me back from the future spelling out the steps each of you took while on your journey to achieve your positive and special outcomes, what will you tell me you did to make that happen?"

Pick the Most Absurd and Outrageous Ideas for Solving Your Problem

With this fun and playful exercise, we have the couple or family write a list of the most absurd and outrageous ideas they could think of for resolving their presenting problem. Next, you have them identify any good or intriguing aspects of these absurd and outrageous ideas that when used separately or combined may serve as potential building blocks for co-constructing solutions to their presenting difficulty.

This exercise not only sparks laughter and great teamwork but couples and families often discover that their most absurd and outrageous ideas they co-generate together have the potential for coming up with some very creative high-quality solutions.

The Couple and Family Solutions Game

This couple or family cooperative game invites the couple partners or family members to pretend to be super sleuth detectives over the next week and carefully looking for clues for what contributes to the times when their presenting difficulties are not happening. With their trusty imaginary magnifying glasses, they are to observe closely on a daily basis daily for what the partners or family members are saying and doing or not doing that contribute to their problems being absent and write down what works. Each night after dinner or later in the evening they are to compare notes about what clues they had discovered that can help increase the non-problem times and serve as potential building blocks for solution construction. This game can successfully move the couple partners and family members away from being trigger happy with one another by anticipating clashes and problems to refocusing their attention on what works and increasing it instead. Once couples and families increase their positive interactions with one another and their viewing of their situations change, their expectancy that more positive changes are going to happen will greatly increase, which will cascade into further changes happening for them well into the future. As the old adage goes, nothing succeeds like success!

Find a Random Trigger Word Game

Have the couple or family bring out a dictionary or turn to any page of a book and take turns blindly picking a word on a page to use as a trigger for at least five ideas related to their presenting problem that involve their selected word. As a couple or family, they can use their trigger words and combine their ideas to co-construct potential solutions to their difficulties.

Construct Your Idea to Spark Solutions

This playful and fun game is great to use with children and their families. The kids and their parents are to use Lego pieces, Cool Crazy Connectors building blocks, wooden building blocks, or STEM Master building toys as a metaphorical solution and for triggering associations to aid them with the co-construction of solutions. They can be asked the following questions:

- "If you were to co-construct together a machine or gadget that would benefit other kids and families just like yours, what special features would it have, and how would it help your family?"
- "What do you call your invention?"

- "(Asking the child) How would your invention help you and your parents get along better?"
- "(The children and parents) What else will it change about your family?"
- "Mom and dad, what other ideas were sparked for you about how your invention will benefit your family?"
- "What was most special and meaningful about doing this activity together?"

Map Your Couple or Family Journey to Possibility Land

The couple or family are to create a map of what their journey to Possibility Land (ideal outcome) will look like. The week before having a couple or family do this art exercise, they are to purchase a large sheet of tagboard from an art supply or office supply shop. They are to draw on a large sheet of tagboard mountains and rugged terrain to represent obstacles and challenges for change and draw creeks, rivers, and lakes to represent movement and transition. Additionally, they are to draw on the map signposts or landmarks that will tell them they are on the right roads or pathways to their ideal outcome and how they will constructively work around mountains, other challenging terrain, rivers and lakes to stay on track and persevere until they reach their ideal destination. This exercise helps foster teamwork and can enhance couples' and families' problem-solving capacities.

Our Couple and Family Miracle Mural

A fun and playful way to have couples and families depict what their ideal outcome pictures will look like is to have a couple or family create a mural that incorporates visually what their miracles will look like. After asking them the miracle question (de Shazer, 1988), they are to show how they have changed individually, how their relationships look different, what they are doing together, in what contexts the changes are happening, what new and pleasurable activities they are engaging in together, and other signs of change on their mural. For our second couple or family tele-health therapy session, I have a couple or family purchase 3–4 large sheets of paper from an art supply store that they can tape together for creating the mural. What is great about this art exercise is that the couple or family have created visually their roadmap for change, which can be posted on a wall in their homes as a reminder of what signs of progress will look like and what will be happening that will tell them that they have made it to their ideal outcome destination.

The Positive Reminiscing for Solutions Game and the Positive Reminiscing Couple/Family Collage

Positive reminiscing has been found to increase positive emotions, reduces negative emotions, bolsters self-esteem, helps to resolve problems and conflicts, and increases warmth and intimacy in couple and family relationships (Osgarby & Halford, 2013;

Bryant, King, & Smart, 2005; Westerhof, Bohlmeijer, & Webster, 2010; Fredrickson, 2009; Coleman, 1974). To begin the game, I give a mini-presentation about all of the mental health and relationship benefits of positive reminiscing. Each couple partner or family member is to is to take turns positive reminiscing about one of the happiest and most meaningful times in their relationships that they can recall. They are to share the following: where in time they went back to; where they were and with whom; what they were doing together and talking about; details about what was most special about the time together; how they were thinking and feeling; and were there any aspects of their past positive experiences they would like to institute in their current couple or family relationships. After a couple partner or family member shares their past sparkling moment experiences, the other partner and family members can reflect on what they shared and what aspects they found special about their shared experiences. Not only does this exercise trigger lots of positive emotions and engender hope and optimism but it helps strengthen the couple partners' and family members' relationship bonds. For therapists, we learn about couples and families past successes as well. This game may extend over a few sessions and we can encourage couples and families to experiment with implementing important elements of their sparkling past relationship moments in their relationships now.

Another option, is to have the couple create a positive reminiscing collage of one of the most meaningful and special times together in the past. It could be a special trip or activity that when they think about it not only puts smiles on their faces but triggers positive emotions for them. They are to get a large sheet of construction paper or tagboard, come up with a title for their collage, cut out words, phrases, and images that capture best their experiences. They could glue on it copies of photos, souvenirs, or other mementos from this special couple or family past experience.

Couple and Family Adventure Missions

During the COVID-19 pandemic, many couples and families felt like prisoners in their homes and paralyzed by all of the restrictions imposed on their lives. However, what was open for them to do was to get out in nature and engage in *couple and family adventure missions*. The couple or family are to come up with some challenging outdoor adventure activity they could do, such as: going on a difficult hike in the woods or on a mountain trail, taking a lengthy and hilly bicycle ride, going for a long run or walk on a forest reserve park path, going on a long kayaking or canoe trip, and so forth. While engaging in their high-quality couple or family adventure, I encourage them to refrain from using their smartphones and instead converse with and stay present with one another. For most of the couples and families I have had do this activity, it not only helped them to rediscover the positive aspects of their relationships but it has helped strengthen their bonds. An added bonus that has grown out of this activity, is that individual partners and family members start to institute in their daily regimes some form of exercise and wanting to get out in nature more often after discovering its healing and relaxing aspects.

"It Would Be Cool if We Did ..."

This game frees up couple and families to inject more excitement and high-quality time into their relationships. The couple partners and family members are to allow their fantasies, dreams, and imagination powers to run wild with coming up with novel, fun, and pleasurable activities they would love to do together. Once they come up with their lists of "cool" activities, they are to choose together one or two that they would like to pursue first, what the necessary preparation would be to set them in motion, and what steps they would have to take to optimize for them to happen. Often, the couple partners and family members co-generate many creative and exciting ideas for future trips and fun activities they could do together.

Stepping Out of Your Comfort Zones

This exercise helps the couple partners and family members to develop more resilience, grit, and develop *growth-oriented mindsets* (Dweck, 2006). Each couple partner or family member is to commit to doing one thing outside of their comfort zones that they have never done before over the next week. While doing there out of their comfort zone activities, they are to pay close attention to what they are telling themselves, thinking, what positive emotions they are experiencing, and the steps they are taking that are helping them to achieve their novel and challenging tasks. They are to write all of this valuable information down and bring it to our next virtual couple or family session. In this session, they are to share with one another what their useful self-talk was, other helpful thoughts they had, what positive emotions they were experiencing, and what steps they took to successfully achieve their tasks. They also are to share with one another what they learned about themselves as a result of taking their courageous risks stepping out of their comfort zones. Next, we can have them decide which aspects of there out of their comfort zones activities could they utilize to conquer their presenting couple or family difficulty. There are no losers in this game, even if one of the couple partners or family members falls short of completing their challenging tasks, what counts is his or her taking the risk and persevering as far as they could go.

Family Guest Consultants' Game

The couple partners or family members are to pick two famous people a piece that they admire and have been inspired by. Next, they are to pretend to enter the minds of their selected people to imagine what they would say and do to resolve their presenting problem. Once they have come up with their famous people's creative ideas for them, the family members can decide which of these ideas they found most useful and apply them to begin tackling their presenting problem over the next week (Selekman, 2017).

Question-Storming

This exercise is great to use with couples and families when we are picking up on certain subjects that appear to be couple or family undiscussables, that is certain subjects the partners or family members seem to be shying away from, innuendos of secrets, and therapeutic brick walls have occurred. The couple partners or family members are to respond first to the following key question: "What are the essential questions we have not yet asked about our couple/family difficulty?" They are than separately to come up with 4–5 questions beginning with: "What?" "What if …?" "How?" or "Why?" After about 20 minutes, the couple partners or family members take turns sharing and reflecting on each other's questions. This powerful exercise can open up space for couples and families to safely share their concerns, hopes, needs, secrets, learn about critical life events that had adversely affected one of the partners or family members, explanations for why emotional cut-offs from certain family members and relatives had occurred, and constraints can be removed that was keeping them stuck in conflict. Often couples and families engage in very meaningful and interesting dialogues that they continue to ponder long after the session and wish to continue responding to each other's questions in subsequent sessions.

In this chapter, I have presented some of the advantages of doing virtual tele-health couple and family therapy. I also have presented several ways therapists can use themselves to make their virtual tele-health sessions much more engaging, upbeat, and fun with couples and families.

7

Resources for Enhancing Your Inventiveness and Expanding Your Therapeutic Range and Style

Outside of the confines of marital, family, and psychotherapy literature lies a gold-mine of rich sources for metaphors and creative ideas from such diverse fields as: art, architecture, film, theater, literature, philosophy, history, music, science and technology, and nature. When I am feeling stuck or looking for some fresh ideas, I go prospecting in these fields for sources of inspiration and creative sparks for crafting intriguing questions and for designing novel and creative therapeutic experiments to offer my clients. Many of the greatest inventors, innovators, and famous people representing the aforementioned fields attributed what had inspired them and their professional success to ideas that were sparked for them from fields outside of their main professional discipline. For example, surrealist artist Salvador Dalí's dream-scape art works were heavily inspired by Freud's theories on the unconscious mind, dreams, and psychosexuality (Taschen, 1994); Buckminster Fuller's geodesic dome, an inverted bird's nest in shape, was inspired by his love of nature, science, and architectural design; and so on. Another resource area when we are feeling stuck or are looking for some fresh ideas that we can tap is what we bring to our clients, our strengths, talents, interests, and life passions. For example, one of my life passions is cooking different cuisines, sometimes fusing them together, and new spins on classic dishes. If a couple or family session has become to humdrum, I will imagine myself spicing it up with some hot chili flakes in an effort to heat the atmosphere up and move the session in a more productive direction.

In this chapter, I discuss practical guidelines for how we can find and utilize metaphors and inspiration for novel ideas from all the fields mentioned above for crafting intriguing questions to pose to our clients and for co-designing high-quality therapeutic experiments to offer our clients. Recent research on *extra-neural resources* provides some empirical support for the value in searching for ideas and identifying certain relaxing, aesthetically appealing, and inspiring contexts where creative ideas seem to spontaneously pop into our minds that are outside of the confines of our brains and professional fields, can greatly enhance our inventiveness and solution-finding capacities. Additionally, I discuss further practical ways we can tap what we bring to our clients, that is our strengths, talents, interests, and life passions to

DOI: 10.4324/9781003334460-7

empower our clients and as another way to enhance our therapeutic inventiveness, range and style. Finally, case examples are provided throughout the chapter.

Stepping Outside of the World of Psychotherapy: Finding Inspiration and Creative Ideas in Unexpected Places

Research in three related areas on extra-neural resources has indicated that they greatly contribute to our thinking processes for generating creative solutions for complex problems and with innovation (Paul, 2021; Clark, 2011; Clark & Chalmers, 1998). The three areas of study are: *embodied cognition*, *situated cognition*, and *distributed cognition*. Embodied cognition has to do with the role our bodies play in our thinking, such as the use of hand gestures, which help us with speech and can deepen our understanding of abstract concepts. Situation cognition examines the role of context or place on our thinking, such as looking at how environmental cues can give us a sense of belonging, a sense of personal agency, and enhance our performance in that space. Distributed cognition studies the effects of thinking with others, how people work in groups and coordinate their areas of expertise and skill, and how groups can collaborate together to co-produce results that exceed members' individual contributions, which is called *collective intelligence* (Paul, 2021; Clark, 2011). It was David Chalmers who came up with the concept of "extended mind" as a description for extra-neural resources (Paul, 2021). Clark (2011) mounted a convincing argument based on his research that the widely believed brain-bound perspective that thinking only occurs inside our brains is incorrect. Instead, he contends that adopting an "extended perspective," which is that resources of our world can and do enter our trains of thought.

Below, I discuss how we can seek inspiration from, prospect for, and tap creative ideas from the fields of art, architecture, film, theater, literature, philosophy, history, music, science and technology, and nature for metaphors, crafting intriguing questions, and designing therapeutic experiments that are in line with our clients' treatment goals. Whatever questions or therapeutic experiments we come up with need to be in line with the clients' talents, interests, life passions, problem views, presenting difficulties, and ideal treatment outcomes. Case examples are provided under each of the different fields.

Art

In the field of art, there are seven major schools of art to prospect for ideas: *realism*, *expressionism*, *impressionism*, *abstract*, *cubism*, *surrealism*, and *pop art* (Cumming, 2020). Major artists who represented these schools typically would paint portraits, depictions of historical or religious events, landscapes, seascapes, dreamscapes, and still life paintings. In 1656, Diego Velazquez, a realist, painted one of the most interesting and light-years-ahead-of-its-time painting called *Las Meninas*. What is most unique about this painting of the royal Habsburg children and their family dog, is that Velazquez paints himself at his easel in the foreground with the children and their dog and in the background, he painted the children's father coming down some steps, providing different perspectives and a festival of realist images (Carr, 2006). Inspired by this great work, Picasso in 1957 painted *Las Meninas* 58 different ways moving from clearly recognizable figures and objects to deconstructing the entire painting into cubist style and unrecognizable abstractions, which is a wonderful example of creativity and improvisation at its best (Planas, 2001)! When it comes to schools of art, I love modern art and particularly the surrealist work of Dalí and Magritte. One of my favorite works by Dalí is *Apparition of Face and Fruit Dish on a Beach*, which was painted in 1938 (Neret, 2022). Dalí had the amazing ability to make objects appear and disappear right before your eyes, depending on what you focused on in the painting. In this particular painting, one can see a face that turns into a bowl of pears, the rugged rocky landscape behind it turns into a dog, and there are a lot of other interesting objects that appear and disappear in this festive dreamscape. A number of my adolescent and adult clients have wanted to share with me reoccurring dreams and nightmares they have been having that appear to be related to past and present traumatic or stressful life events and difficulties they were currently struggling with. For some of our clients, they may have grave difficulty talking about traumatic past or present painful life events or other unpleasant struggles they are grappling with, however through the use of art therapy methods, can safely provide them and us with access to their unconscious dream state minds to help externalize on paper their negative emotions and thoughts connected to their painful life events and the contents of their dreams or nightmares, which can have a liberating effect for them.

The case example below illustrates the use of my art therapy experiment *surrealist art solutions* with a 14-year-old Caucasian boy, Charlie, who was suffering from post-traumatic stress disorder and anxiety symptoms related to his repeated exposure to his out-of-control alcoholic father's violent and threatening behaviors towards him and his mother (Selekman, 2017, 2009). He also was being bullied at school. The father eventually was arrested, was court-ordered to alcoholism treatment, and the parents divorced. Since Charlie loved art, I presented him with my surrealist art solutions experiment during our individual session time in family therapy with his mother and 10-year-old brother. To get his creative juices flowing, I showed him some Dalí and Magritte art books to provide examples of surrealist style art and shared with him what inspired their work (Taschen, 1994; Whitfield, 1992).

Charlie for the first time drew a surrealist work that depicted his reoccurring nightmare he was having about his father and what the family had endured over a two-year period. To show how scary and powerful the father was, he drew him as a giant fire-breathing dinosaur in the foreground. Charlie drew himself as a scorpion with a large stinger to defend himself. His mother was running toward their car but the road was a dead-end street, so there was no escape. He drew his brother as a shark in his bedroom not only so he could defend himself against the father but because he was constantly taking things out of the bedroom without permission and losing them, which really upset Charlie. Charlie did a beautiful job with the art exercise and this was first time he got out his thoughts and feelings about the family violence, his fears, and how all of this was not only fueling his anxiety but he made the connection about how he was setting himself up to be bullied at school due his past traumatic experience and distorted views of himself. For the longest time, his father's verbal abuse towards him and not spending time with him made him feel unlovable and deserving of punishment. This was an "Aha!" experience for Charlie. His mother was really proud of him and was impressed with his insightfulness. As a result of the surrealist art solution experiment, not only did it help reduce his post-traumatic stress disorder and anxiety symptoms but he stopped setting himself to get bullied at school.

With couple and family case situations, where one or more partners or family members are familiar with the different schools of art or do artwork themselves, I will ask them the following questions:

- "If your couple relationship/family were a painting, what school of art or style would it represent?"
- "Why cubist?"
- "How does the painting look?"
- "How come you decided to arrange the objects in your painting that way?"
- "What else does that mean or represent for you?"
- "What themes or messages would observers of your painting pick up on?"
- "If you could change your couple relationship/family into a different style or school of art painting, how will it look?"
- "How would that new painting of your relationship/family make a difference to you?"
- "How will this new style of painting benefit you/your relationship/your family?"

Since a lot of kids today are into the Marvel superhero craze and can't wait to check-out new movies with their favorite superheroes, I developed a therapeutic experiment that I call *my superhero comic strip* (Selekman, 2017; Selekman & Beyebach, 2013). On a large sketchpad sheet of paper, I first have the child or adolescent draw large cartoon boxes connected to one another. I ask them the following questions:

- "If you were a new Marvel superhero, how would you look and what special powers would you have?"
- "If the problem you/your parents think you have (ADD, anxiety, depression, etc.) could transform into a super villain, how would he/she/it look and what special powers would he/she/it have?"

Next, I have the child or adolescent in the first box introduce themselves as their new Marvel superhero. In the second box, they are to introduce the externalized problem in the form of a super villain. In the subsequent boxes, they are to show how they will use their super powers, including details about specific weapons, techniques, and strategies they will use to conquer the super villain. They also need to display in one or two of the boxes the clever counter moves the super villain will make to thwart his or her efforts to defeat him or her as well. Where children's and adolescents' creativity and imagination powers really shine is how they use certain aspects of their superheroes' special powers to help them to better cope with and resolve their difficulties, albeit pretending in areas of their lives where they are experiencing difficulties. For example, Charlie (see case example earlier in this Art section) loved Marvel comic superheroes and became the new superhero the Blue Lantern in his drawing. He externalized his anxiety into the super villain the Green Ghoul, which looked like a giant Godzilla head that had razor-sharp teeth and blew fire at its victims. The Blue Lantern had two special powers, a giant sledgehammer that he could control with his thinking or use as a combat weapon in his hand, and an invisible, impervious sphere he could put up around himself to defend against laser beams and the fire from the Green Ghoul. In the last box of his comic strip, he hammered to death the Green Ghoul with his large and powerful sledgehammer. Charlie came up with the brilliant idea of using the invisible sphere to ward off name-calling and bullying from mean peers at school and when he would have to visit his recovering alcoholic father and worry that the Green Ghoul might strike. This art experiment helped Charlie to completely stabilize his anxiety symptoms, feign off school bullies, and feel more in control when having visitations with his father.

Architecture

Like art, I find the architectural masterpieces designed by Antoni Gaudí and Santiago Calatrava to be highly inspiring. Both architects went outside their professions prospecting for ideas and shared a love for nature, which greatly inspired the designs of many of their buildings. One can see both in the exterior and interior design of Gaudí's beautiful Casa Batlló building in Barcelona strong undersea life and nautical influences. The building is organic and feels alive when you walk through it. For Calatrava, he is greatly influenced by the shape and movement of butterflies and birds. Like Gaudí, Calatrava's buildings have a dynamic aliveness quality to them. His buildings can be seen all over the world. Some of his most popular buildings can be seen in Valencia, Spain at the *City of Arts and Sciences*. In 2008, in New York City, right next to the World Trade Center, Calatrava built the *Oculus*, which is an indoor shopping mall that looks like a giant dove. The public enters the mall through the breast of the dove-shaped building. When I am working with families where they are reporting structural and organizational issues, such as there is an inequity of parental involvement with the children and each other, or that they report that the family atmosphere is chaotic, and it's not clear who is charge, I begin to think about how Gaudí or Calatrava would approach these families and redesign how they live together so it is more adaptive and aesthetically appealing to them. The case example below illustrates how we can use the work of Gaudí and Calatrava and architectural language and metaphors to transform structurally a family with a 16-year-old Caucasian acting out boy with ADD and abusing marijuana.

David had a long history of behavioral problems at home and school. He had a 17-year-old sister, Melissa, who got most of her father's love and attention because she was an "A" student and never got into trouble.

Meanwhile, David was getting "D" and "F" grades in school. There was a long history of favoritism shown by the father toward Melissa, which both the mother and David were upset about. I also had discovered during my time alone with the parents that there was a Grand Canyon of emotional distance in the marital relationship, partially because the father had to travel a lot with his business job. When the father was around, he would spend high-quality time with Melissa and neglect both his wife and David. Even David's valiant attempts to demand his father's attention by getting into trouble at school and at home would only lead to a short-lived lecture or his getting yelled at by him and then he would walk away. There were times when even Melissa would voice to her mother and David that her father should spend time with her brother. In a session alone with the parents, I created intensity with them about the importance of their serving as the co-architects for their family and redesigning it in a way that all members equally enjoy its shape and how they move through it. I further added that when you look at great modern architecture there is a flow and aliveness to it. I encouraged them to check out on-line the architectural works of Gaudí (Casa Batlló) and Calatrava to see what I mean. Next, I pointed out to them that failing to take the necessary steps to transform the family foundation, organization, and how family members can flow better together, David could potentially spiral further downward behaviorally and much more serious consequences with him could occur, such as his moving into more heavy drug use and failing out of school. Both parents became animated and asked me what they could do to prevent this dire situation from occurring. The mother chimed in using my architectural language to share that their family organization was out of whack and not only did her husband have to balance his time out better with both kids but that they needed to add an addition to the family foundation, which was their carving out some high-quality time together as a couple. I used the strategy of unbalancing to support the mother and get the father to step up and agree to work on better meeting both her and David's needs. The father agreed to be a better co-architect with balancing out his time with his wife and with both kids. I reiterated to the father that unless these changes happened soon, it was only a matter of when David's dire future reality could start to occur. Once the father instituted the necessary changes that needed to happen, David started functioning much better at home and at school. David was a talented basketball player and he had not played one-on-one with his father in years. He had a great outside shot but according to him his father only made baskets when he would be close to the basketball rim. I decided to put David in charge of mentoring his father for a week on the basketball court to serve as his coach and teach him how to have a better outside shot in an effort for them to have fun together and strengthen their relationship bond. The father smiled and agreed to do this in family therapy. Not only did the father and son have a great time playing basketball together but he had complimented David on being a very patient and good coach.

Film

One of the most popular pastimes that people like to engage in during their leisure time is watching movies. Movies cover every aspect of the human condition. They can emotionally touch, excite, entertain, scare us and can have many surprising twists and turns. My experience watching foreign and arthouse independent films is that they tend to go more in-depth with character development and in general have more substance and meaning to them then popular mainstream movies. Not only can we see ourselves as characters and our important relationship themes in movies but some of the movies capture best our clients' situations as well. Some of my favorite film directors are Michelangelo Antonioni, Luis Buñuel, Alfred Hitchcock, Michael Haneke, Woody Allen, Wes Anderson, Pedro Almodóvar, and Steven Spielberg. Since I am a big movie buff of most genres of film, I am always on the lookout for films and clips from movies I can use in sessions with clients or encourage them to see the movies looking for key themes, roles, relationship dynamics, and messages that parallel their situations and resonated with them. The nature of the clients' presenting problems will determine what film clips I will show in the session or movies I will recommend they check out. If I am working with couples where one or both partners are clinging to a rigid and narrow view of their problem situation and like to watch movies, I will have them watch Austrian film director Michael Haneke's French film, *Caché* (Haneke, 2005). The movie is about a journalist named George Laurant played by Daniel Auteuil who has a popular talk show on TV and suddenly started receiving packages in the mail, which contained surveillance-like videotapes of him and his family members exiting and returning to their home, along with child-like drawings with violent themes. Needless to say, George and his family were quite anxious about receiving these packages. The local police department's investigation was not helpful and George decided to conduct his own investigation to try and solve this mystery and stop the perpetrator(s) behind their fear-inducing harassment. George had a hunch that the perpetrator behind the harassment was his adopted brother Majid who he never had connected with because the latter's cruelty to animals and difficulties adjusting in the family.

Majid was jealous of all the love and attention George had received from his biological parents. However, George could not prove with absolute certainty that Majid was the perpetrator. At the very end of the movie, a strange man approaches Pierrot, George's young teenage son, as he is leaving his school for the day. They talk for a short while and then walk off together. The movie ends with this scene leaving the viewer guessing. We ask ourselves the following: Who is this man? Is he the perpetrator? If so, will he kidnap Pierrot and worse yet, torture or kill him? Was this man a drug dealer and he and Pierrot agreed to meet after school so he could purchase drugs from him? We are left hanging. On the DVD, in an interview extra following the movie, Haneke shares with the interviewer that he deliberately wanted viewers to be left with the uncertainties and ambiguities of reality. He also alluded to how life is not about happier ever after clean endings, that this is not what reality is about (Haneke, 2005). Another film that drives home the fact that for any event or problem situation there can be multiple explanations for why and how it happened, is Akira Kurosawa's excellent film *Rashomon* (Kurosawa, 1950). The story is about a rape and murder as described by four different characters, each having their own unique interpretation of the tragic event. Both of these movies drive home the point that unless we have hard facts and evidence to back up our explanations and beliefs, having absolute certainty and truth about anything is an impossibility.

The case example below is of a family going through a divorce transition process with a depressed 17-year-old Caucasian boy named Sam and his 15-year-old brother George. Although the parents, Jack and Betty had legally worked out a joint custody arrangement, each boy was split-off and in a coalition with one of the parents, which had existed prior to the divorce. Sam was in his father's corner and greatly disliked having to spend time with his mother and George did not want to spend time with his father. This problem created a lot of friction and conflict between the parents when they tempted to co-parent and the boys were bickering a lot.

I tried initially to work with the whole family together but after two sessions it proved to be futile in that the parents would get into blame-counter-blame exchanges and the boys would say things to push each other's buttons. I then started seeing each parent separately with the boys, which proved to be more productive. While working with each subgroup of the family, the boys would take turns complaining about all of the idiosyncrasies and faults of each parent and why did not want to have their visitations with the other parents. Although I had sought the advice of each of the boys regarding what adjustments the parents could make that could help make their visits more enjoyable, they were skeptical that their parents would be able to deliver. Apparently, both parents in the past had made a lot of empty promises to them and they had not changed. Both parents agreed to commit during their visitation times with the boys that they would work on cutting back on their lecturing, nagging, and incessant inquiries about whether or not they completed their school homework. As a way to normalize all that the family was going through with the highs and lows of the divorce transition process, I had them get a hold of the Noah Baumbach movie *The Squid and the Whale* and watch it together as a family (Baumbach, 2005). The movie parallels a lot of the couple's co-parenting struggles, the parent-child coalitions, the challenges with visitations, and the tension between two brothers having to endure a challenging divorce transition process. They agreed to watch it, discuss it among themselves, and be prepared to share both what resonated with them and what the key takeaways were from the movie. In our next session, all family members were in agreement that the movie accurately captured the impact of divorce on both individual family members and their relationships with one another. What hit home for the boys was that their nice cozy coalitions with each of the parents was not working, only fueling more conflict for their parents' relationship, and that their sibling relationship had become strained and negative. Both boys agreed to work on repairing their relationship and giving each parent a fair shake and another chance to have a better relationship with them. The parents agreed to work on being more civil and respectful towards one another and improve their co-parenting. They all agreed that this movie had a profound impact on them because it paralleled and normalized their divorce transition situation in many ways. I spent a few more sessions improving the family's communications, working with the couple on their co-parenting teamwork, and helping the family to resolve their conflicts. Once all of the family structural and communications changes occurred, Sam's depression uplifted, both boys were happier with the family situation and getting along better, and the parents became a more solid co-parenting team.

Many years ago, I was inspired by the Woody Allen film *The Purple Rose of Cairo*, where Jeff Daniels plays a film star who steps out of a cinema screen and into the real world, to spend time with Cecilia (played by Mia Farrow), who was a big fan of his. The film follows the highs and the lows of their time together (Allen, 1985). Based on Woody Allen's creative idea and for solution-finding, I have asked clients the following questions:

- "If your favorite actor/actress could step out of the screen of your favorite movie with him or her in it and you could spend the day together, what would you talk about or do together?"
- "What have you been dying to ask or say to him or her?"
- "What would you want him or her to know about you?"
- "How would this experience hanging out together make a difference in your life?"
- "What advice would Al Pacino have for you to help resolve your difficulty?"
- "What would Charlize Theron recommend you try that might help you with your relationship with your husband?"

For couples and families that enjoy making their own movies of vacations and special events, I will have them make their own documentary, which I call *Our Happiest Moments* documentary (Selekman & Beyebach, 2013). As part of the documentary, they are to include photos, film clips, mementos, share their happiest memories together and what was most meaningful about those experiences for each couple partner or family member, and put together a soundtrack of their most favorite and meaningful tunes. This fun and meaningful therapeutic experiment can benefit couples and families where they are overly focused on problems, there is a doom and gloom couple or family atmosphere, and there is emotional disconnection in their relationships. While making their documentary it triggers positive emotions for them, engenders hope, underscores their past successes, and it is a reminder of the love in their relationships and all that they share together. Once they have made their documentaries, I encourage couples and families to look at them periodically as a positive emotional booster and during rough patches in their relationships, as a reminder to be grateful for all that they do have in their couple and family relationships.

Theater

Five of my favorite playwrights, who have greatly inspired me by their brilliant scripts and theatrical productions, are Tennessee Williams, Anton Chekhov, Edward Albee, Eugene O'Neill, and Henrik Ibsen. Some of their most popular plays cover major couple and family themes, issues, and human struggles, such as: sibling rivalry, being locked into rigid couple or family role behaviors, family secrets, intense relationship conflicts, infidelity, alcoholism, greed, grief and loss, and so forth. Like the use of film clips and recommending that clients see certain movies for us to discuss, I do the same with these playwrights' theatrical works in sessions with couples and families. The most popular theatrical works of these playwrights can be a rich source of creative ideas when we our feeling stuck or looking for great lines or powerful scenes from these plays to share with our clients to offer them either something to reflect on or a new way of looking at their situations. The case example below mirrors Ibsen's *A Doll's House* play in many ways (Ibsen, 1992).

> Katarina and William had been married for 10 years. Katarina had immigrated here from Lithuania and they had met and fell in love in Paris after a conversation they had had in a popular department store. He was in Paris on business and Katarina was on vacation. After a year of corresponding back and forth, and some brief visits in each other's countries, William proposed to Katarina and she quickly accepted. What Katarina was not aware of was that not only did he grow up in a traditional home where his mother did not have a lot of independence and his father expected her to cook, clean, take care of all household matters, including everything that involved the children, as well as William had a long history of being unfaithful with past girlfriends. Within two years of their marriage and after they had had twin boys, Katarina found herself trapped in the same rigid traditional role as William's mother was expected to play and he would get angry with her if she requested any kind of free time away from the kids.

Katarina also had discovered from seeing texts on William's phone and e-mail exchanges with multiple women that appeared to indicate that he was having affairs. After a big argument, William vehemently denied that he was fooling around with other women and claimed that at times at work there was mutual flirting going on with his female work colleagues and him, but nothing more. Katarina accepted his explanation and decided to give William the benefit of the doubt. Several years had passed where Katarina had not seen any signs of William's being unfaithful, however she had become depressed about not having a life outside their home and there was a lack of emotional and sexual intimacy in the relationship. William agreed to go for couple therapy because he was worried that Katarina's depression would have an adverse effect on their children and because of the lack of sexual intimacy in the relationship, which was upsetting to him. Once I had built rapport with both partners and elicited their views on the problem situation, I began to reframe the problem as a depressing situation for both of them, rather than Katarina being the depressed problem person. I shared with them that they both felt unfulfilled in different ways. William wanted to bring back the affectionate and spontaneous wife that he was madly in love with that used to enjoy regularly being sexual intimate with him. Katarina wanted to bring back some of her former life before having the children, where she worked out regularly, saw friends, and expand the meaning and purpose in her life beyond parenthood and tending to the home. I took a risk and shared with the couple that their relationship paralleled a famous Henrik Ibsen play called *A Doll's House*. Neither partner had heard of it but seemed to be intrigued by my bringing this up. Interestingly enough, Katarina chimed in that she felt like a "doll trapped in a house." While crying, she shared how unfulfilled she felt and how she no longer liked her body because she was overweight. The latter was one of the reasons she had withdrawn from being intimate with William. William moved from his corner of the couch right up against Katarina and put his arm around her to comfort her. I had them talk to one another about what adjustments they could make so that they would both feel less down and more up about the relationship situation. Katarina voiced her desire for them to get a nanny or reliable sitter who could watch the kids a few days a week so that she would be free to exercise again and re-connect with old girlfriends for a lunch or time-limited get togethers that she used to see before their children were born. William voiced a desire to bring back the woman he had fallen in love with, more affectionate, sexually active with him, and happier. They came up with a plan to look for a nanny or a reliable sitter three days a week, have a weekend date night, and carve out daily evening time after the kids went to bed to try and rekindle the pre-marital and early marriage happiness they used have in their relationship. Before the couple left my office, they asked how they could see the *A Doll's House* play. I pointed out that unless a local theater is putting on a production of the play, the best bet would be to try and stream it online or take out of the public library the DVD of the 1973 movie version of it, which starred Jane Fonda as Nora and David Warner as Torvald (Losey, 1973). In our next meeting, the couple had been successful at not only implementing their plan but one night they watched the DVD of *A Doll's House*. I asked them how they thought their marriage was similar to Torvald and Nora's marriage. They both saw a lot of parallels and Katarina strongly identified with Nora's plight, that is being boxed into the dutiful wife and mother roles but not having a life beyond those roles. William did not like the way Torvald treated Nora. However, what scared William the most was Nora's decision to leave both Torvald and the children at the end of the play/movie. Katarina had asserted herself with William and shared with him after watching the movie that she had considered leaving him more than once if their marital relationship had not changed. William agreed to do whatever it took to prevent this from happening. At this point in the therapy, not only did the balance of power and control in the relationship dramatically change but William was honoring her voice more and Katarina had shared that she "no longer felt like a doll trapped in the home." Due to their great progress, I gave them a two-week vacation from counseling as a vote confidence. Two weeks later, they reported being more sexually intimate and feeling like they brought back the love and happiness in their relationship. Similar to the positive impact of using films in couple and family therapy, recommended plays that parallel couples' and families' lives in terms of their presenting difficulties, rigid role behaviors, and other relationship dynamics helps them to gain a meta-outsider's perspective looking in at their relationship difficulties from a distance, discovering that they don't like what they see and hear occurring in the interactions between the lead characters that closely resembles them and their situation, which can lead to altering their outmoded beliefs and disrupting their problem-maintaining interactions. This was the case for Katarina and William and with Sam and his family going through a rocky divorce transition process (see case example under the Film section).

Literature

Like movies and with great theater productions, there are many wonderful fiction, nonfiction, science fiction, biography books and passages from these works we can use in couple and family therapy. Some of the books that I often use passages from and recommend to clients are: Maya Angelou's *I Know Why the Caged Bird Sings* (Angelou, 2009); Ralph Ellison's *The Invisible Man* (Ellison, 1995); Miguel de Cervante's *Don Quixote* (Cervantes, 2003); Viktor Frankl's *Man's Search for Meaning* (Frankl, 1992); Pablo Neruda's *The Book of Questions* (Neruda, 2001); George Orwell's *1984* (Orwell, 1961); Sarah Bakewell's *How to Live or A Life of Montaigne in One Question and Twenty Attempts at an Answer* (Bakewell, 2010); Epictetus's *The Art of Living: The Classical Manual on Virtue, Happiness, and Effectiveness* (Epictetus, 1995); Grayling's *History of Philosophy* (Grayling, 2019); Doris Kearns Goodwin's *Team of Rivals: The Political Genius of Abraham Lincoln* (Goodwin, 2005); David

Blight's *Frederick Douglas: Prophet of Freedom* (Blight, 2018); Robin D. G. Kelley's *Thelonious Monk: The Life and Times of an American Original* (Kelley, 2009); Aidan Levy's *Saxophone Colossus: The Life and Music of Sonny Rollins* (Levy, 2022); Marcus Aurelius's *Meditations* (Aurelius, 2002); Aristotle's *The Nicomachean Ethics* (Aristotle, 1987); Buckminster Fuller's *Critical Path* (Fuller & Tanaka, 1982); J.M. Barrie's: *Peter and Wendy* (Barrie, 2017); Lewis Carroll's *Alice in Wonderland and Through the Looking Glass* (Carroll, 2018); Paulo Coelho's *The Alchemist* (Coelho, 1993); Umberto Eco's *The Name of the Rose* (Eco, 1983); Kurt Vonnegut's *Slaughter-House Five*; H.G. Wells's *The Time-Machine* (Wells, 2005); Robert Heinlein's *Stranger in a Strange Land* (Heinlein, 2018); Philip K. Dick's *The Man in the High Castle* (Dick, 2012) and *Do Androids Dream of Electric Sheep?* (Dick, 1996); Walter Isaacson's *Benjamin Franklin: An American Life* (Isaacson, 2003); Michael Puett and Christine Gross-Loh's *The Path: A New Way to Think About Everything* (Puett & Gross-Loh, 2016); Joan Halifax's *Standing at the Edge: Finding Freedom Where Fear and Courage Meet* (Halifax, 2018); Jay Shetty's *Think Like a Monk: Train Your Mind for Peace and Purpose Every Day* (Shetty, 2020); and Ed Catmull's *Creativity, Inc.: Overcoming the Unseen Forces that Stand in the Way of True Inspiration* (Catmull, 2014).

When exploring with clients what their hobbies and interests are, if they happen to share that they love to read, I will find out who their favorite authors are and what genre of books they like to read the most. If I am familiar with their favorite authors and the characters from their books, I will bring what we know about these characters into our conversations and explore with the client how they would approach and try and resolve their difficulties. Doing so often sparks for clients fresh and creative ideas for potential solutions to experiment with. One expressive writing exercise I have clients who like to read and write do is called *my favorite author rewrites my story* (Selekman, 2017; Selekman & Beyebach, 2013). Once clients identify their favorite authors, they are to imagine the following: how the identified author would rewrite their story; would it be a novel, drama, mystery, an adventure story; what kind of character would they be, including talents and skills; what would the other characters be like; would family members and close friends be characters in this story and how would they be different; what would be the main themes of the new story about them; and would it be contemporary or take place during a different time period. I only ask clients to write the first page of the first chapter of the new story about them. Some of my clients in one week's time wrote an entire first chapter! Once they have completed the writing exercise, we can ask them to consult with the new character they have become for advice about how to resolve their current difficulty. For many clients, looking at their situations through the eyes and minds of someone else can help them to gain a new perspective on their problem situations and not only see more clearly what they need to stop doing that is unproductive but that pathways to solutions do exist that they had not thought of, seen before, or can pursue. The case below illustrates how to use an imaginary time machine, inspired by the creative mind of H.G. Wells in his classic book *The Time Machine* to co-create possibilities with a substance-abusing 17-year-old Japanese boy named Kiyoshi and his highly pessimistic parents Hiroto and Hana. Hiroto was a highly successful brain surgeon and Hana was an attorney. Kiyoshi was an incredible anime artist, had created his own video games, and thought it would be cool to work for a top video game design company in the future (Wells, 2005).

Kiyoshi had been referred to me by a colleague who had worked with him in her hospital-based adolescent substance abuse intensive outpatient program. He had been in this program for six weeks. Prior to that, Kiyoshi had participated in a summer wilderness program for substance-abusing youth and had been in an inpatient adolescent chemical dependency program that had been court-ordered for his being caught at school dealing marijuana, which put him on court super-vision for nine months. Kiyoshi had seen a number of outpatient therapists both individually and in family therapy three times before. Needless to say, the parents were highly pessimistic and could not think of one thing positive to say about Kiyoshi. In our first two family sessions, the parents would take turns pointing out how their son was a big disappointment, how he had a bad attitude, that he was failing in school and disruptive there, and what upset Kiyoshi the most, was criticizing him about not being like his two success story siblings who were "A" students. The older son Hiroshi was 21 and in pre-medical studies at a top university and their 14-year-old daughter Keiko who was a member of a swim club team and an outstanding swimmer. Apparently, Kiyoshi used to be a top student until he began high school and got involved with an unsavory group of peers that were heavily into substance abuse. According to the parents, Kiyoshi's second family (the negative peer group) disempowered them and they no longer had any leverage with him. Hiroto made it very clear to me that seeing me was their last-ditched effort with counseling before sending him off for a year to a residential treatment center. No matter what I tried to do, seeing the parents and Kiyoshi separately, trying to disrupt the destructive family interactions, and engender hope with the parents, nothing was making a difference in eliminating the parental negativity and pessimism. During an inter-session break in my third family session, the light bulb had lit up over my head, that when we are stuck in the present moment in problem-saturated quicksand with clients, one should adopt a future-oriented approach where the possibilities are endless. When I reconvened the family, I had Kiyoshi hop into my imaginary time-machine and take into the future when he was well on his way to achieving his future career goals as a professional animator, video game designer, and finishing his last year at an art and design school. When he stepped out of the time-machine he was now 22 years old and having Sunday night dinner at his parents' house. The parents looked stunned to hear for the first time that Kiyoshi had a positive vision for himself in the future. I asked Kiyoshi, "What will you be the most excited to share with your parents that is now going on in your life?" He shared with his parents that he had an internship with Nintendo and they had an inter-est in possibly hiring him after he graduates. Again, the parents were smiling and thrilled that Kiyoshi could picture in his mind being successful in life and doing meaningful work. Another important future change that he wanted to share with his parents was that he gave up using drugs. For the first time, the three of them were interacting in a positive way with one another and the parents shared with him that they were proud of him for getting serious about his future. Next, I had Kiyoshi walk us back from the future spelling out the steps that he took to achieve a successful future for himself. First, he would force himself to completely give up his drug use and stay away from his drug-using friends; second, he would meet with all of his teachers to come up with catch up plans to help pull up his grades; take an advanced placement art class; and he would have taken at the local art center both an animation and two video game design classes to further improve his skills and to help better position himself to get into a good art and design school. The parents were very impressed with Kiyoshi's plan and I offered to collaborate with all of his teachers to help support his efforts to pick up his grades and perform better in school. I also offered to teach Kiyoshi relapse prevention tools and strategies to help him to maintain his abstinence from drugs, which included bringing in two former substance-abusing clients who had been abstinent for a year, were regularly attending a young person's Narcotics' Anonymous group, and had been accepted at the colleges of their choice, to help provide further support for him and share their expertise about what has worked for them. Both the parents and Kiyoshi gave me written consent to bring in my former clients. The parents and Kiyoshi thanked me for offering to do these things. I pointed out to both parties that slips do go with the territory of change when one is attempting to kick a long-term drug habit, and if they do occur, rather than viewing them as being disastrous, view them instead as being a great opportunity for resilience-building comeback practice and learning about where we need to tighten up with the structure. I also offered to collaborate with Kiyoshi's teachers to help him get back on track there if he needed further support with this. Again, the family thanked me. Finally, I asked Kiyoshi what adjustments he would like to see his parents make that will help optimize for his future success. He shared the following: "Stop comparing me to my brother and sister, stop treating me like a loser, stop threatening to put me in a residential treatment center, and I would like to spend time with my dad like we used to do in the past on the weekends hanging out." I put Kiyoshi in charge of giving his parents feedback on their parenting at the end of each week regarding how well they were doing with him in the parenting department, both positive and negative. I encouraged the parents to accept Kiyoshi's feedback with their hearts, do more of what works, and make the recommended adjustments in order to help him be all that he could possibly become. We ended up seeing each other four more times with longer time intervals between each meeting as a vote of confidence to them. With the help of the imaginary time-machine, not only were we able to unstick our treatment system but it opened up space for profound second-order level changes with Kiyoshi individually, it changed the parents' problem-saturated view of him, and their family interactions became much more positive. Kiyoshi gave up his drug use, made new friends, and picked up his grades to a high enough level to be able to get into three of the art and design schools he had applied to.

Philosophy

During the COVID-19 pandemic lockdown period, many people were struggling with nihilistic fear about the future, experiencing various levels of existential crisis, there was a worldwide rise in anxiety, depression, alcohol and substance abuse, children and adolescents' grades declined and their social offline lives and extra-curricular activities were completely eliminated. Parents were forced to juggle their work role responsibilities with supporting and monitoring their kids with school classes on Zoom, with little breaks to take care of themselves (Selekman, 2021). I experienced low grade depressed mood, anxiety, and nihilistic fear about the future regarding my in-person training and consulting business and no longer being able to travel, which is one of my passions in life. One day, while on a long walk, I had an epiphany, which was one of radical acceptance (Brach, 2004). By embracing the fact that COVID-19 and the lockdown were things I had no control over and I had to embrace them as the new reality, I suddenly felt liberated from my catastrophizing and rumination, which was fueling my depressed and anxious moods. The sunlight had broken through the clouds and I began to see the upside of having to contend with constraints, such as new possibilities with tele-health therapy and training and consulting on Zoom for myself and all of the great benefits of spending more high-quality time with my family. I also turned to adopting a daily mindfulness meditation practice, useful Buddhist principles, and the wisdom of Thich Nhat Hanh, Lama Zopa Rinpoche, Pema Chodron, Tara Brach, 2004; and Mark Epstein (Hanh, 2019, 1998, 1991; Rinpoche, 1993; Chodron, 2009; Epstein, 2022, 2018, 2013). The Buddhists offer us many useful principles on how to live our lives and view life's peaks and valleys, such as: embracing each other with loving-kindness and compassion, this includes self-compassion; the *Middle Path* (staying centered and refraining from emotionally over-reacting negatively to setbacks or disappointments or living in extremes); detachment, that is not allowing your thoughts and feelings to own and control you; life is suffering; problems are transitory and not fixed; change is a continuous process; there is no self and scientific proof for it, that it is a fictional story that we author about ourselves based on our life experiences and how we perceive ourselves and how we think others perceive us, but in reality, our stories are constantly evolving, which means the sky is the limit in terms of the future possibilities for ourselves; and radical acceptance (Hanh, 2019, 1998; Neff, 2015; Brach, 2004; Berns, 2022; Garfield, 2022; Epstein, 2022). I re-read Viktor Frankl's *Man's Search for Meaning* as a reminder of how we are all capable of bouncing back from trauma and adversity, how these life experiences make us emotionally stronger, more resilient, and that we will eventually find the light in the darkness. I also turned to the leading figures in the Stoicism, Utilitarianism, and Existentialism schools of philosophy for wisdom on the following: constructively managing stress, conflict, and problems; critically examining our thinking and striving for clear reasoning; finding meaning and purpose in our lives; being ethical and having good values which we uphold; being authentic, nonjudgmental, and open-minded; and ways to increase our happiness and improving the quality of life (Grayling, 2019; Aurelius, 2002; Seneca, 2007; Bakewell, 2010; Marinoff, 2003; Nisker, 1990). Depending on the couple or family's presenting problems, how they get stuck, and what their goals are will help determine what philosopher's wisdom and quotes I will bring into our conversations. When well-timed and right on target, a philosophical bit of wisdom or quote can be transformative in altering clients' narrow and rigid ways of viewing their situations. The case example below illustrates how the use of philosophical wisdom opened up space for a couple to view their situation differently and led to a change in their interactions with one another.

Larry and Sandra, an African-American couple, sought therapy for their communications and conflict-resolution difficulties. They were arguing daily. During the COVID-19 pandemic lockdown situation, Larry had to close down his highly successful breakfast restaurant that had been in existence for ten years. He was angry and frustrated about being unemployed and having to give up his restaurant that had been like an institution in his town. Sandra was the director of a nursing department at a hospital. She had made enough to help support them and put no pressure on Larry to get another job. The situation was a real existential crisis for Larry because had no clue what he was going to do work-wise. I normalized for Larry what he was going through and self-disclosed the negative emotional impact the COVID lockdown had on me with my training and consulting business. Larry was struggling with finding meaning and purpose in life after closing his restaurant. In listening to Larry's struggles, I thought about the existentialists and Camus's quote, "Do the right thing even if the universe is cruel or meaningless" (cited in Marinoff, 2003, p. 342). I took a risk and shared this quote with the couple regarding Larry's situation and stressed the importance of no matter how painful the loss of his business was and being at a crossroads about what to do next work-wise, doing the "right thing" is to remember that Sandra loved him unconditionally and was on his team. Larry broke a smile and gazed into Sandra's eyes and she smiled back. He apologized for dumping his anger and frustration on her and shared with Sandra that he wanted things to be better between them. Sandra accepted his apology and acknowledged that she too wanted them to work together and get along. We discussed ways that Sandra could support Larry while he figured out what he planned to do work-wise. Since the COVID situation had greatly improved when I had begun to see the couple, Sandra felt that Larry should re-attempt to open up his restaurant. She truly believed that he had a huge fan base of customers and they would return if he re-opened. Sandra further added that Larry should consider adding take-out and delivery services to his restaurant, which had worked for a number of restaurants during and after the lockdown had uplifted to help them to stay afloat financially. Larry thought these were great ideas and started to get excited about the prospect of re-opening his restaurant with the additional services Sandra had recommended. In response to Larry's newfound excitement about bouncing back from adversity and attempting to re-open his restaurant and albeit he was worried that it may not be as successful as it was in the past, I shared with the couple a great quote from the Stoic Marcus Aurelius's *Meditations* about how obstacles or impediments are the way to overcoming adversity and one's life challenges. Like the great hypnotist Milton H. Erickson, Aurelius believed that all humans possess the necessary strengths and resources to master life's challenges and hardships (Aurelius, 2002; O'Hanlon, 1987; Havens, 1996).

Both Larry and Sandra found this quote to be very inspiring. Larry shared, "I guess the way is the obstacle and I need to take action." I responded with, "You already have the recipe for success within you, a combination of resilience, perseverance, and grit that made your restaurant the go-to breakfast spot in your town, you will do it again!" I ended up seeing Larry and Sandra four more times. The couple were no longer arguing and they were working better together as a team. The best news was that Larry drummed up the courage to take the risk and re-open his restaurant. He also added the take-out and delivery services, which ended up making his business much more profitable thanks to Sandra's great idea. He also succeeded at getting most of his original staff and his regular customers back.

History

History has always been one of my favorite subjects. I love reading about famous historical figures like Ben Franklin, Theodore Roosevelt, Gandhi, Martin Luther King, Abraham Lincoln, Frederick Douglas, to name a few. There were certain time periods in history that I have found to be most interesting like the Italian Renaissance period, which was rich in ideas and innovation in the fields of art, philosophy, architecture, and science. The wealthy Medici family regularly held dinners with experts and accomplished professionals from different fields as a context for exchanging their creative and innovative ideas and to contract with them to help fund their professional endeavors (Hibbert, 1999). In undergraduate college, I took three courses on Civil War history with my favorite professor who was a scholar in this area and had the amazing ability to transport us back in time, as if he lived back then. He put us in the minds of Abraham Lincoln, Frederick Douglas, General Ulysses S. Grant, General Robert E. Lee, Jefferson Davis, and other key figures during this time. He also regularly reminded us that the aftermath of slavery and racism was still alive and well in our present day and the importance of being sensitive to this fact and being racial justice allies in the world. When I am looking for fresh and creative ideas, I often think about the aforementioned famous historic figures and entertain in my mind how they would approach my clients' difficulties.

Lucinda, a 16-year-old Latina girl, was depressed and struggling with peer acceptance and rejection and taking out her frustration and anger on her single-parent mother Raquel in the form of snapping at and swearing at her, not cooperating with her, and she was doing poorly academically. Her father lived out of state and had very little contact with her. He was now remarried and had two children with his new wife. Lucinda was new to her high school and came in as a junior. The family had moved from the big city to the current suburb they were living in. Lucinda used to be popular at her former high school. However, at her new suburban high school the majority of the girls had grown up together and had very close relationships. Lucinda had made a valiant effort to try and build relationships with some of the girls that she had met in her classes and while eating in the school cafeteria. They were hot and cold with her, sometimes nice and sometimes would give her the cold shoulder. Two out of the seven of these girls she was trying to become friendly with seemed to like her and became faithful friends with her. However, the other girls were much more popular and were considered high status socially in the school. Lucinda tried everything she could think of to get in the door with them but nothing worked, which greatly frustrated her. Some of her attempted solutions were to dress like them, be willing to experiment with alcohol and marijuana with them at parties even though she did not like doing this, and flirting with popular boys to try and get their attention. The attention she would get from them tended to be of the negative variety such as two of the popular girls calling her "a slut." In my first family session, I had learned that Lucinda's best subjects in school were history and art. I shared with her that history was my top subject too and that I was a Civil War buff. Lucinda shared that she also found Civil War history interesting and really liked Abraham Lincoln. During my individual session time with Lucinda, I told her about Delores Kearns Goodwin's book *Team of Rivals: The Political Genius of Abraham Lincoln*, which is about how Lincoln found a way to foster cooperative and better relationships with other politicians that he had run against for the presidency, who did not like him, tried to undermine him behind his back, and how not only did most of them end up serving as his cabinet members but they became close colleagues and friends. Lucinda was curious about how Lincoln had pulled this tremendous feat off. I shared with her Lincoln's recipe for success. First, he decided to look past whether they liked him or not or their behind-the-scenes shenanigans and see their strengths. Second, he would not allow himself to get defensive with his foes and steered clear from what did not work with them. Third, by complimenting and staying positive with them even when they were being sarcastic or cold to him, it proved to be disarming, neutralized their venom, and eventually helped foster cooperative partnerships with them, and they became loyal and competent cabinet members for his administration. Apparently, what would happen with Lucinda and the five popular girls was that she would worry too much about whether or not they liked her or if she was cool enough, which included doing things she would not normally do, such as experimenting with substances and flirting with boys. Sometimes she would personalize when they would give her the cold shoulder or say something sarcastic to her by visibly showing them that it was getting to her. Lucinda thought it was so cool how Lincoln handled so well a very difficult situation and that maybe she needed to try a different approach with the five girls. As an experiment, I offered Lucinda the *do-something-different* strategy whenever she interacted with any of the five girls, she is to blow their minds by responding differently to anything they may throw her way, no matter how negative, as long as it is different than anything they have ever encountered with her. Lucinda thought this was a cool idea. I offered the caveat that sometimes in spite of our best-efforts interactions and relationships don't change immediately, to be patient, to not blame herself if in the long-run she does not achieve the outcome she was hoping for. I further added that the important thing was that she drummed up the courage to try. We shared with Raquel the experiment that were going to try over the next week. Raquel shared with Lucinda that she was proud of her and that she would put forth the effort to be more supportive and not arguing with her over the next week. One week later, Lucinda came in smiling that not only did she seem to win over three of the five girls by staying positive, joking around with them, but when they would be sarcastic or cutting with her, she would respond with, "You're right. I am surprised you didn't call me a _____ or a _____!" According to Lucinda, this really blew their minds! They were expecting that she would get upset and be their scapegoat. In fact, they laughed at her off-the-wall responses and one of the girls said to her, "You're tripping me out, girl!" Another positive change was that four of the five girls invited her to have lunch with them in the school cafeteria, which was a first for Lucinda. She had found that Lincoln's tactics worked well with them. I amplified and consolidated Lucinda's gains, encouraged her to do more of what works with the four girls, and shared that the fifth girl might come around do to peer pressure. I also wanted to let her know that there will always be peer drama and shifting alliances and if, anything negative should occur, to shake it off and know that it was not her doing. I further added to stay true to herself and don't ever feel she needs to do things out of character or against her values to please others. Two other important changes that occurred over the week was that Raquel and Lucinda did not clash once and Lucinda had met with her math, science, and English teachers to get some extra help and to come up with catch-up plans with her backlogged homework. Raquel was highly pleased that Lucinda was taking her schoolwork more seriously. I ended up seeing the family four more times. The best news was not only that Lucinda had pulled up all of her grades to A–B level but that she had won over the fifth girl that she was trying to connect with. All five of the girls were treating Lucinda with more respect and they all grew closer together.

Music

With adolescents and young adults, it is helpful to find out what music they like. Music says a lot about our clients, their personalities, interests, passions, and the emotional effects they get from listening to their favorite musical artists and popular tunes (Rogers & Ogas, 2022). I like to ask them what their *theme songs* are, those tunes that lift their spirits and get them fired up. For myself, Led Zeppelin's "Ramble On" and Peter Gabriel's live version of "In Your Eyes" are two tunes that rapidly lift my spirits and pump me up before giving a workshop or just for listening pleasure (Led Zeppelin, 2014; Gabriel, 1994). We can have our clients play their theme songs in their minds while trying out proposed therapeutic tools and strategies as a way to inspire and motivate them with the implementation process. If I have adolescent clients who play instruments, I will have them bring them in and I will bring my djembe drum in and we will jam together. While co-creating new music together we can talk about what is important to them, they could come up with lyrics that capture the difficulties they are struggling with, and lyrics and music that would capture what ideal outcomes of their situations would look and sound like. The adolescents take the lead in directing what notes, chords, or sounds they would like us to play but also provide us with some leeway for our own creative expression and improvisation as well. In my sessions with adolescents, young adults, and couples in conflicted relationships, I sometimes will sing some lines from a song that best captures their situations. For example, if my clients are stuck in a redundant pattern of being on and off again in their intimate relationships, I will share with them how their situation reminds me of one of the Stylistics' most popular songs, "Break Up to Make Up," and sing for them some of the main lines from the song (Stylistics, 2013). Hearing this often resonates with individual partners and/or couples and sometimes they become more receptive or fired up to break-up this longstanding pattern, learn more constructive ways of resolving their conflicts, or in a healthy constructive way decide to part from one another on good terms.

When I am feeling stuck in a session with a difficult couple or family, during my inter-session break I will imagine some of my favorite jazz heroes showing up for an impromptu consultation to offer me some novel and fresh ideas to get unstuck. The case example below with a challenging therapy-veteran family helps illustrate the power in imagining what famous musicians or other people who have inspired us would share with us as guest consultants to help us to get unstuck with difficult clients.

The Johnsons, a Caucasian family, had been to nine therapists before me for help with their daughter Cynthia's bulimia and self-injuring behaviors. The parents had felt that the past therapists had failed to resolve their relationship conflicts, give Cynthia the right coping and problem-solving tools and strategies to stop her bulimia and self-injuring, and that her grades in school had not improved. With most of the past treatment experiences, Cynthia had been seen individually and the parents had been peripherally involved in her treatment. The parents were high achievement oriented and put a lot of academic pressure on Cynthia to pull in "A" grades and over-scheduled her in too many extra-curricular activities, which she had disclosed to me during our individual session time that all this pressure and stress fueled her bulimia and self-injuring behaviors. When asked how come she had not brought this to her parents' attention, Cynthia responded with, "I have … but it doesn't go anywhere. They just say, 'You are capable of getting straight A grades.'" It sounded like Cynthia had been repeatedly invalidated by the parents and had resigned herself to keeping a lid on her thoughts and feelings about the pressure they had been putting on her. During my private time with the parents, their theory was that Cynthia's bulimia and self-injuring was started and is being maintained by her association with a group of girls she was friends with. They were totally oblivious to their part in contributing to the problem-life-support-system Cynthia's bulimia and self-injuring behaviors were embedded in. My efforts to reframe the parents' viewing of Cynthia's difficulties, attempts to disrupt their problem-maintaining interactions, or have the parents experiment with interacting in new ways with Cynthia, both in session and at home, went absolutely nowhere. I felt completely stuck. In our fourth family session, during my inter-session break, I imagined that if Thelonious Monk, Miles Davis, Ornette Coleman, and drummer extraordinaire Roy Haynes were to visit me as guest consultants what improvisational advice would they have for me about what I need to do differently with the Johnson family when we reconvene. I imagined that Coleman might say, "You are failing, this is good. You might be on to something original here, so fail faster." I thought Monk might say, "You need to be more playful, with a twist of surprise." I imagined that Davis might say, "Don't play what's there, play what's not there." Finally, Haynes would probably say, "You've got to get a better beat going, man! Punctuate anything that feels and sounds good with *time bombs*" (they help to keep time and mark transitions into something new on the drums). After this imaginary consultation session, lots of ideas had been sparked for me, such as: the session conversations are too problem-focused, therapy has become too serious and I need to inject some humor and playfulness into the session to loosen things up, and was reminded of Einstein's thinking, that solutions lie outside of the original problem explanations and attempted solutions. Armed with a lot of new ideas and fired up to operate differently with the Johnsons, I opened up with a playful and fun question, "Let's say today's session proved to be helpful to all of you beyond your wildest dreams. When you are driving home from here what will you each of you notice that is better with your situation?" Cynthia responded first with, "My mom won't be on my case about picking up my grades, pushing me to get straight 'A's,' and reminding me to meet with my teachers for extra help." She went on to add while shedding some tears that this would help her to be "less stressed out and less likely to binge and purge and cut myself." For the first time, Cynthia had opened up to her parents about this and they responded to her in a supportive way. The parents shared that Cynthia will have stopped her bulimia and self-injuring and would be happier. After ten more minutes of describing in great detail everyone's beyond their wildest dreams scenarios, I inquired with, "Sometimes pieces of one's wildest dreams had started to spontaneously happen out of the blue, has that happened for any of you?" Cynthia had surprised all of us by sharing that she had gone five days without bingeing and purging or cutting herself! The parents responded with smiles and were shocked that she was able to pull this off on her own. After hearing Cynthia's noteworthy accomplishment, I used Haynes's advice by punctuating it with time bombs to help transition us into a new direction in the session. I asked Cynthia, "Are you aware of how you did that?" Cynthia responded with, "I was worried about my throat being sore from throwing up too much and had read about how bulimics can potentially rupture their esophagus wall," which had scared her. She also had looked at her cutting scars on her arms and legs and told herself that she needed to stop disfiguring herself. Cynthia asked if her mom could take her to a skin specialist to try and cover up some of her worst scars. I had shared with Cynthia and her parents how impressed I was with her resourcefulness and how on her own she came to the realization that the time was now to stop her self-harming habits and embrace herself with loving-kindness and compassion. I also pointed out that often when self-injurers arrive at the place of wanting to cover up their scars and move on with their lives, it is an important turning point for closing the doors on their self-injuring habits. Finally, I gave Cynthia the experiment of writing her own *my self-compassion letter* to use during those dark moments when she might be emotionally triggered or highly stressed out as a reminder of all of her strengths and goodness, and to not take it out on herself but embrace herself with loving-kindness and compassion. Cynthia and her parents thought this was a great idea (Neff, 2015). Miles Davis's and Thelonious Monk's advice about "playing what's not there" and "being more playful, with a twist of surprise" had paid off big time with this family. The family left the session in great spirits and more hopeful about their situation. Future sessions focused on helping the parents and Cynthia learn more constructive ways of communicating with one another. I used family enactments as a teaching tool to help the parents practice listening, validating, soothing, and asking Cynthia if she needed anything else from them to comfort her after she had been emotionally triggered or highly stressed out. Another important change was the parents stopping their putting too much pressure on Cynthia for high academic achievement and allowing her to get out of all four of her extra-curricular activities. We also eventually got to a place where Cynthia could count more consistently on her parents to soothe her when she would experience emotional distress, rather than like in the past, where she felt invalidated by them and would have to take matters into her own hands with a razor blade to comfort herself.

Science and Technology

Today, we are so hooked on our digital devices and gadgets that they have become much more important than having human contact or spending high-quality time with our partners and families. We can't wait for the next hot digital device or gadget to be out on the market. With the rise of artificial intelligence, some are fearful that humans will be eventually replaced by machines in many different professional areas and industries. On a cautionary note, and as psychologist Sherry Turkle put it best in the title of her provocative book, *Alone Together: Why We Expect More from Technology and Less from Each Other*, she raises the important question as her main thesis, are we connected or disconnected from one another today (Turkle, 2011)? I was in a Starbucks recently and saw a couple sitting across from one another, and each partner had Apple AirPods in their ears, talking on their I-phones, and working on their MacBook laptops, and I asked myself are they connected or disconnected from one another? What happened to looking at your partner's eyes and listening intently to what he or she was saying? In my work with couples and families and when I am hearing that digital devices are being used excessively and as an escape from problems and at the expense of having meaningful human connections with one another in the offline world, we work together to find that on and offline balance, including instituting a weekend digital-free day where they could do something high-quality together in the offline world.

When I am working with clients who are interested in science and technology and possibly work in these professional areas or like reading about these areas, we need to intersperse in our conversations with them metaphors and language from their specialty science and technology areas, which can aid in our therapeutic alliance building with them. Also, I have found the use of my *invisible couple or family inventions* therapeutic experiment to work well with clients that are interested in science and technology or work in these fields (Selekman, 2017; Selekman & Beyebach, 2013). The case example below illustrates the use of invisible family inventions with an adolescent to help transform his relationship with his parents.

Tommy, a 14-year-old Caucasian boy who was under-achieving academically, was driving his parents crazy with getting poor grades in most of his subjects except science and math, where he was getting "A" grades. Tommy would push his parents' buttons by not staying on top of his school assignments, fail to turn completed homework in, and he was angry with them about their incessant nagging and lecturing about doing his schoolwork. His father Conrad was an engineer and his mother Hilda worked for a pharmaceutical company as a scientist. Tommy was very interested in artificial intelligence and quite skilled with computer technology. In our second family session, while meeting alone with Tommy, I gave him an in-session experiment to do, which I call the *invisible family inventions* exercise (Selekman, 2017). He was given the following instructions: "If you were to invent a machine or gadget that would benefit you and families like yours, what would you call it, how would it look, and what unique and special features would it have?" Next, I had him make a prototype sketch of it on large sketchpad sheet of paper, come up with a name for it, and draw its special features and explain what each one does. He came up with *The Anti-Parent Hassle Hand Changer.* Tommy's gadget was the size of a smartphone, was a digital device, and had six colored buttons that would appear on the screen. The device used artificial intelligence and advanced logarithm rules with determining what parents' facial expressions and postures indicated, in terms of what they were thinking and feeling, and assessing through the use of probability what the parents' next moves would be when approaching their kids. Another button that could be used to counter parental hassling was Tommy's version of the *stupefying charm or spell* that Harry Potter would use to defend himself, which would stun a person and render them unconscious (Rolling, 2000). Tommy changed the stupefying charm to just stunning or stopping his parents in their tracks like statues when they were about to lecture, nag, or yell at him, and when they would come out of the spell, they would not remember the original reason why they were approaching him and leave his bedroom or the family room where he was relaxing. One of the other buttons would offer him a wide range of strategies with a high probability of working that he could employ to change negative interactions with his parents. The last cool feature was that Tommy could take a photo of any school assignment and his device would provide quickly answers to questions, paper outlines, annotations for reading assignments, and so forth. I said to him that just this feature alone would be a hot sell for kids all around the globe! He laughed. Tommy agreed to show his parents his special invention. They were very impressed with Tommy's creative invention. For the first time, he shared with his parents if they would just stop nagging and lecturing him about doing his schoolwork, picking up his grades, and putting pressure on him to get straight A grades, he would commit to completing his backlogged school assignments, stay on top of new schoolwork, and pick up his grades. We tried this as an experiment over the next week as a way to disrupt their longstanding power struggles over doing schoolwork and the importance of getting "A" grades. Not only did Tommy get all of current schoolwork done but he had completed a great deal of his older assignments. I encouraged the parents to reward him for his hard work and fund something fun Tommy would like to do with a friend over the weekend. They thought this was a great idea. In future sessions, we worked on establishing more positive family interactions and carving out some fun family time together.

Nature

There are many health and psychological benefits to being out in nature. I often encourage couples and families to institute one digital-free day on the weekends to do something together out in nature. There is so much beauty and splendor out in nature that we lose sight of because we spend way too much time on our digital devices and are caught up in our rat race existences. I have taken many mental and real photos of being in awe with what I had discovered while hiking, running, biking, and boating out in nature. For example, I had a fabulous multi-sensory cruise on the Milford Sound fjord in New Zealand, which was like a Zen Buddhist experience. There were beautiful waterfalls on either side of the boat, the water was crystal clear, there were adorable-looking *Blue Penguins* on the reefs jutting out into the water that are the world's smallest penguins (25 centimeters tall), and schools of dolphins swimming alongside our boat for part of our cruise. One day on a long bicycle ride on a path that was snaking upward along a long lagoon, I caught out of the corner of my right eye a long green object that was resting on a large water plant leaf. I rode back because I was intrigued by what I had caught a glimpse of. It was the largest *Praying Mantis* insect I had ever seen. It was approximately 5 inches in length, had big bulging eyes carefully watching every move I made as I studied it in awe, it was completely still, and had small moving hairs on it. It had a beautiful shade of green coloring that helped it to camouflage itself from predators. Its stillness reminded me of the Chinese principle of learning to attain *wu wei* or actionless action (Tzu & Watson, 1968). In couple and family sessions, when my intuition is telling me not to talk or do anything, I think of the Praying Mantis and adopt a position of actionless action. With both of these special experiences out in nature, brought back my child-like sense of wonder and awe. Research on awe and self-transcendent experiences like the ones described above have been found to make us wiser, more likely to take others' perspectives, improve our critical reasoning, have humility, and be more empathetic (Kim, Nusbaum, & Yang, 2022; Keltner, 2023). Thoreau viewed nature as affording us with endless sources for healing, wisdom, beauty, and spiritual nourishment. He believed that trees alone could be our spiritual companions (Thoreau & Cramer, 2004). I have found that most of my best ideas for future journal articles and book topics or new things to try with my more challenging clients spontaneously popped into my mind on a long walk, run, or bike ride. This is why I keep handy in a pocket a piece of paper and a pen or if I have my smartphone with me, I type the ideas down on the memo page. Ideas are like birds on a window sill – if you don't notice them and write them down, they will fly away!

When I have clients that love doing things out in nature like hiking, mountain-climbing, canoeing, white-water rafting, fishing, and camping, I like to use metaphors in my conversations with them related to these activities and encourage them to reminisce with me about past positive experiences they had doing these activities where they were in awe with the beautiful scenery and wildlife and impressed themselves with their physical strength and endurance engaging in physically challenging outdoor activities. I encourage clients to go back and relive these special life experiences by *visualizing a movie of joy,* which consists of having them close their eyes, and using all of their senses, including color and motion to create a movie that they could play on a blank screen in their minds for 12–15 minutes of their most joyous times out in nature (Selekman, 2017). This visualization can be quite effective as a coping strategy to prevent our clients from lashing out with anger and engaging in self-destructive behaviors because it triggers positive emotions, which helps calm the inner emotional storms they may be experiencing (Selekman & Beyebach, 2013). I have had couples and families use my imaginary time machine and take it back to a special outdoor adventure vacation they were on together, describing in great detail with all of their senses and color and motion and what activities they engaged in. While processing their time travel experiences, we can learn about their past successes of what works in their relationships that we can use to help empower them to resolve their current difficulties. During the COVID-19 pandemic I had couples and families experiment with *family adventure missions* (Selekman, 2021). Although traveling was quite limited and mostly on the ground, our clients did have available to them mountains, hiking trails, country roads, forest preserve paths, lakes, rivers, and larger bodies of water for hiking, climbing, biking, and boating. I had the couple and family pick what their outdoor adventure mission would be and where they would do it. The couple or family adventure mission had to be challenging, be outside of their comfort zones, and would require solid teamwork. What I have had heard consistently from couples and families who tried this outdoor experiment was that their relationship bonds grew stronger, they learned new things about each other's competencies and resourcefulness, and most importantly, they had such a great time together that wanted to do it more fun and challenging outdoor adventures together. During the COVID-19 pandemic, clients discovered that this activity helped to liberate them and be free to be out in the world and enjoy life again.

I often use metaphors of animals and insects in my sessions with couples and families. From encouraging a client to soar like an eagle when he or she is about to give a big presentation at work or school or perform musically, in a theater production, or sports event, to describing an adolescent who isolates himself in his bedroom being like a trap-door spider, which spends most the day deeply hunkered down in an underground tunnel and comes up to hunt in the night time, pushes its little door out of the way, finds prey, brings it back, and covers the tunnel hole with the door until the next day. The beauty in the use of nature metaphors is that our clients can picture what we are sharing with them, which can be emotionally uplifting or indirectly challenge the way they are choosing to live that is unproductive and may be costing them. The case example below is of a 17-year-old Saudi-Arabian depressed boy named Ahsan. Ahsan had begun to apply to universities and was interested in going to a school that offered a career track of courses in bio-design work. He always had a strong interest in the life sciences, engineering, math, and art. Ahsan had three pets, an iguana, a box turtle, and a Golden Retriever dog that he loved dearly.

What had been depressing Ahsan was that his parents used to argue a lot in front of him and his 15-year-old sister Fatima and had decided to separate. Since Ahsan's father Ayaan had moved out, they did not have much contact, partially because of his having many business trips and his spending more time with his friends playing squash rather than wanting to spend quality time with him and his sister. I found out that Ahsan and his father used to spend a lot of time together when he was younger but since he had landed a high-powered CEO position with an international company that became his main priority. His father worked long hours and had to travel a lot. His sister Fatima and mother Farah spent a lot of time together. There were times where Ahsan felt all alone in the family. When I first started family therapy with them, Ayaan had agreed to try a session with Farah, Ahsan, and Fatima. When Farah brought up that Ahsan was depressed and missed not seeing him, Ayaan got defensive and angry with her for blaming him for Ahsan's problems. They started to argue and I decided to divide the session up where I would see each parent separately with the kids. Being sensitive to the cultural dynamic that the father often wields the most power and is the main authority in an Arabic family and I was worried about him possibly dropping out of treatment, I decided to meet with Ayaan and the kids first. Both kids were happy that their father had come to the family meeting and expressed how they missed not seeing their father more often. Ayaan shared with them that he had a lot of business trips during this time but that when it slowed down in a few weeks he had planned to not only spend one-on-one time with each of them and that if he could work things out with their mother, he wanted to take them on a trip to London over spring break. The kids had never been to London before and were quite excited about the possibility of having this special vacation with their father. When I met with Farah and the kids, I could tell she was still upset with how Ayaan had treated her in front of them. She was particularly upset to hear that their father was making travel plans for them without consulting her. I said that if she wished and if Ayaan would participate, I could have a meeting with just the two of them to discuss co-parenting issues and the trip situation. Farah agreed to try another session with Ayaan. One week later, Ayaan came in to meet with Farah. The session started off well when we were discussing how they can work together around the kids better but when the London trip was brought up, they started to argue about it. Ayaan felt that it was his right as the father to be able to do whatever he wanted to do with the kids, including taking them on a special trip to London. Farah raised her voice and said, "You don't think I would have wanted to take them on a trip!" At this point, Ayaan stormed out of the session. I went after him to see if he would be willing to come back and try and work things out with Farah. Ayaan shared with me, "She doesn't respect me and this is why I'm going to divorce her!" When I returned to my office, Farah was crying and shared with me that she was done with the marriage and could no longer live with Ayaan, let alone do another session with him. She also liked the idea of seeing each parent separately with the kids in the future. I provided empathy and support and requested that I see Ahsan individually for the next meeting to begin building an alliance with him. Ahsan and I had a wonderful individual session. He opened up to me about the major stressors in his life that were depressing him, such as: their years of arguing in front him and his sister, the parental separation, not spending enough one-on-one time with his father, and at school being harassed by three racist members of the football team who were calling him: "A terrorist," "a nerd," and "a sissy." I asked him what he and his parents had attempted to do about this problem with school administration and apparently nothing had been done about it. As a racial justice ally and advocate for Ahsan, I felt it was my responsibility to go to the school and meet with Ahsan's dean and principal to find out why these boys were not be reprimanded for their racist comments and bullying behavior. Both Farah and Ahsan signed off on a consent form so I could collaborate with the school. I also learned all about Ahsan's interest in bio-design and how we can design and create products and architectural structures based on living organisms and their unique features. He was fascinated with undersea life, particularly the octopus. I asked him if he saw the great documentary *My Octopus Teacher* (Foster, 2020). Ahsan loved it and found it to be quite touching and the cinematography to be amazing. He shared with me that octopuses have many unique features like: being able to camouflage themselves by changing their colors to blend in with the environment around them, spray ink as a smokescreen to protect themselves and escape from predators, and using their strong suction cups on their long tentacles to pry open shelled animals. Ahsan asked if I had a sketchpad so he could draw for me a prototype of a new product he was trying to design, which was inspired by his love of the octopus. It was a plastic and rubber octopus jar opener that had special suction cups on the upper parts of the tentacles, so when you pushed downward on the head of the octopus, it would adhere tightly to the jar top, and the consumer would hold tightly the head portion of the device while turning the opener until the top came off. He called it the *Octo-Jar-Opener*. I shared with him that this was a cool idea and probably would sell well because there is nothing like this on the market. Since a lot of the products his father's company made used plastics and were household type products, I recommended that we do a session with his father so he could share his great idea with him and see what his thoughts were about if this could be built and how best to do it. Ahsan really liked this idea. I thought this would be a great way to strengthen their bond and work together on this project. I learned that the father had both an MBA and a Master's in engineering. I also learned that the two of them had gone on some wonderful scuba-diving trips together in the past. One week later, I met with Ahsan and his father and put him in charge of sharing his prototype drawing of his innovative Octo-Jar-Opener and explain to him how it worked. He shared with his father what had inspired him to create this product and how most jar-openers don't work very well and are not as aesthetically pleasing to look at as his proposed invention. Ahsan thought it could be made out of a combination of plastic and rubber. Ayaan was very impressed with Ahsan's creative idea and he offered to run this by his research and design colleague at his company to see if something like this could be made and work. Ayaan also thought that Ahsan's device could be made to be wireless and work on voice-command like an Alexa Amazon device once positioned correctly on top of the jar with a turning mechanism built into the Octo-Jar-Opener. I also shared with the two of them that I had met with Ahsan's dean and the school principal to address the racist and bullying behavior of the three boys that continue to harass him and are getting away with it. I learned that the three boys had just been given a number of detentions and were suspended for bullying. Ahsan and Ayaan thanked me for advocating for them and were happy to hear that they were finally being held accountable. Towards the end of our session, Ahsan opened up about missing not seeing his father more often. Ayaan hugged his son and made a commitment to be more present in his life. After the session, they went out for dinner and agreed to meet with me in two weeks once Ayaan got back from his business trip. When I had met with Farah, Ahsan, and Fatima, I discovered that Ayaan had apologized to Farah and they were able to work out an arrangement for future vacations with the kids. Farah was now okay with the kids going to London with their father because he agreed for her to take them on the next vacation in the upcoming summer. Both parents had agreed to resume conjoint family therapy sessions and be civil and respectful towards one another in front of the kids and start to prepare them for their mutual decision to divorce. Future sessions focused on supporting the kids during the divorce transition, helping the parents be a better co-parenting team, and Ayaan committing to spending more time with his kids. Ahsan's depression had uplifted and he and his father rekindled their strong father-son bond. The last I heard about Ahsan's Octo-Jar Opener was that his father's research and design colleague thought his idea was great but will take time to figure out the proper materials and getting it to work in a user-friendly efficient way. By the time I had terminated with the family, both parents were no longer clashing and were co-parenting better, and Ayaan had found that balance of spending high-quality time with each of his kids.

Other Strategies for Becoming More Inventive and Expanding Our Therapeutic Range and Styles

For most of this chapter, I have shown practical and creative ways we can draw from the fields of art, architecture, film, theater, literature, philosophy, history, music, science and technology, and nature to co-construct with our clients' solutions for their presenting difficulties. What we have not covered thus far are other ways we can expand our therapeutic range and style such as: idea-generating strategies for getting unstuck when working alone to generate novel and creative ideas, using a consultation team of colleagues, and tapping into our own inner resources, skills, and life passions to bring to our clients for co-creating possibilities. I describe each one of these strategies briefly below.

Idea-Generating Strategies When Working Solo and Feeling Stuck

To help get my creative juices going and spark some novel ideas, there are seven major idea-strategies I may try:

1 changing perspectives on the problem;
2 pretending to have a consultation team of famous people who have inspired us offering us novel ideas at inter-session breaks or when reflecting-on-action after sessions;
3 mind-wandering and incubating;
4 immerse yourself in your cherished flow state activities;
5 tapping into our own inner resources, talents, and life passions to co-create possibilities;
6 the use of the solutions and famous philosophers' quotes recipe boxes; and
7 using the collective intelligence of colleagues serving as a consultation team to co-generate novel ideas and help you to get unstuck.

Changing Perspectives on the Problem

Sometimes when we look at a problem from a different perspective, we see important things that we missed, ideas are suddenly sparked in our minds, and new locus points for intervention start to appear. Some questions I might ask myself to gain new perspectives on my clients' problem situations are as follows:

• If I were to hop into my imaginary helicopter looking down at this couple or family from high above, what do I see that I might have missed?
• If I were to pick up the front page of the Sunday edition of the *New York Times* newspaper and in big bold letters is a headline that best describes this couple or family, how would it read?
• What would be a popular song that best captures this couple or family's problem situation?
• What do I find aesthetically pleasing about this couple or family's presenting problem?
• If this problem were to come to me for counseling, what might I learn from it that I don't know and what questions would I ask it?
• If this problem transformed into an animal, what kind of animal would it become and why?
• What is this problem a solution for in this family?
• Why this problem and not another one?
• If the problem were to pack its bags and leave town, what impact would it have on this couple's relationship?
• What would they miss from its absence?

Questions like the above can help give us new ways to view our clients' difficulties and help co-create possibilities with them.

Pretending to Have a Consultation Team of Famous People to Inspire and Offer Us Novel and Creative Ideas

When I am feeling stuck in a couple or family session, at the inter-session break at 40–45 minutes before the hour, I will imagine if Sonny Rollins, Gandhi, Theodore Roosevelt, and René Magritte were to pay me a visit and offer their insights and creative ideas about what to do differently with the couple or family, what would they share with me? Because each of the famous people come from different professional backgrounds and are well-known for their contributions in their respective fields and in history, by pretending to put ourselves in their minds and what they were famous for, could potentially offer us a goldmine of associations, metaphors, insights, and creative ideas and help us to get unstuck with the couple or family and move in a more productive direction with them. This thought exercise also can be used after completing a session with a challenging couple or family while doing reflection-on-action, and offer us many novel ideas and potential solutions to bring into the next couple or family session with them.

Mind-Wandering and Incubating

Bar (2022) has found in his research that allowing daily for our minds to naturally wander and free associate can elevate our moods, enhance our creativity, and improve our social functioning. Our minds naturally wander or drift because we are not hard-wired to focus on one thing for long periods of time, so he believes we should take advantage of these moments to allow our minds to wander and see where they go and what we come up with. Closely related to mind-wandering, is giving ourselves time to incubate and reflect on your thoughts about or what best to do when faced with a complex and challenging couple or family case situation. Nobel Prize winner Daniel Kahneman recommends that we use *system 2* thinking when faced with complex and challenging problems, which involves giving oneself an adequate amount of time to reflect and allow your ideas to marinate before taking action. He recommends that we consider multiple options in terms of how to best intervene with a difficult problem situation and reminds us that just because we may have dealt with a similar problem situation successfully in the past does not mean that the same strategies that were employed will produce the same results with the current problem situation. Finally, he recommends that we compare and contrast the differences of the past problem case situations with the current one to help determine the best course of action from what you learned from this comparative analysis (Kahneman, 2011).

Immerse Yourself in Your Cherished Flow State Activities

In addition to mind-wandering and incubating, we can pursue our flow state activities to take our minds off of a complex and challenging client problem situation we are struggling with. Flow was discovered by the psychologist Mikhail Csikszentmihalyi who was studying the creative process of artists and found that they would enter a zone in their minds and while expressing themselves through their art activity where they completely lost track of time and feeling and reported they were coming up with their most creative ideas at this time (Csikszentmihalyi, 1997, 1990). My flow state activities are cooking, writing, and when I play my djembe. I completely lose track of time and feeling. Flow state activities can be dancing, reading, acting, playing an instrument, engaging in artwork, wood-working, and so forth. They provide meaning and purpose for us and are healthy activities to pursue that bring us pleasure and help to prevent burn-out from our stressful jobs as therapists. I have found that sometimes after being immersed in my flow state activities that creative ideas start to flow in my mind to bring to some of my most challenging couple and family cases.

Tapping into Our Own Inner Resources, Talents, and Life Passions to Co-create Possibilities

Throughout this book, I have stressed the importance of our making maximum usage of all that our clients bring to us, which are our allies, their strengths, resources, past successes, epiphanies, interests and life passions to empower them to resolve their difficulties. What I have not discussed as a resource is what we can bring to them when feeling stuck. Our inner resources that we may be regularly deploying in other areas of our lives may be the following: our courage, resilience, being a risk-taker, being highly optimistic, being playful and a jokester, and so forth. Our talents and passions in life might be: doing art, playing tennis, martial arts, doing outdoor adventure activities, going to live jazz concerts, gourmet cooking, singing or playing an instrument, watching and going to football games, and so forth. When we are feeling stuck with our clients, this is a ripe time to tap into the same courage, resilience, and risk-taking we may be regularly using in tennis competitions, when conducting seminars, when performing musically or theatrically. We need to give ourselves permission to be daring and take more risks outside of our comfort zones using our inner resources, talents, and life passion activities as potential sources for metaphors, storytelling, and as building blocks for potential therapeutic experiments that can grow out of what we bring to our clients. The important thing to remember is that we need to be purposeful with what we choose to bring to our clients and it has to be in line with their theories of change and goals.

Use of the Solutions and Famous Philosophers' Quotes Recipe Boxes

A number of years ago, I started two recipe boxes to have handy at my office desk, they are: the *solutions recipe box* and the *famous philosophers' quotes recipe box*. Not only did I start saving on index cards creative self-generated solutions of my clients but solutions for different types of couple and family difficulties my colleagues and I came up with that worked. When I am at a loss for ideas and potential solutions, during my inter-session break, I look through my alphabetized by problem solutions box for ideas. Often, clients' problem situations may spark in our minds quotes from particular philosophers that we can use to inspire them, offer them new ways of looking at their problem situations, and can potentially spark an epiphany or can open up space for possibilities. In these situations, I will consult with my famous philosophers' quotes recipe box at an inter-session break. One of my favorite quotes I like to share with clients who are clinging to narrow and rigid ways of looking at their problem situations or abandoning unproductive attempted solutions is from Emile Chartier, a French existentialist philosopher, who once said, "Nothing is more dangerous than an idea when it is the only one you have" (cited by Goolishian & Anderson, 1988). I find Chartier's nineteenth century wisdom to be timeless, in that when I find myself clinging to one way of looking at a client's problem situation or continuing to use a particular therapy approach that is not working and my need to be therapeutically flexible.

Three or More Heads Are Better Than One: The Power of Collective Intelligence

Another way we can get unstuck with challenging couple and family cases, is to have a consultation team of 3–4 colleagues observing us in a session and offering our clients and us some fresh and novel perspectives on the presenting problem and current therapeutic dilemma. They may observe how we are getting stuck, our blind spots, and include something about this in their reflections. There are different team strategies that I like to use, they are: the *reflecting team,* a *solution-focused brief therapy team* approach, and the *therapeutic debate strategic team* approach (Andersen, 1995, 1991; Lax, 1995; Miller, 1997; de Shazer, 1991, 1988; de Shazer et al., 2007; Sheinberg, 1985; Papp, 1983).

The *reflecting team* method consists of the team offering the family and I reflections 35–40 minutes into the hour for approximately 7–8 minutes dialoguing with two central themes that were touched on in the first half of the session by the couple or family and the therapist. The team members begin their reflections with qualifiers like: "I wonder if …?" "Could it be …?" "I was struck by …" All reflections are presented in a tentative way, team members use either logical (it makes sense what is shared) or positive connotation (positive relabeling of negative behaviors or interactions) when describing behaviors and interactions, and need to offer reflections or constructions of the couple or family's problem situation or the current therapeutic dilemma that is neither too similar nor too different from how the clients perceive their situation. The therapist than asks the couple or family to share their thoughts about what the team had to say, particularly ideas that they found useful or resonated with them. This can lead to a change in their viewing of their situation, which in turn can lead to new and more positive interactions happening in the room, or opening up space for a couple partner or family member to share a secret or other undiscussables that have served as constraints for change (Andersen, 1995). A variation of the regular reflecting team method I use with adolescents and their families is a peer reflecting team (Selekman, 1995, 1991). After having the parents, adolescent, their closest friends, and the friends' parents give me written consent to have at least three friends participate in a family therapy session, I will have them serve as the reflecting team and share their ideas with the family and I 35–40 minutes into the hour. The family will then share their thoughts about the peer consultation team's reflections. Often, the peers offer us helpful and creative ideas for resolving parent-teen power struggles, conflicts, and improving their communications, which worked in their relationships with their parents. Both adolescents and parents have found the use of peer reflecting teams very insightful and helpful.

The solution-focused brief therapy team approach consists of the therapist joining three or four of his observing colleagues approximately 40–45 minutes into the hour pulling their heads together to co-construct a message that will be read to the couple or family. The therapist writes out the message from the team that consists of the following: compliments for each couple partner or family member underscoring their resourcefulness, resilience, and creative self-generated coping and problem-solving strategies, positively relabeling negative behaviors (an angry parent is a concerned parent), and one or two therapeutic experiments to try over the next week that are in line with the clients' goals (Miller, 1997; de Shazer, 1991, 1988).

The therapeutic debate strategic team approach is particularly useful with couples and families that are rigidly entrenched in their problem-maintaining patterns of interaction, the presenting problems or symptoms have become intractable, and they are highly challenging to work with (Sheinberg, 1985; Papp, 1983). With the therapeutic debate, one team member takes the side of the couple partner/parents, another team member takes the side of the other couple partner/adolescent or young adult identified client, and the therapist remains neutral or supports a pro-change position with the couple or family. Approximately 35–40 minutes into the hour, the team members join the couple or family and have a debate in front of them about the dilemmas of change. The couple partners or family members are free to join the conversation, challenge and dispute team members' points of view, and share new views about their problem situation that were sparked for them. I have added a new member to the therapeutic debate, that is having a team member put himself or herself into the shoes and mind of the presenting problem and represent the problem's perspective on the couple or family situation, which has added a unique and interesting voice to the therapeutic debate process (Selekman, 2006). Three or more heads are better than one in terms of brain power and creativity. The collective intelligence that occurs between the therapist and his or her experienced team members cannot be matched by any individual, no matter how seasoned or skilled he or she is as a therapist (Paul, 2021; Clark, 2011). When using a team approach, it is best to have a team of colleagues that operate from different theoretical orientations and come from different cultural backgrounds, which offers us multiplicity of views and pathways for intervening. Both working with and participating as a team member affords us the opportunity to further expand our therapeutic range, knowledge bases, and increase our practice wisdom by learning from one another how to manage specific types of clinical presentations of couples and families. Finally, having a team offers us a wonderful support system when struggling with complex and challenging couples and families.

In this chapter, I have presented a plethora of resources couple and family therapists can tap to expand their therapeutic ranges and ways of using themselves as the catalysts for change. Additionally, both therapists and their clients alike will find the use of ideas from outside our field to co-design creative solutions will make their work together more upbeat, fun, and meaningful.

8

The Therapist's Use of Self Developmental Framework

From Beginning Couple and Family Therapist to Master Level and Beyond

The Use of Self Developmental Framework

Throughout this book, I have presented a plethora of ways we can use ourselves as being an integral part of co-creating solution-determined realities with couples and families. What we have not covered is a developmental framework for the therapist's use of self from being a novice couple and family therapist to achieving master level and beyond. Similar to human developmental theories, there are some important steps therapists need to take and tasks they need to master to advance to the next stage of development with their use of themselves as the catalysts for change with their clients. At each stage of the use of self-developmental framework, there are important theoretical concepts and principles they need to grasp and sets of skills in three major areas they need to achieve mastery, which are: *conceptual*, *perceptual*, and *executive* skills. With each of the three major skill areas, I discuss what theoretical concepts and principles, use of self-developmental tasks, self of the therapist personal work that needs to be done, and specific therapeutic tools and strategies that beginning, intermediate, advanced, and master-level couple and family therapists need to develop solid grounding in and competency with (see Figure 8.1). Once therapists move into the advanced and master levels of use of self-skill-development, they possess the necessary knowledge and skills for using themselves on higher levels and in newer ways, such as: being trainers, supervisors, mentors, consultants, publishing, presenting workshops at major national and international conferences, serving as consultants for social service agencies, mental health clinics, and treatment programs, teaching for graduate schools in marital and family therapy, psychology, and social work, and doing research. Finally, I close out the chapter with training exercises and activities for honing therapists' use of self-skills and inventiveness, which I have used in the contexts of individual and group supervision, consultation in social service and mental health settings, and as workshop skill-building exercises.

In the following sections, I present under each of the four developmental stages the important theoretical concepts and principles therapists need to grasp and

DOI: 10.4324/9781003334460-8

Stages	Developmental Tasks
Beginning Level	<ul><li>Begin working on your signature themes, the three-generational family genogram of own family, critically examine your own racist biases and prejudicial ideologies, stereotypical views, and homophobic reactions to LGBTQ individuals.</li><li>Develop a courageous mindset and reducing risk aversion.</li><li>Cultivating a curious mind and bringing back your childhood sense of wonder and awe.</li><li>Inquiring about and listening for clients' self-generated pretreatment coping and problem-solving strategies.</li><li>Interviewing for possibilities: Knowing when to ask the *right* question at the right time.</li><li>Setting short- and long-term skill development goals.</li><li>Using the therapeutic brilliance scale.</li><li>Using reflection-in-action and reflection-on-action.</li><li>Soliciting feedback from couples and families: using the session rating scale and the outcome rating scale.</li><li>Covering the Back Door: Goal-maintenance and regularly consolidating couple and family gains.</li><li>Collaborate with referral sources, involved helping professionals, key resource people from clients' social networks.</li><li>Receptive to live supervision, videotaping sessions, and being observed by a consultation team.</li><li>Serving as a consultation team member.</li></ul>
Intermediate Level	<ul><li>Learn to view your mistakes and failures as great opportunities for gaining wisdom and professional growth.</li><li>Integrative thinking and cultivating a synthesizing mind.</li><li>Learning how to tailor-fit your couple and family therapy approach to best meet the needs of your clients.</li><li>Cultivating the abilities to sit with client silence and practice actionless-action.</li><li>Start a daily mindfulness practice.</li><li>Find mentors highly skilled in a particular therapy approach or specialization area you want to learn more about.</li><li>Establish cooperative partnerships with highly pessimistic and pathology-minded involved helping professionals.</li></ul>
Advanced Level	<ul><li>Allowing your choice couple and family therapy approach to evolve.</li><li>Prospect for ideas outside of the couple and family therapy field to expand your therapeutic range.</li><li>Challenge yourself: Work with treatment populations and presenting problems you have limited experience with.</li><li>Beware of the risks of being too overconfident and the shortcomings of becoming a specialist.</li><li>Expand your horizons: Attend workshops on new therapy approaches and on subjects outside our field.</li><li>Serve as a trainer and/or supervisor.</li><li>Get published.</li><li>Give workshops and present at major local, national, and international conferences.</li></ul>
Master's Level	<ul><li>Never settle, keep pushing the limits for what is possible.</li><li>Mentoring and supervising advanced level couple and family therapists.</li><li>Serve on the faculty of a family therapy institute, marital and family therapy program, or other graduate school programs.</li><li>Expand the possibilities with your signature therapy model by applying it to an existing but unexplored treatment issue/problem, or a new emerging issue/problem of contemporary couples and families.</li><li>Consider doing treatment outcome research.</li><li>Keep publishing and presenting your cutting-edge clinical work.</li><li>Serve as consultant for a treatment program, youth and family service agency, or mental health clinic.</li><li>Maintain a small-to-medium size private practice to keep up with families' ever changing problems of the day.</li><li>Therapeutic Humility: Continue to cultivate this important virtue.</li></ul>

Figure 8.1 Use of Self Developmental Framework

specific skills they need to master with their conceptual, perceptual, and executive skills. Like all developmental theories, personal growth, learning, and the mastery of skills is rarely a smooth sailing process and often therapists may need further work, can benefit from the support, wisdom, and expertise of outside mentors, and more professional experience to advance to the next stage of their use of self-development.

Beginning Couple and Family Therapists

New couple and family therapists often come to the field with some basic under-standing of or are well-grounded in a wide-range of individual therapy approaches, such as: cognitive-behavioral therapy, psychodynamic therapy, dialectical behav-ior therapy, and so forth (Barlow, 2001; Beck, 2011; Kendall, 2011; Summers & Barber, 2010; Rathus & Miller, 2015; Miller, Rathus, & Linehan, 2007; Linehan, 1993). They are used to diagnosing their clients and using their choice model's theo-retical framework and concomitant sets of therapeutic tools and strategies to restore them back to health with their thinking, feeling, and doing, like expert repairmen or women. One of the biggest challenges for beginning couple and family therapists who have done individual therapy for a long time or new graduates from social work, psychology, counseling, or medical school programs is making what I call the *systemic relational leap*, that is that emotional and behavioral difficulties develop and are maintained in a relational context. Furthermore, when we enter a conversation with clients about their identified "problem" voiced by them or involved concerned others, we not only become part of the same problem system, but we are part of the same observation vis-à-vis the clients (Selekman, 1995; Anderson, Goolishian, & Winderman, 1986; von Foerster, 1981). We can never find an outside place or God's eye view in which to look at our clients from nor can we separate how what we think, feel, and do influences their behavior, which can either hinder or promote change (Hoffman, 1988).

Another important theoretical principle to remember in terms of the use of self is that all couples and families have the strengths and resources to change and are the true experts on their lives. This is supported by psychotherapy treatment outcome research on the common factor *client extra-therapeutic factors*, which indicates what counts the most for positive treatment outcomes is the clients that are the true heroes and the therapist's expertise is at utilizing to the maximum degree all that their clients bring to them: their strengths and resources, life passions, language (key words), metaphors, beliefs, pretreatment self-generated coping and problem-solving strategies, past successes at resolving other difficulties, their theories of change, best hopes and expectations of us and are work together, and epiphanies, serendipitous practices (Bohart & Tallman, 2022, 1999; Greaves, 2022; Duncan & Miller, 2000; Duncan, 2010; Wampold, 2010; Sprenkle, Davis, & Lebow, 2009; Selekman, 2017). Couple and family therapy is a collaborative enterprise and the clients determine their goals, their treatment blueprints for change, who partici-pates in sessions, how often we meet, and when they are ready to stop. Closely related to the importance of utilizing the clients' expertise collaboratively is to invite them to determine the *relationship-of-fit*, that is how each couple partner and family member would like us to use ourselves with them in our sessions with them, such as being more interactive in sessions, offer lots of tools and strategies to experi-ment with between sessions, or be more reflective than past therapists they had seen (Norcross & Lambert, 2013). The therapeutic relationship has been found to be highly predictive of positive family treatment outcomes and is reported by clients as the key ingredient for why they had strong therapeutic alliances with their therapists. Clients have indicated the following in couple and family treatment outcome studies about their relationships with their therapists: they had great relationship and structuring skills (were competent and took charge in sessions when necessary), and felt both emotionally safe and had strong emotional connections with them (Levy, 2023; Diamond, Diamond, & Levy, 2014; Friedlander, Escudero, Heatherington, & Diamond, 2011; Szapocznik & Hervis, 2020; Duncan, 2019; Alexander, Waldron, Robbins, & Neeb, 2013).

Two other important theoretical principles beginning couple and family therapists need to grasp are based on the core assumptions of the solution-focused brief therapy and MRI brief strategic therapy models respectively. No problem no matter how severe or chronic is happening all of the time, there are always exceptions to the rule (de Shazer, 1988, 1991; de Shazer et al., 2007). As the Buddhists pointed out centuries ago, problems are transitory and in a constant state of evolutionary flux (Epstein, 2022; Hanh, 1998; Rinpoche, 1993). Therefore, couple and family therapists need to inquire about clients' exception patterns of thinking, feeling, and doing when the problem is not occurring, which can serve as building blocks for solution construction. In fact, these exceptions are often occurring well before we see clients in our offices or online for the first time, usually in the form of client self-generated coping and problem-solving strategies (Selekman, 2017; McKeel, 2012; Weiner-Davis, de Shazer, & Gingerich, 1987). One of the major theoretical assumptions of the MRI brief strategic therapy model is that it is the clients' attempted solutions that is the problem, which extends to involved and concerned key resource people from their social networks, involved helping professionals from larger systems, and treatment program staff (Watzlawick, Weakland, & Fisch, 1974). These attempted solution problem-maintaining patterns are what needs to be disrupted, which are perpetuating the couple or family's difficulties. Beginning couple and family therapists need to take the time in their first sessions with their clients to inquire about both their exception-oriented and problem-maintaining patterns, particularly a detailed inquiry about what all of the couple partners', parents', adolescents', concerned relatives', and past and present therapists' and treatment program staff's attempted solutions have been, so they don't replicate what has not worked.

As far as conceptual skill development goes and the use of self, it is important that beginning couple and family therapists are exposed to and familiarize themselves with the major therapeutic techniques and strategies of a wide range of systemic therapy approaches and find the couple or family therapy approach or approaches that resonate with them the most and is in line with the person of who they are in terms of their personality, values, beliefs about the change process, and the style of working as a therapist that feels most comfortable for them. They need to become familiar with how therapists use themselves differently in the therapeutic process with different couple and family therapy models. For example, a structural therapist is highly active in the beginning of family therapy and assumes a leadership role in transforming family interactions, belief systems, and challenging the symptom-bearer. When supervising and training couple and family therapists, my bias is that being flexible and integrative as a therapist is most advantageous in that one can view couple and family difficulties through multiple theoretical lens and have multiple pathways for intervention. If trainees or supervisees wish to become integrative, it is important that the trainer or supervisor helps them to select couple or family therapy approaches that can logically fit together and offer some guidelines for them regarding with what clinical situations it may make the most sense to use more therapeutic tools and strategies and ways of using oneself in the therapeutic process from a specific model or a combination of the integrated models. No couple or family therapy approach is a panacea for all client presenting problems. Most of the major empirically supported couple and family therapy approaches are integrative and they offer therapists clear guidelines for when to do what, which is one of the reasons why they had great outcome data to support their efficacy (Smith & Meyers, 2023; O'Farrell & Fals-Stewart, 2006; Henggeler & Sheidow, 2011; Alexander, Waldron, Robbins, & Neeb, 2013; Levy, 2023; Szapocznik & Hervis, 2020). Finally, beginning couple and family therapists need to familiarize themselves with the role family life cycle changes play in the development of couple and family difficulties. For example, the tumultuous adolescent years can put a tremendous strain on parents' marital relationships.

In order to be truly present and not emotionally reactive to couples or families that mirror their intimate couple relationships, their parents' marriage, or the family that they grew up in, which will inevitably occur at some point in their careers, beginning couple and family therapists need to do their own personal work during their free time. One of the most emotionally growth-producing experiences I ever had in my own therapy with a Bowenian therapist was to take a voyage home and co-construct with my parents a three-generational family genogram (McGoldrick & Gerson, 1986; Bowen, 1978). Although it was anxiety-provoking for both my parents and I when they shared with me intimate details about their family-of-origin politics, some of which were quite negative and traumatizing, I learned a lot about why they related to me the way they did when I was growing up. I also learned about patterns, rigid role behaviors, triangles and cross-generational coalitions that perpetuated themselves throughout the generations. Aponte's *signature themes* work discussed earlier in Chapter 2 is a nice compliment to doing one's own three-generational family genogram and offers us further insights about ourselves and family-of-origin experiences, which help us to be truly present with and less likely to experience negative emotional reactivity to our clients. Some common signature themes are as follows: like to be in control at all costs, fear of rejection and not being good enough, highly reactive to criticism, or have difficulty with constructively managing stress (Aponte, 2016; Zeytinoglu, 2016; Aponte et al., 2009). A variation of the signature themes work I like to use is to have the trainees or supervisees identify their positive signature themes as well, such as: being resilient and having grit, being daring and like to take on challenging tasks, being authentic, caring and compassionate, having a good sense of humor and are playful, to name a few. Trainees' and supervisees' can utilize both their negative and positive signature themes to normalize their clients' struggles, strengthen their therapeutic alliances, and use them for co-creating a context for change with them.

Two other important areas beginning couple and family therapists need to increase their awareness of and critically examine is their own racist biases and prejudicial ideologies and beliefs that they may still carry from their family-of-origins, primary social groups, and the communities they grew up in (Hardy & Laszloffy, 2005). Once they make a commitment to eliminating these racist biases and prejudicial ideologies, they need to adopt a mindset of cultural humility and serve as racial justice allies and advocates for their clients of color (Tervalon & Murray-Garcia, 1998). They also need to critically examine their stereotypical views and homophobic reactions to LGBTQ people that also may have emanated out of their family-of-origin, primary social group, and the communities they grew up in and make a commitment to eliminating them as well. All of the above deep and personal self-work should continue throughout their professional careers. We, like our trainees and supervisees, are works in progress in terms of emotional growth, further honing and learning new skills, and striving to be our best possible selves.

As part of their training in the use of self, I encourage beginning couple and family therapists to participate in their own couple or family therapy to be able to experience the process and to know what it is like to sit in the other chair in a relational context. This can occur with them and their partner and/or family or even with members of their family-of-origin to resolve longstanding conflicts, disrupt destructive patterns of interaction, or to be liberated from a role that they may continue to play in their own family drama as an adult.

When it comes to perceptual skills in the beginning couple and family therapist stage, they need to work on developing solid listening and observation skills. As a metaphor for working on becoming a good listener, I like to share with trainees and supervisees how the Hindu elephant God *Ganesha* has very large ears and a tiny mouth, as a reminder that we need to listen more and talk less. In initial couple and family therapy sessions, trainees and supervisees need to be able to sit back, talk less, and listen and observe for the couple or family's interactive dances, which are the *what* and *how* of both exception-oriented (non-problem behaviors and patterns) and problem-maintaining patterns. Once these patterns begin to repeat themselves, they can seize the opportunities that exception-oriented patterns provide for amplification and co-constructing solutions. With the couple and family problem-maintaining attempted solution patterns, they can locate in second and subsequent sessions locus points for intervening to disrupt them through the use of pattern intervention strategies (Fisch & Schlanger, 1999; Fisch, Weakland, & Segal, 1982; O'Hanlon, 1987).

Beginning couple and family therapists need to be able to assess the stage of readiness for change each couple partner and family member is in so as to guide how them in how they should use themselves and how best to intervene (Prochaska

& Prochaska, 2016; Prochaska, Norcross, & DiClemente, 1994). Closely related to the stage of change assessment framework is assessing the cooperative response patterns of each couple partner and family member with us (de Shazer et al., 2007; de Shazer, 1988; Fisch, Weakland, & Segal, 1982). For example, often court-ordered clients are coming to us under duress and would be considered *visitors* or *pre-contemplators* because they don't think they have a problem and are not armed with goals to change anything but concerned others have a problem with their behavior or the trouble they may be in. Ultimately, the beginning couple and family therapist must determine who in the client system or social network is the true *customer* for change or in the *action* stage of readiness for change who we can partner up with as the agent of change who is ready and willing to do anything to improve their couple or family relationships or change the identified client's problematic behaviors (de Shazer, 1988; Prochaska & Prochaska, 2016; Fisch, Weakland, & Segal, 1982). Finally, the beginning couple and family therapist must assess with the couple or family what they consider to be the *right* problem to change first, negotiate the problem into smaller and realistic behavioral terms with them, and what their theories of change are in terms of how they envision their work together to look and how they will know they are completely satisfied with the treatment process and have identified what their ideal positive outcomes will look like.

With executive skill development, beginning couple and family therapists will need to work on becoming competent in *interviewing for possibilities* with their clients, that is familiarize themselves with different categories of questions from different brief and family therapy approaches, such as solution-focused brief therapy (Selekman, 2017; de Shazer et al., 2007; Lipchik, 2002; Miller, 1997; de Shazer, 1988, 1985); the MRI brief strategic therapy approach (de Shazer, 1999; Fisch & Schlanger, 1999; Fisch, Weakland, & Segal, 1982); the Milan systemic family therapy approach (Boscolo & Bertrando, 1993; Boscolo, Cecchin, Hoffman, & Penn, 1987; Tomm, 1988, 1987), narrative therapy (White, 2007; White, 1995, 1988a; White & Epston, 1990a); the collaborative language systems therapy approach (Anderson & Gehart, 2007; Anderson, 1997), and the reflecting team approach (Andersen, 1995, 1991; Lax, 1995). Beginning couple and family therapists can begin to learn and practice using these different categories of questions and when to use them by observing their trainers and supervisors working live or on videotapes with couples and families, through role-playing, and watching DVDs of the pioneers of the aforementioned brief and family therapy approaches. Having the intuitive sense and developing the skill of when to use what category of questions comes with lots of practice and experience. There is no expectation that beginning couple and family therapists will quickly achieve mastery with how and when to use certain categories of questions.

In my mind, the solution-focused brief therapy approach offers the best sequencing of categories of questions for efficiently setting goals with and empowering demoralized and highly pessimistic clients out of all of the above-mentioned family therapy models. The goal-setting process begins with asking couple and families the *miracle question*, expanding the possibilities with clients regarding how things will change individually and in their couple, family, peer, school, and work relationships and the positive affects the reported changes will have on them and their relationships; exploring with them if any pieces of the miracle had already started to happen, even a little bit; how the clients account for those pieces of the miracle that occurred (useful self-talk and action steps taken by them and significant others); and from miracle land, asking the *miracle scaling question* on a scale from 10 to 1 (1 being taking the courageous step to call and set up an appointment and 10 being the day after the miracle happened) to find out post-miracle where they would rate their situation (rated situation at a 7) and what the couple partners or family members are *going* to do over the next week to try and achieve their initial treatment goal (to get one step higher on the scale to an 8 (de Shazer et al., 2007). The majority of the beginning couple and family therapists I have trained or supervised were able to quickly master this solution-focused brief therapy goal-setting process. Even with demoralized and pessimistic couples and families the solution-focused brief therapy model offers guidance and questions (coping, pessimistic, and sub-zero scaling questions) that help engender hope and invite them to compliment themselves on their resourcefulness and resilience (Selekman, 2017; de Shazer et al., 2007; Lipchik, 2002; Miller, 1997). An important aspect of interviewing for possibilities is embedding in questions pre-suppositional words like *when, will, going* to do and in conversations with clients speaking the language of change or *solution talk*, which is not only using pre-suppositional language with them but inquiring what specifically they are thinking, feeling, and doing during the times when the problem is absent and finding out about their past successes. By doing so, it raises the clients' expectancy levels that the changes they desire are already starting to happen and it is only a matter of *when* they *will* happen more often.

As far as the purposeful use of self goes with executive skill development, below I present thirteen developmental tasks that I have found to greatly benefit beginning couple and family therapists to empower them to become more confident, daring, and courageous with taking risks, keeping an open mind and staying therapeutically flexible, and be more playful and enjoy their work with their clients more. I describe under each of the developmental tasks what trainers and supervisors can do to help their trainees and supervisees to achieve mastery with each of the tasks.

Beginning Couple and Family Therapist Developmental Tasks

There is no expectation or pressure on trainees and supervisees to master all thirteen of the developmental tasks during this beginning couple and family therapist stage of their careers, it will take time for them to overcome the following common struggles of new therapists: being too cautious and second guessing themselves; having a strong aversion to uncertainty and silence; being afraid of making mistakes; being too much in their heads and preoccupied with performance; and viewing therapy as serious business! Through lots of practice with use of self-skill development in sessions, gaining more experience working with culturally diverse couples and families with a wide range of presenting problems, and on the spot supervisory support and encouragement, they will begin to make great headway in removing the aforementioned constraints that are blocking them from taking risks in sessions and achieve mastery with each of the developmental tasks over time.

Developing a Courageous Mind-Set and Reducing Risk Aversion

We can develop courageous mind-sets in our trainees and supervisees by encouraging and giving them the confidence to practice taking risks in each of their couple and family sessions so that their self-efficacy, hope, open-mindedness, and resilience becomes more stable and will be habitually activated in the face of fear or when being daring trying a new therapeutic technique or strategy out (Hannah, Sweeney, & Lester, 2010; Lester et al., 2010; Pury, Lopez, & Key-Roberts, 2010). Once trainees and supervisees learn through practice and experience what they can control in sessions and are confident that their trainer or supervisor will do all that they can to help them to become more skilled clinicians, and prevent crises from occurring in sessions, will give them the power to manage uncertainty (Wucker, 2021). Research indicates that successful past or current performance enhances future performance (Bandura, 2000, 1997). Therefore, the more exposed trainees and supervisees are to situations that elicit fear and require constructive action does contribute to them becoming more courageous (Boag & Pury, 2022; Lester et al., 2010; Bandura, 2000, 1997). Wucker (2021) contends that risk perception and response are like muscles that complement one another and strengthen the more we are exposed to challenging situations and the more you use them, the better we will become with making good decisions and take smart therapeutic actions in sessions. Bandura (2000) developed a training method for skill development called *cognitive mastery*, which consists of teaching trainees or supervisees how to visualize or mentally rehearse in their minds seeing themselves making good decisions and performing at a high level with challenging tasks. Inspired by Bandura's work, I use my *visualizing my best possible session* with trainees and supervisees in supervision meetings prior to seeing a challenging couple or family that they want help with. They first are to close their eyes, picture blank movie screens in their minds, and create movies (using all of their senses, including color and motion) that will be projected onto their mind screens in which they see themselves with their most challenging couples or families conducting their best possible sessions with them. Next, I have them describe in great detail what techniques and strategies they picture themselves using successfully to promote change with their clients. Finally, once it becomes crystal clear for them what they envision that will have a great shot of working with their clients as far as the use of self and certain techniques and strategies they will be using, they can enter their sessions with confidence and taking risks outside of their comfort zones to make those changes happen. This visualization strategy helps co-create a positive self-fulfilling prophecy for the trainee or supervisee. Pury (Boag & Pury,

2022) found in her research on courage that it is all about "taking a worthwhile risk" and deciding what we want to accomplish and taking the risks to make it happen because we care about it and find it meaningful to us.

Another way to optimize for trainees and supervisees success and further bolster their courage and confidence with challenging couples and families is to do couple and family simulations of clinically difficult couple and family scenarios they will inevitably face, such as: working with angry and hostile and demoralized and highly pessimistic parents; working with a high-conflict couple deadlocked in an intense and rigid blame-counter-blame interaction that occurs in session, engaging a reluctant adolescent who refuses to talk, and so forth. The therapists in the couple and family simulations are to come up with at least three therapeutic moves they can make in their use of self in the different scenarios, which includes therapeutic techniques and strategies they may want to try, and practice reflection-in-action or stepping outside of themselves watching how the clients are responding to what they are saying and doing. By having trainees' and supervisees' practice exposing themselves to challenging couple and family scenarios as described above, they will be much better prepared to confidently and constructively manage these clinical dilemmas when they occur in the future because they have experienced them before.

An exercise I like to use with beginning couple and family therapists is having them write their own *courage stories*. They are to write about a time in their lives where they were courageous in mastering challenging situations or where they used their courage to benefit or help other people. I encourage them to close their eyes and transport themselves back to the courageous act and try and access using all of their senses, including color and motion, and what they were telling themselves and the steps they took to act courageously with a high level of self-confidence. This exercise reminds beginning couple and family therapists that they already possess this inner strength that they can access and use in any given couple or family session.

Cultivating a Curious Mind and Bringing Back
Your Childhood Sense of Wonder and Awe

With my trainees and supervisees, I encourage them to cultivate curious minds and come armed with lots of questions not just about their clients but the theoretical underpinnings of and the therapeutic process of different couple and family therapy approaches that we can discuss in both individual and group supervision. I want them to bring back their old childhood sense of wonder and awe about their clients' resilience, problem stories, and what they find aesthetically pleasing and interesting about the couple and family drama and the cast of characters they are working with. I have them use their own curiosity and creativity to craft intriguing and bold questions using the *question-storming* exercise (see Chapter 6) that they can pose to their clients. When they report feeling stuck or confused with a particular couple or family, I encourage them to ask their clients open-ended questions from a position of respectful curiosity, rather than continuing to use known questions from particular therapy models, which has been unproductive. Sometimes I ask trainees and supervisees to pretend that they are 10 or 11 again and tapping into their former childhood sense of wonder and awe, and I ask them the following questions:

- "What would you be curious to learn more about with a challenging couple or family they are feeling stuck with?"
- "What questions have you not asked them about their couple or family situation that could be helpful to pose to them?"
- "What questions do you think the couple or family are hoping you might ask them or have been surprised that you had not asked up to this point?"

I encourage beginning couple and family therapists to allow their curiosity to run wild in their sessions reminding them that there is always more to know and many chapters to their clients' stories. I have them avoid at all costs locking down on the first two explanations for couples' and families' problem situations and instead, allow themselves to be curious about the third, fourth, and fifth possible explanations for what might be contributing to what is maintaining their difficulties.

Inquiring About and Listening for Clients' Self-Generated Pretreatment Coping and Problem-Solving Strategies

Couples and families often take constructive step towards better coping with and trying to resolve their difficulties well before we see them for the first time (Selekman, 2017; McKeel, 2012; Weiner-Davis, de Shazer, & Gingerich, 1987). As mentioned in Chapter 1, the clients are the true heroes in the solution-determined stories we co-author with them. They are resilient, resourceful, and creative with coming up with their own unique coping and problem-solving strategies. This is why it behooves therapists to give their new clients a pretreatment change experiment to do before they come in for their first appointments with them. We can have the help-seeking couple partner or parent keep track on daily basis and write down the various things they are telling themselves or doing to either reduce the frequency of the complaint or problem from happening or not occurring at all. Additionally, they can be asked to also keep track and write down the times when their partner or children are being more responsible, respectful, and loving towards them. The help-seeking partner or parent is to bring into their first appointment their lists of what is working and that they would like to continue to have happen (Selekman, 2017). As a result of using this pretreatment change experiment with new clients, we can utilize what they are already doing that works, amplify and consolidate their gains, and rapidly co-construct solutions with them using their expertise about what works. Beginning-level couple and family therapists will find that once they master this skill it will not only reduce clients' lengths of stay in treatment but it will remind them that all clients have the strengths and resources to change and they are the true experts!

Interviewing for Possibilities: Knowing When to Ask the Right Question

Earlier in the chapter, I discussed the importance of beginning couple and family therapists learning how to use the miracle and scaling questions with their clients to elicit both their short-term and ideal treatment outcome pictures when their problems are solved and small realistic initial behavioral goals with them. With practice, they will become increasingly more skilled at successfully negotiating both short- and long-term outcome goals with their clients. However, what is more challenging for beginning couple and family therapists is when they have demoralized and highly pessimistic therapy veteran couples and families that cannot identify any past successes, self-generated pretreatment changes, or entertain the idea of a miracle ever happening with their intractable problem situations. Both beginning and even more experienced solution-focused therapists can make the mistake of pushing too hard for these clients to play around with or pretend the miracle happened like pushy salespeople, which leads to the clients feeling invalidated, becoming defensive, and frustrated (Nylund & Corsiglia, 1994). Instead, in order to better cooperate with their pessimism, the therapist needs to shift gears and ask them *coping questions* (Selekman, 2017; de Shazer et al., 2007) like:

- "It sounds like your daughter really pushes your buttons at times. Tell me, how have you prevented the situation from getting much worse?"
- "(Parent reports going for three days without yelling at her daughter, which lead to more cooperation from her) Are you aware of how you pulled that off?"
- "What else are you doing to prevent things from getting much worse with her?"
- "(Mother shares that she is avoiding getting into power struggles with her daughter) Are you aware of how you came to that realization?"

By better cooperating with the mother's pessimism and negativity, it produced important self-generated coping and problem-solving strategies the mother was coming up with that prompted more cooperation from the daughter and reduced her need to yell at her. In situations where the clients continue to be pessimistic and negative, two other options are the use of *pessimistic* or *sub-zero scaling questions* (Selekman, 2017; de Shazer et al., 2007). Some examples of these questions are as follows:

- "Some couples in your situation would have thrown in the towel with counseling a long time ago. After all I am the eighth therapist you have been to! What keeps you hanging in there?"
- "What would have to be the tiniest change that would have to happen over the next week that would give you a glimmer of hope that your situation can improve a little bit?"
- "Some parents in your situation would have given up on counseling a long time ago, would have put their son in a boarding school, residential treatment, or better yet, put him up for adoption, what has stopped from pursuing that option?"

- "On a scale from -10, being that your situation is totally hopeless and irresolvable and -1 you have an inkling of hope that you may be able to improve your situation a little bit, where would you have rated your situation a month ago?"
- "At a -8. How about two weeks ago?"
- "At a -6. Are you aware of what you did to get two notches higher on the scale?"
- "What are you going to do over the next week to get up to a -5?"

Both these questions often produce important client information regarding self-generated coping and problem-solving strategies and engender hope and optimism for them. The sub-zero scaling question also invites clients to compliment themselves on their resourcefulness, perseverance, and resilience.

Other categories of questions that we should expose beginning couple and family therapists to when faced with clients that have been oppressed by their problems for a long-time or have experienced many losses, traumas, and where we may be detecting secrets, are *externalizing questions* and *conversational questions* respectively (White, 2007, 1995; Anderson & Gehart, 2007; Anderson, 1997). Externalizing questions are particularly useful with clients describing their problems as being oppressive, intractable, and having a life of their own. What is most important when externalizing clients' problems is that it has to be based on the clients' descriptions or beliefs about it. For more on externalizing questions, see chapter one under Michael White. Conversational questions are open-ended questions and are asked from a position of not-knowing and respectful curiosity. These questions are constructed and asked in response to the clients' telling and retelling the chapters of their problem stories, so as to gain access to the *not-yet-said* such as secrets or open up space for new ways of looking at their situations. The last category of questions I like new couple and family therapists to become familiar with are future-oriented questions (Boscolo & Bertrando, 1993; Tomm, 1988, 1987). When the treatment system has come to a standstill and we are feeling stuck, the future yields all kind of possibilities, in that it has not happened yet. Some examples of future-oriented questions are as follows:

- "Let's say we were to run into one another six months down-the-road at the Williams Shopping Mall, long after we successfully completed counseling together, what will the three of you be most eager to share with me that changed that I will be the most surprised to hear about?"
- "How have those changes made a difference in your relationship (the mother and daughter)?"
- "What else will you (the daughter) share with me that is much better in your relationship with your father?"
- "If the three of you were to walk me back from our conversation at the Williams Shopping Mall, what will be the steps that you told me you took to make all of these great changes happen?"
- "When will you quit bulimia, in one week? One month? One year?"

- "One week from now after you quit bulimia, what will you tell me you are doing instead that is helping you stay quit and preventing slips from happening?"
- "Let's say that tomorrow the two of you wake up and you are completely amnesiac to what you used to argue about all of the time, what are you doing instead that is making your relationship go much better?"

Through lots of practice, good supervision, and increased experience using the aforementioned categories of questions, beginning couple and family therapists will get better at knowing when to ask the right question at the right time.

Setting Personal Short- and Long-Term Skill-Development Goals

Just like with clients, beginning couple and family therapists should take the lead in defining their short- and long-term learning and skill development goals for supervision. I often begin with soliciting from them what their ideal long-term outcome skill-development pictures will look like at one-year, six months, and in three months. I ask trainees and supervisees the following questions to secure this important information:

- "Let's say our supervision together over the next year proves to be professionally fulfilling for you beyond your wildest dreams, what will you have become more knowledgeable about and what specific skills will you have mastered?"
- "How about at six months, what have you further increased your knowledge about and what skills are you honing that you are pleased with?"
- "How about at three months, what have you become more knowledgeable about and what specific skills are you getting better at using with couples and families?"

The answers to these questions will guide the trainer or supervisor on the focus of their work together at different time periods in their professional skill-development process. As far as short-term goals go, we need to solicit from them one-two specific skills they wish to focus on developing competency with using over the next week or two with their couple and family clients. For example, if a supervisee says that he or she would like to work on more skillfully using the miracle and scaling questions with soliciting ideal treatment outcomes and negotiating solvable short-term goals with their new clients in first sessions, I would ask her the following questions:

- "If I were a fly on your office wall watching you achieve your skill-development goal, what steps will I be seeing you consistently take to make this happen with your clients?"
- "What else will you be doing that will tell you that you are making good progress with using the miracle and scaling questions?"
- "How will you know that you have really succeeded at achieving your goal?"

An instrument that I use with trainees and supervisees to gain a quantitative measurement of their progress over time in their selected skill-development target goal areas and other things they are doing that works in couple and family therapy sessions, is the *therapeutic brilliance scale.*

Using the Therapeutic Brilliance Scale

The therapeutic brilliance scale is a highly positive and empowering tool that therapists can use for identifying specific skills they wish to develop or further hone with their couple and family clients, secure a quantitative measurement of their progress in their skill-development goal area, and keep track of what works, that is their sparkling moments and what they would call their therapeutic brilliance in a given session (see Figure 8.2). The therapeutic brilliance scale ranges from a 10 being the best session of my career to a 1 being the worst session of my career. Therapists are to use the therapeutic brilliance scale as a rating for assessing their progress weekly in their identified skill-development target goal areas until they have achieved them with their couple and family clients. For example, a supervisee rated themselves at a 7, which stands for it was a good session in terms of using more humor and being playful with the clients (skill-development target goal area). I would than ask the supervisee the following questions:

- "What are you going to do in your next session with the Smith couple that will move you one step upward to an 8 on the scale?"
- "What else will you do to help you to get up to that 8?"

What is great about the therapeutic brilliance scale is that we and our trainees and supervisees know where we stand in terms of progress in their skill-development target areas, as well as other things that they are doing that is making a positive difference in sessions with their clients. Once we discover what works, we want them to continue doing more of what is works.

Using Reflection-in-Action and Reflection-on-Action

As far as the use of self goes, learning how to step outside of oneself in the midst of the therapeutic process, gain a double-vision of ourselves in relationship to a couple partner or family member, can help us to determine how well we are connecting with him or her and what impact our questions or in-session therapeutic strategies are having on the client. This therapeutic operation is known as *reflection-in-action* and can aid us in being more therapeutically flexible and help us become more aware of when to shift gears in the therapeutic process in order to find better fit with trying out specific techniques and strategies with our clients and meeting their unique needs (Schon, 1983). *Reflection-on-action* consists of critically reflecting on what we did in a given couple or family session and asking oneself, "If I had the opportunity to do

THE *THERAPEUTIC BRILLIANCE SCALE*

10 = Best session of my career

9 = Outstanding session

8 = Excellent session

7 = It was a very good session

6 = It was a good session

5 = It was an average session

4 = It was a sub-par session

3 = It was a bad session

2 = It was a terrible session

1 = It was the worst session of my career

Instructions: Keep track of in this week's couple/family session with the _____ what specifically you did to make further progress in your target skill development goal areas and your brilliant therapeutic moves in sessions that appeared to have a positive impact with your clients. At the end of each couple/family session, rate using the scale above how well you fared in your session, including writing down below what you did that were examples of your therapeutic brilliance and sparkling moments in your sessions.

Session Rating: _____

Session #: _____

Therapeutic Brilliance and Skill Development Sparkling Moments:

_____

_____

_____

Figure 8.2 The Therapeutic Brilliance Scale

this session all over again, what would I have done differently?" In response to this question, I have trainees and supervisees create a checklist of adjustments they need to make to strengthen their alliances with one of the couple partners or with a disengaged father, specific questions that might be worthwhile asking and techniques or strategies worth trying. Reflection-on-action helps us to stay therapeutically flexible, be curious about what has not been talked about, and keep an open mind with our hunches and formulations about our clients' problem situations (Schon, 1983).

Soliciting Feedback from Couples and Families: Using the Session Rating Scale and Outcome Rating Scale

There is a growing body of research that indicates that therapists who session-by-session solicit feedback from their clients on the quality of their therapeutic relationships with them and their perceptions of the change process in major areas of their lives not only can prevent premature client dropouts and treatment failure from occurring but can help optimize for treatment success (Duncan, 2019; Maeschalck & Barfnecht, 2017; Schucklard, Miller, & Hubble, 2017; Swift & Greenberg, 2015; Lambert, 2010; Duncan & Miller, 2000). There is no better way to secure this information for strengthening our therapeutic alliances with couples and families and optimizing for their treatment success than administering at the end of each session the *session rating scale* (SRS) and the *outcome rating scale* (ORS) (Duncan, 2019; Miller, Mee-Lee, Plum, & Hubble, 2005). With the SRS, couple partners or family members are to rate by drawing an X on a horizontal scale where they would rate the following regarding four major areas: the relationship (from not feeling heard, understood, and respected to totally feeling heard, understood and respected); goals and topics (we did not work on or talk about what I wanted to work on and talk about to adequately addressing this); approach or method (from the therapist's approach is not a good fit for me to it is a good fit for me); overall (there was something missing in the session today to overall today's session was right for me). Once the clients complete the scale, the therapist can solicit feedback from them about what adjustments they need to make to strengthen his or her alliances with them and better tailor fit his or her approach or methods that they would find more useful to them.

Using a similar horizontal scale, the ORS has couple partners and family members place an X on the scale where they would rate the change process in the following four major areas: individually (an increase or a decrease in personal sense of well-being); interpersonally (improvements or no change in intimate couple and family relationships); socially (improvements in friendship, school, or work relationships; overall (from no general sense of well-being to total improvement in this area). Similar to the SRS, the therapist and couple partners or family members need to discuss what specific adjustments he or she could make to help them to make further progress in the four major areas and explore if there are any constraints that may need to be removed that are keeping the change process at a standstill. Together, the therapist can collaborate with the clients in identifying the constraints and problem-solve on how best to remove or work around them. Both the SRS and ORS are easy to use and even beginning couple and family therapists will appreciate knowing from their clients that they have strong alliances with them and they are satisfied with the changes occurring in all areas of their lives. If therapeutic alliances are deemed weak by one or both couple partners or with certain family members, and/or changes are not occurring in major areas of the clients' lives, the therapist needs to inquire with them what specific adjustments he or she has to make to better deliver therapeutically what they need and expect from him or her. For readers interested in securing copies of the latest versions of the SRS and ORS scales, go to: https://betteroutcomesnow.com.

Covering the Back Door: Goal-Maintenance and Regularly Consolidating Couple and Family Gains

Another important executive skill area beginning couple and family therapist must master is what I call *covering the back door*. Once their clients start making good headway towards achieving their goals and helping their clients make important relationship changes, trainees and supervisees must prepare them for the inevitability of unexpected slips occurring, normalize them, and offer them goal-maintenance strategies to stay on track and consolidate their gains. We can have them do *worst-case scenario planning*, which consists of having the couple or family identify four possible triggering worst case scenarios that could occur, the steps the identified client will take to not cave into having a slip, what his or her partners or parents will take to support them, and the steps concerned and involved key resource people from their social network will take to help them to feign off the slip. Some great goal-maintenance and consolidating questions to ask are as follows:

- "What would you have to do to go backward at this point?"
- "Let's say you have a slip, what steps will you take to quickly get back on track?"
- "Slips are like sages and valuable teachers for us. So, what did you learn from that slip yesterday that you will put to immediate use the next time you are faced with a similar stressful situation?"
- "(With a crisis-prone family) What will be the next crisis?"
- "Where and what time of the day do you think it will happen?"
- "Who will be involved with the crisis?"
- "Now that we got all of the details about the next crisis, what steps will each of you immediately take to quickly stabilize the situation?"
- "If I were to work with another couple just like you, what advice would you have for them for how best to stay on track?"
- "Let's say we had a one-year anniversary party in my office, what further changes will each of you be eager to share with me that you made happen that I will be the most surprised to hear about?"

Not only can these questions help consolidate clients' gains and prevent client relapses from occurring, but they increase their awareness levels about the steps they need to take if slips should occur.

Collaborating with Referring Persons, Other Involved Helping Professionals, and Key Resource People from Clients' Social Networks

Since the referring person, other involved helping professionals from larger systems, and involved key resource people from clients' social networks are all both part of the problem and solution-developing, solution construction system, it is critical that beginning couple and family therapists learn how to build cooperative partnerships with them (Selekman, 2023, 2017, 1995). I like to share with them that the referring person, involved helping professionals, and the key resource people from their social networks can become important allies that possess a wealth of strengths, are resourceful, creative, and can help advocate for their clients in larger systems that they are experiencing difficulties dealing with. I also stress to new couple and family therapists that we need to treat the helping professionals with the same level of respect that we do with our clients, that is listening generously and deeply to what their co-collaborators have to say. When facilitating collaborative meetings with the referring person and other involved helping professionals, they need to ask questions from a position of not-knowing and respectful curiosity to learn from their co-collaborators their stories of involvement with their clients, what their concerns and problem explanations are, and how they will know that the clients' difficulties have been successfully stabilized. After the beginning couple and family therapist has heard from all of the meeting participants, he or she can share his formulations about the client's problem situation in a tentative way. The therapist needs to avoid at all costs trying to parade his or her problem views and proposed change strategies as if he or she has some hold on the truth for what is best for their clients. Instead, he should adopt a both/and perspective and use multi-partiality, which is siding simultaneously with everyone's different perspectives on the client's problems situations and proposed solutions (Anderson & Gehart, 2007; Anderson, 1997; Goolishian & Anderson, 1988). They should look for ways to cross-fertilize and connect proposed ideas and solution strategies. Finally, whenever possible I encourage beginning couple and family therapists to have their clients be part of these collaborative meetings so that they convey to the involved helping professionals and their key resource people from their social networks what their unique needs and best hopes are and how they can help them in the best way possible.

Receptive to Live Supervision, Videotaping, and Being Observed by a Consultation Team

There is no better way to train or supervise couple and family therapists than doing a combination of live supervision, videotaping sessions, and allowing oneself to be observed and receive feedback from an observing consultation team of colleagues. I remember back in 1984 when I was in that grey area of being between a beginning and intermediate-level couple and family therapist and had to do my first live supervision family therapy session in front of my wonderful supervisor John Schwartzman and six of my fellow trainees who were behind a one-way mirror. We were part of a one-year family therapy training program in working with families with alcohol and substance abuse problems at the Family Institute of Chicago, which helped me to make my own systemic relational leap in treating clients with alcohol and substance-abusing difficulties in a more efficient and effective way. I was quite anxious about exposing myself in front of others. I even began to have catastrophic thoughts like: "What if they think I am a lousy family therapist?" "What will I do if the session completely spirals out of control?" The family I was working with that I had brought for the consultation was extremely challenging in that there were multiple symptom-bearers: the father had a drinking problem, the parents fought all of the time and never could agree on how best to manage their marijuana-abusing psychotic 18-year-old son, and the mother and son were in a cross-generational coalition where she would protect him from her angry and frustrated husband. The first phone-in call I had received from Schwartzman had me ask the son who was sitting right next to his mother and would distract her whenever the father started talking was to have the son go sit out in the lobby. Every time I attempted in the session to get the parents while meeting alone with them to work together around expectations for their son like trying to get a low-stress job (a bagger at the local grocery store), stop smoking marijuana, taking his medication regularly, the conversation would digress into an intense blame-counter-blame exchange. The second call I had received from my supervisor was to break up the destructive interaction between the parents and see each parent separately to make the situation more manageable, help strengthen my alliances with both parents, and try and establish separate goals and work projects with each parent. Believe me, there were many times in this session where I had wished Scottie the engineer from the popular TV show *Star Trek* had beamed me up to the *Starship Enterprise*. At our inter-session break, my supervisor and team of colleagues were enormously supportive and complimented me on my perseverance and resilience to hang in there with this challenging therapy-veteran family. I was the eighth therapist they had been to. After the team break, I went back in there with the family more confident and able to establish some realistic goals and offer them some small doable change strategies that the parents agreed to implement. Once I broke the ice and drummed up the courage to perform live in front of my supervisor and a consultation team, I became a big believer in this training method and found it be enormously helpful in my professional growth and skill development as a couple and family therapist.

While in this training program, I found videotaping sessions and reviewing them with my supervisor and team to be highly beneficial for learning about my blindspots, what I was doing that was unproductive, seeing opportunities I had missed seizing, and what I was doing well at using particular techniques and strategies in my supervision meetings. I also learned about how we can use videotapes with couples and families as a teaching tool in sessions, helping them see how they get stuck with one another and what they are doing that helps them to get along better and should increase doing.

Serving as a Consultation Team Member

As great ways to learn about how to collaborate with colleagues, the power in collective intelligence, and how other therapists think and work clinically, it is helpful for beginning couple and family therapists to participate as a team member and offer their thoughts regarding a couple or family's problem situation and what might be useful for the consulting therapist to try with them. I like to expose beginning couple and family therapists to two different team strategies: the solution-focused brief therapy team approach (de Shazer et al., 2007; Miller, 1997) and the reflecting team approach (Andersen, 1995, 1991; Lax, 1995). When serving as a solution-focused team member, the therapist needs to carefully listen for examples of couple partners' and family members' resourcefulness, resilience, great teamwork, and creative self-generated coping and problem-solving strategies that they are to be complimented on. Negative behaviors are relabeled into positive qualities or behaviors, such as: angry parents are relabeled as concerned and committed parents, a quiet or withdrawn adolescent is relabeled as a respectful listener, a so-called "ADD" child is relabeled as being energetic or as being *active, determined,* and *dynamic.* Together, the team will construct a message for the couple or family composed of compliments for each partner or family member, limited use of positively relabeled negative behaviors, and one-two therapeutic experiments for the clients to try over the next week that are in line with their goals. For beginning couple and family therapists, the key takeaways from serving on a solution-focused team is looking and listening for clients' strengths and resources, important anomalies or exceptions, and the positive intent behind negative behaviors.

When serving as a reflecting team member, the beginning couple and family therapist will rely more on his or her curiosity and wonder about what is not being talked about or the constraints that are contributing to the consulting therapist and couple or family being stuck. Team members are to begin their reflections with qualifiers like:

- "I wonder if ..."
- "Could it be ..."
- "I was struck by ..."

Reflections need to be shared with a suspension of disbelief and as tentative thoughts, not definitive explanations for the client's difficulties. Since change cannot occur under a negative connotation, the reflections should use either positive or logical connotation (Lax, 1995; Andersen, 1991; Boscolo, Cecchin, Hoffman, & Penn, 1987).

Reflections also need to fall somewhere between being too similar to and too unusual than how the clients already view their problem situation. The team deliberates in front of the clients exchanging their thoughts with one another for 7-8 minutes. The clients will be asked by the consulting therapist to reflect on the team's reflections in terms of what ideas resonated with them or offered them a new way of looking at their situation. With the reflecting team method, there is no end of session therapeutic experiments offered to the clients, instead they are asked to continue to reflect on and talk about over the next week the specific ideas that were offered by the team that they found useful. The key takeaways for beginning couple and family therapists serving on a reflecting team are: there are many ways to view a couple or family's problem situation and that change can happen when clients' viewing of their situations change, which can lead to new meanings and interactions.

Intermediate-Level Couple and Family Therapists

During the intermediate stage of use of self-skill development, couple and family therapists are continuing to work on honing their major conceptual, perceptual, and executive skills. In the conceptual skill area, they are working on getting better at logically integrating therapeutic tools and strategies from different couple and family therapy approaches and finding their unique voices as the next generation of couple and family therapists. On the perceptual skill level, they are getting better at doing the following: more accurately assessing at what stages of readiness for change couple partners and family members are in and matching what they do with their unique stages; identifying key client exception patterns worth seizing; identifying problem-maintaining patterns and beliefs and other couple and family dynamics that are contributing to the maintenance to the clients' difficulties; and at observing themselves vis-à-vis the clients and the role that they may be playing with their thinking and therapeutic actions in inadvertently contributing to the maintenance of their clients' difficulties. As far as their executive skill-development goes, they are working on further honing the following: alliance-building and finding the relationship-of-fit; their interviewing skills; being more daring and taking more risks in sessions with the use of humor, playfulness, curiosity, and taking charge in sessions when necessary; using reflection-in-action and reflection-on-action, soliciting feedback from clients using the SRS and ORS, and making the necessary adjustments; using the therapeutic brilliance scale; developing more confidence with videotaping their sessions, having live supervision, and serving as a team member; doing goal-maintenance work and consolidating clients' gains once they make progress; and strengthening their collaboration skills with involved helping professionals from larger systems. Finally, they need to continue working on their personal signature theme work, their three-generational family genogram, and come to terms with and eliminating their racist biases and prejudicial ideologies and stereotypical views and homophobic reactions to LGBTQ individuals. Below, I present important use of self-developmental tasks intermediate-level couple and family therapists need to work on mastering.

Intermediate-Level Couple and Family Therapist Developmental Tasks

Below, I present seven important use of self-developmental tasks intermediate-level couple and family therapists need to work on mastering. For each of the developmental tasks, I explain how they can strengthen their conceptual, perceptual, and executive skills.

Learn to View Your Mistakes and Failures as Great Opportunities
for Gaining Wisdom and Professional Growth

Throughout our professional careers, we are all bound to make mistakes, have clients' dropout on us, and experience treatment failures, which has been the case for even the master couple and family therapists. I will never forget, back in 1986 in the context of a four-day live supervision training in strategic family therapy with Jay Haley and Chloe Madanes, I had made what I had thought was a big mistake. I had brought in a frustrated single-parent mother and her poly-substance abusing son Roger (Haley & Madanes, 1986). She was constantly getting into power struggles with Roger about cutting his long hair, doing his school homework, stopping his drug use, and getting a job. Haley observed that it was counter-productive to allow the mother to continue with her litany of complaints about Roger and that she needed to lighten up and called me on the phone from behind a one-way mirror and first complimented me on how well I had connected with Roger and then gave me the following directive, "Have Roger share with his mother a joke or something funny that will help her to lighten up." Instead, I shared a funny and true story from my adolescence. I first shared with them that Roger was lucky because when he grows his hair long it grows down and when I grow my kinky curly hair long it grows up! They both laughed. I went on to share that my friends placed bets with me that if I would keep growing my hair longer over the next month that eventually it would flop over. Not only did my hair not flop over but it grew into a big afro and I won $50 from my friends! Again, Roger and his mother laughed. At the inter-session break, Haley and the eight other participants were smiling and laughing. Haley used this as a teachable moment and pointed out that mistakes can yield great results, they can offer the clients and us something novel to work with, and he further shared how clients are forgiving once we have a relationship with them. After the inter-session break, I decided to meet alone with Roger and make purposeful use of self-disclosure again since it produced great results before the break. I shared with Roger that once I cut my afro down to a lower and more respectable level, put on more dressy clothes, I had landed my first job. Roger made a commitment to cut his hair, dress differently, and look for jobs over the next week. In my next session, the mother and Roger had come in smiling. Roger not only had cut his hair but he had landed his first job!

Another beautiful example of how mistakes can serve as great opportunities to do something novel that I like to share with intermediate-level couple and family therapists occurred with the great jazz pianist Herbie Hancock. Hancock had been recruited by Miles Davis to join his quintet on a European tour. At the time,

Hancock was just a teenager and was thrilled by being given this wonderful career-boosting opportunity with the great Miles Davis. While performing in Stockholm, Sweden, Hancock had played the wrong note on one of Davis's well-known tunes and this triggered intense anxiety and catastrophic thoughts inside of him. Davis being one of jazz's grandmasters of improvisation, took Hancock's wrong note and turned it into something special and his other bandmates did creative things with it as well. When the song was over, they received a standing ovation from the audience (Hancock & Dickey, 2014).

With client dropout situations and failures, it can be quite helpful to look at videotapes of sessions that led up to these situations occurring and do a deep dive and analyze what the contributing factors might have been such as: relationship ruptures that were not repaired or the therapist waited too long to begin the repair work; unresolved and unidentified constraints that were blocking the change process from occurring; there was a mismatch in terms of the treatment approach being used and the stages of readiness for change couple partners or the family members were in; the therapist therapeutically was replicating what previous therapists had tried that had not worked; and the true customer for change in the client system was not identified or invited to participate in the treatment process. Research indicates that if change does not occur by the third session this has a demoralizing effect on the client and often leads to premature dropout occurring (Swift & Greenberg, 2015; Duncan, 2010). In Chapter 3, I discussed the salient analogies cognitive bias, which is how just because a current family looks very similar in their presentation to other families you had successfully treated in the past, does not mean that the same treatment regimen or approach will be equally effective with every similar family. When we fall prey to this bias and one-size-fits-all logic, this may be some of the reasons why couple partners or family members prematurely dropout or worse yet, leads to treatment failure. In response to these dire treatment outcomes, we can do a deep dive and look at the similarities and differences between all the past similar couples and families and the one we just failed with to learn about what we could have done differently with them if we had another shot at working with them again (Kahneman, Lovallo, & Sibony, 2015; Kahneman, 2011; Schon, 1983).

Integrative Thinking and Cultivating a Synthesizing Mind

Becoming skilled with using integrative thinking and cultivating a synthesizing mind are therapist skills that take time to cultivate and need to be worked on well into the master level of their professional development (Martin, 2007; Gardner, 2008). With integrative thinking, therapists learn how to hold in their mind three or more different perspectives on a couple or family problem situation and how to resolve it without locking down on any one perspective or solution. Intermediate-level couple or family therapists learn how to play with these different ideas in their minds and see how they can be connected in such a way that high-quality solutions can be co-constructed in the contexts of group supervision with their supervisor or trainer and/or colleagues while serving on a consultation team with them. I strongly encourage intermediate-level couple and family therapists to serve as much as possible on a consultation team or be teamed by their colleagues, which is an ideal setting to play with different ideas, learn about alternative ways of viewing clients' difficulties, and look for ways to connect them.

Having a synthesizing mind, consists of developing the skill of preparing before a couple or family session what questions might be worthwhile asking or therapeutic tools and strategies from specific approaches that may be useful to try in the next session based on your prior sessions with them. Synthesizing also includes making use of new and important information that you learned about the client's situation or some new therapeutic strategies that you learned about in supervision or heard about at a workshop that is supposed to be effective with the specific presenting problem your client is struggling with and adding it to your therapeutic armamentarium. Finally, being able to know what therapeutic approaches can be logically integrated, or when to work in a more-pure way with a particular therapeutic approach, comes from using your synthesizing mind and with more practice experience (Gardner, 2008).

Learning how to Tailor-Fit Your Couple or Family Therapy to Best Meet the Needs of Your Clients

An important executive skill that intermediate-level couple and family therapists need to cultivate is how to tailor-fit their couple or family therapy approach to the unique needs, stages of readiness for change each couple partner and family member is in, their theories of change, the nature of their presenting problems, their key couple or family dynamics that serve as the problem-life-support-system, and their treatment goals (Selekman, 2017). By using a flexible and integrative couple or family therapy approach and matching what we do therapeutically with what couples and families need and expect from us we can optimize for their treatment success. To further enhance our integrative couple or family approach, with some couples and families we may want to incorporate empirically supported therapeutic tools and strategies from mindfulness-based approaches, dialectical behavior therapy, or cognitive-behavioral therapy (Marlatt, Bowen, Chawla, & Witkiewitz, 2008; Miller, Rathus, & Linehan, 2007; Rathus & Miller, 2015; Beck, 2011; Kendall, 2011). Similar to getting more skilled at using integrative thinking, we get better at tailor-fitting our couple and family therapy approaches by participating on a consultation team and hearing what therapeutic tools and strategies one's colleagues thinks might be of great benefit to our clients based on their success with having treated similar couples and families in the past. However, as mentioned earlier, we need to be mindful of the fact that every couple and family is unique and make sure that the clients are similar enough that the proposed therapeutic tools and strategies have a good shot at working. If the therapist continues to be concerned about whether the proposed tools or strategies have a good shot at working, he or she can return to the clients after the inter-session break and ask them, "I just learned about some therapeutic tools and strategies that my colleagues have recommended to me that I should propose to you to experiment with, would you like to hear what they are?" Ultimately, the clients should decide what's best for them and they could choose whether or not to try out the team's proposed tools and strategies. Getting more skilled with the tailor-fitting process comes with experience and this use of self-mastery skill-development task should continue well into one becomes an advanced-level couple and family therapist.

Cultivating the Abilities to Sit with Client Silence and Practice Actionless-Action

Beginning and intermediate couple and family therapists are not alone with being able to sit with client silence in sessions, even advanced-level therapists struggle with this at times. It feels uncomfortable not knowing what is going on with the silent couple partner or family member(s). They may start to go inward and question their abilities to successfully engage the couple partner or family member(s) or their competence as a couple or family therapist. From a position of respectful curiosity, they can check in with them to explore is there something they said or did that might have contributed to a relationship rupture or if they have some concerns about their approach or the change process moving too slowly. The use of the SRS and ORS can be helpful with gathering more information about the quality of the therapeutic relationship and the change process and lack of improvement in key areas of their lives that we can attempt to remedy (Duncan, 2019; Maeschalck & Barfnecht, 2017; Schucklard, Miller, & Hubble, 2017).

Silence can also be used by couple partners or family members as a power play tactic to frustrate or stonewall their partners or other family members, particularly if they are mired in conflict or want to keep the situation at status quo (Gottman & Silver, 2015). I recently had a couple in my office where the husband was stonewalling his wife with silence because of longstanding anger and unresolved conflicts with her regarding his belief that she was still communicating with a past boyfriend of hers with absolutely no proof that this was occurring. The wife was working really hard to keep the focus on improving their relationship in the here-and-now. To try and prevent this from happening, he sat quietly wedged on the opposite end of the couch maintaining his silence and protest. To break up this unproductive interaction, I used *unbalancing* and temporarily sided with his wife (Minuchin & Fishman, 1981). Not only did he get defensive but for the first time he opened up with his wife and I about the specifics of what was fueling his anger with her and his strong desire to resolve this longstanding conflict with her. Together, they worked hard both at home and in future sessions to resolve the conflict and move forward in a better direction as a couple.

Actionless-action or *wu wei* is a skill that we need to cultivate throughout our professional careers (Tzu & Watson, 1968). At times, we need to talk less or remain quiet and have our clients practice new ways of communicating and work through conflicts directly together in sessions. As intermediate-level couple and family therapists gain more practice years of experience, they will get better at knowing intuitively and in what clinical situations in sessions it would be best to remain silent.

Start a Daily Mindfulness Practice

Intermediate-level couple and family therapists can greatly increase their therapeutic presence and their awareness levels with their clients by adopting a daily mindfulness practice. By learning how to sit with strong negative thoughts and feelings that are triggered in their interactions with their clients or in response to what they observe or hear in sessions without flinching, they can be truly present with them, not be distracted, and seize ripe opportunities that may spontaneously present themselves. With the help of mindfulness meditation, therapists will see and hear things in sessions that non-meditators will miss because their awareness levels have been greatly heightened. All intermediate-level couple and family therapists need to do is either sitting daily in silence for 15-20 minutes somewhere quiet or going for a 30–40-minute mindful walk on a forest preserve park path paying close attention to all that they see, hear, and smell, as their daily mindfulness practices and over time, will discover its healthful benefits in mood and spirit, concentration, self-awareness, and feeling more relaxed and centered (Fredrickson, 2009). Finally, maintaining a daily mindfulness practice also will enhance their ability to tolerate client silence and uncertainty in sessions and get better with using actionless-action.

Find Mentors Skilled in a Particular Couple or Family Therapy
Approach or Specialization Area they are Interested in

To help expand their therapeutic range, go more in-depth with a particular couple or family therapy approach, or when wanting to learn more about creative ways to work systemically with challenging couple or family problems like addictions, eating disorders, self-injury, trauma, high-conflict couples, aggressive and violent behaviors, and so forth, intermediate-level couple or family therapists should seek out one or two mentors based on what their unique training needs are. At this point, I would like to share briefly three of the most positive experiences I had had as an intermediate-level couple and family therapist with mentors that had greatly contributed to my skill development and whose practice wisdom had a profound impact on me to this very day. Because I was interested in systemic family therapy approaches to alcohol and substance abuse problems, I had sought out Thomas Todd as my first mentor. Todd, along with M. Duncan Stanton had served as supervisors and researchers in the first family therapy treatment outcome study with adult heroin addicts and their families while at the Philadelphia Child Guidance Center with Salvador Minuchin and Jay Haley in the seventies (Stanton & Todd, 1982). Together, they had developed the structural-strategic family therapy model that was used in the study. Although Todd was well-versed in this therapeutic approach, his earlier strategic family therapy training with Jay Haley was more his strong suit and I had learned many major strategic therapeutic tools and strategies while training and receiving supervision with him. He encouraged me to be more playful, use more humor, how and when to use indirect strategic change strategies, and to give myself permission to take more risks in sessions with couples and families presenting with alcohol and substance-abuse difficulties. Over time we became friends and colleagues, presenting and writing together, and co-edited the book *Family Therapy Approaches with Adolescent Substance Abusers* in 1991, which showcases eleven different family therapy approaches and important family treatment outcome research findings for working with this challenging treatment population (Todd & Selekman, 1991b).

My second mentor, Michele Weiner-Davis, was the director of training and research at our youth service agency. Weiner-Davis had provided me with a year of videotape and live supervision in solution-focused brief therapy. The added bonus of serving as the program director of our substance abuse program was that Weiner-Davis, our clinical director, and I got to go up to the Brief Family Therapy Center in Milwaukee, Wisconsin and receive supervision-of-supervision with Eve Lipchik, who along with Steve de Shazer and Insoo Kim Berg were co-developers of solution-focused brief therapy interviewing questions. Weiner-Davis taught me about the short road to change by seizing client self-generated pretreatment changes and utilizing to the maximum degree clients' strengths and resources and past successes to co-construct solutions. She helped me discover the elegance of simplicity and how clients are the true experts on their stories and know what is best for them. Her great supervision and practice wisdom helped me to become a competent strengths-based clinician and optimize for my clients' treatment success.

The third mentor I had was Harry Goolishian who I had participated in a short-term intensive training experience in collaborative language systems therapy with him, along with his wonderful colleague Harlene Anderson. They taught us about the importance of honoring clients' stories and avoiding at all costs being narrative editors. Goolishian had tremendous warmth and charisma and embraced all of the training participants, no matter what our theoretical persuasions were, as if we were part of his family. All the clients that came in for daily consultations felt the same way about Goolishian. Unlike many well-known pioneers in the family therapy field, Goolishian offered to correspond with me via letters for almost a whole year regarding the challenging family I had brought in for a consultation with him that had three generations of schizophrenia, suicides, and an extensive trauma history. His expert guidance and great support helped me to successfully stabilize the son's schizophrenic symptoms and help him to function well enough to secure a job. I also learned from him and Anderson how to collaborate with involved helping professionals from larger systems in a respectful and effective way.

At some point in the mentoring relationship process, therapists often want to take the practice wisdom and skills they learned from their mentors and build off it to develop their own versions of the models they learned or new techniques and strategies for working with specific treatment populations that had been inspired by the teachings of their mentors. Finally, as intermediate-level couple and family therapists accrue more practice experience and become more self-confident and wiser, they will start to see that their mentors and the treatment approaches they espouse have their limitations, which can be a powerful incentive for them to look for creative ways to fill the gaps in their mentors' choice models and expand the possibilities with their approaches by integrating techniques and strategies from other models as they move forward in their professional careers.

Establishing Cooperative Partnerships with Highly Pessimistic and Pathologizing-Minded Involved Helping Professionals

One of the biggest challenges for beginning and intermediate-level couple and family therapists is attempting to collaborate with highly pessimistic and pathologizing-minded involved helping professionals. Three collaborative tools and strategies that can be helpful in establishing cooperative partnerships with them are as follows: *suspension, persuadability and reversing your position,* and *"yes … and"* (Bohm, 1996; Selekman, 2017, 2010; Pittampalli, 2016). For intermediate-level couple and family therapists, being in collaborative meetings with highly pessimistic and pathologizing-minded helping professionals is often challenging for them to refrain from trying to defend their clients or wanting to try and convince them that they are wrong and their clients not only want to change and are doing so. If they get lead-footed and react this way to these helpers, they and the other meeting participants may get defensive or worse yet, decide that it is not safe to contribute one's opinions and choose to not attend future meetings. Therefore, intermediate-level couple and family therapists can use the collaborative tool of suspension to better manage their emotional reactions and unproductive ways of thinking about the highly pessimistic and pathologizing-minded helpers. Suspension consists of taking a pause, and imagine like a cartoon character having a cloud over his or her head that he or she will fill with all of his or her negative emotions and thoughts (Bohm, 1996). Next, the therapist needs to craft questions from a position of respectful curiosity to pose to the helpers they are having a negative reaction with, such as the following questions:

- "Can you help me understand how you came to the conclusion that Marjorie is a borderline personality disorder?"
- "Have you worked with similar clients before?"
- "As far as I can tell, she has not self-injured for two weeks, which was confirmed by her and her parents. Do you think there may be a cover-up here between Marjorie and her parents and that it still may be happening behind the scenes?"
- "If you have been faced with this situation before, what did you do to get at the truth?"

By turning one's negative thoughts and feelings toward a particular helping professional into the above questions, highly pessimistic and pathology-minded helpers will feel validated and respected by the therapist and want to help him or her out with his or her clients.

Just like we expect and hope helping professionals we collaborate with will be open to adopting new and more positive views of our clients, we too have to be willing to opening up our minds to the helping professionals varied problem views and proposed solutions for our clients' difficulties. We need to demonstrate to highly pessimistic and pathology-minded helping professionals that we can be persuaded and reverse our original positions on the client's situation and entertain their perspectives (Pittampalli, 2016). Finally, intermediate-level couple and family therapists need to move away from "yes ... but" or "I'm right, you're wrong" ways of thinking about highly pessimistic and pathology-minded helping professionals' views, and instead, adopt the mind-sets of both/and or "yes ... and." They need to remind themselves that we and the helpers are in this together and need to look for useful ways to make sense of the client's problem situation and cross-fertilize their ideas to co-construct solutions.

Advanced-Level Couple and Family Therapists

Advanced-level and couple and family therapists have become solid and well-rounded with their conceptual, perceptual, and executive skills. They now possess a high level of confidence and courage to take risks in sessions being more daring, provocative, playful, using humor and absurdity, storytelling, and have cultivated an intuitive sense for knowing what question or therapeutic strategy might have a great shot at working in a given moment in a session. They also have great timing for when to take charge in sessions, knowing when to work with the couple partners and family subsystems separately, and trying certain therapeutic techniques and strategies. Advanced-level couple and family therapists have no problem working outside of their comfort zones, have growth-oriented mindsets, and have a strong thirst for learning (Dweck, 2006). They are now ready to use themselves as the catalysts for change on higher and newer levels, such as: working with new treatment populations and different types of couple and family presenting problems, serving as trainers and supervisors, presenting workshops, and publishing their clinical work.

Advanced-Level Couple and Family Therapist Developmental Tasks

Below, I present eight use of self-developmental tasks that advanced-level couple and family therapists need to work on mastering. For each of the developmental tasks, I explain how they can further strengthen their conceptual, perceptual, and executive skills.

Allowing Your Choice Couple and Family Therapy Approach to Evolve

Although advanced-level couple and family therapists have cultivated strong conceptual, perceptual, and executive skills using a particular couple or family therapy approach, they need to allow their choice approach to evolve and look for creative ways to strengthen it. This could include adding therapeutic tools and strategies from empirically supported or clinically promising individual and other couple and family therapy approaches. For example, with my collaborative strengths-based family therapy approach I found it quite beneficial to add mindfulness meditation practices, art, experiential, and expressive writing tools and strategies to my base model to have a broader therapeutic armamentarium, which led to better treatment outcomes with my clients (Selekman, 2017, 2009). Another major advantage of allowing one's choice model to evolve is that gives us both multiple lens for viewing couple and family difficulties and many more therapeutic tools and strategies to intervene with. If we become too wedded to our choice couple and family therapy approaches and fail to be therapeutically flexible and allow them to evolve, we can easily fall prey to one-size-fits-all thinking, which can lead to a mismatch with our treatment approaches and couples' and families' unique needs and theories of change.

Prospect for Ideas from Outside of the Couple and Family Therapy Field to Expand Your Therapeutic Range

In Chapter 7, I presented several ways we can prospect for novel ideas outside of our field. From fields as diverse as art to nature, there is a goldmine of metaphors and creative ideas we can tap for crafting bold and intriguing questions, co-designing with our clients' therapeutic experiments that taps there inventiveness, and inspiring stories and great quotes from well-known and famous figures representing these different fields to share with our clients that can provide new ways of viewing their presenting difficulties, help disrupt problem-maintaining patterns, and improve their relationships. By prospecting from and using creative ideas from these different fields, we can expand the possibilities with our choice couple and family therapy approaches and can increase our therapeutic range and ways to use ourselves' in the therapeutic process.

Challenge Yourself and Work with Treatment Populations and Presenting Problems You Have Limited to No Experience with

To further grow professionally as advanced-level couple and family therapists, they need to devote some weekly time stepping out of their comfort zones and begin working with client treatment populations and types of couples' and family presenting problems they have limited to no experience working with. This is a great opportunity to operate from a position of not-knowing, using respectful curiosity, and honing their listening skills to become better educated about the nature of the clients' presenting problems, what has not worked with former therapists, their unique cultural values, customs, and practices, and how best to help them in the most meaningful way. This also encourages advanced-level couple and family therapists to challenge themselves, grow their mental storehouse of patterns, and expand their therapeutic range and knowledge bases.

Beware of the Risks of Being Too Overconfident and the Therapeutic Shortcomings of Becoming a Specialist

Although advanced-level couple and family therapists have gained thousands of hours of practice experience, have begun to cultivate a good intuitive sense, a high level of competence with their conceptual, perceptual, and executive skills, they still need to be careful with allowing their over-confidence and expertise and good reputation for being a specialist with a particular type of client problem or treatment population to get in the way of carefully tailoring their couple or family therapy approach to the unique needs, theories of change, and goals of the clients. As mentioned earlier about salient analogies cognitive bias, we have to be mindful of the fact that every couple and family we treat is unique and just because we have met with success quite a bit in the past with particular treatment populations and specific types of client problems, does not mean that the same approach or set of therapeutic tools and strategies will work with every similar couple and family.

Expand Your Horizons: Attend Workshops on New Marital, Family, and Individual Therapy Approaches and on Subjects Outside of Our Field

As part of one's professional growth and as a way to expand the possibilities with their choice couple and family therapy approaches, it is important to open up their minds to learning about new couple, family, and individual therapy approaches that are either empirically supported or are showing great clinical promise with particular treatment populations and types of problems that might be worthwhile integrating into their choice approaches. Additionally, there are lots of great and creative ideas in other fields like business, science and technology, and art that can be integrated into their couple and family therapy approaches that they can learn about in the contexts of workshops and conferences.

Serve as a Trainer and/or Supervisor

As advanced-level couple and family therapists, a great way to give back their knowledge and skills is to train and/or supervise beginning and intermediate-level couple and family therapists. It can be quite rewarding to empower them to become increasingly more skilled with developing their conceptual, perceptual, and executive skills and be a part of their professional growth. They can use self-disclosure to normalize their trainees' and supervisees' struggles with mastering certain skills, share their early mistakes and failures as couple and family therapists, show videotapes of themselves bungling as a beginning or intermediate-level therapist with couples and families, as an opportunity to discuss in the contexts of training or supervision groups what they could have done differently. It also is helpful to have their beginning and intermediate-level trainees and supervisees serve as a consultation team observing them struggle with a difficult couple or family case and offer input both during the inter-session break and after the session in terms of future directions to pursue with this couple or family.

Get Published

Advanced-level couple and family therapists can make their unique voices known through publishing journal articles or even a book. It is a great way to bring together their practice wisdom, creative ideas, and new techniques or strategies that they developed to other therapists nationally and worldwide. Publishing articles and books will give them credibility, are viewed as scholarly contributions to the field, can increase their private practice referrals, and lead to invitations to guest lecture at universities and be a workshop presenter on the local, national, and international levels. On their websites or in the form of podcasts, they can share specific therapeutic techniques and strategies that they had developed and have invited thought leaders from the couple and family therapy field to publish their ideas and share their clinical practice wisdom in those contexts as well, which will help increase their Internet visibility to a worldwide audience as well.

Give Workshops and Present at Major Local, National, and International Conferences

Another great way for advanced-level couple and family therapists to get their message out and market their work is to present workshops on the local, national, and international levels. One of the great benefits of presenting is learning from participants not only what therapeutic tools and strategies they had taught them that they found helpful and creative, as well as learning from them about the concerns they had about using some of their tools and strategies with specific treatment populations and types of client problems, certain gaps in their couple or family therapy approach, and hear from them their recommendations about how to further improve what they do therapeutically.

Master-Level Couple and Family Therapists

Master-level couple and family therapists are never satisfied with status quo. They are always looking for ways to improve their skills and expand their choice couple and family therapy approaches by integrating new therapeutic ideas, using curiosity, asking themselves and colleagues questions, actively experimenting with new techniques and strategies they developed, and critically evaluating what works, what needs to be modified, or discarded. They view and attack problems from different angles without allowing themselves to prematurely lock down on one way of looking at a client situation and instead, are curious about the second, third, or fourth possible explanation for what is going on. Like having a sixth sense and a third ear, their high level of awareness allows them to zoom in and see and hear client anomalies that most therapists would miss that are worth seizing as opportunities for creating possibilities in sessions. They can zoom out to capture a big picture view of the couple or family system to see what they may be missing or what might be worthwhile trying with them. When faced with highly complex and challenging couple and family situations, they can intuit quickly patterns that they recognize and solutions quickly in the form of flashes of insight. Those ideas and solutions they think are the most useful to try they will act upon (Greene, 2012; Klein, 2013, 1998; Kanter, 2023).

The next professional step for master-level couple and family therapists with their high level of knowledge, skills, and clinical practice wisdom is to take it to the macro-level, such as: changing whole treatment populations through broad-scale research and prevention work; regularly presenting their new clinical ideas in the forms of publications and at national and international conferences; serving as mentors and supervisors for advanced-level couple and family therapists; serving as a senior family therapy consultant to a treatment program, family service agency, or mental health clinic; organizational consulting and executive coaching in corporate settings; and constantly looking for new ways to further evolve their signature couple and family therapy approach and use it with new types of presenting problems that contemporary couples and families are struggling with.

Master-Level Couple and Family Therapist Developmental Tasks

Below, I Present nine use of self-developmental tasks that master-level couple and family therapists should consider working on further honing and using their practice wisdom and knowledge to make additional contributions to our field on higher levels. This includes the following: mentoring and coaching, teaching and presenting, consulting, doing research, and publishing.

Never Settle, Keep Pushing the Limits for What is Possible

Master couple and family therapists are rarely satisfied with complacency and status quo. They are always looking to take their approaches to the next level and beyond their offices. Be it finding therapeutic tools and strategies from other couple and family therapy and/or individual therapy approaches to further expand the possibilities with their model to using their signature treatment approach with a challenging treatment population or type of client problem situation that they have written or presented on before. Minuchin put his structural family therapy approach to the test by attempting to use it to transform the state of New York's foster care delivery system. He and his colleagues intervened on multiple systems levels. One of their missions was to reunify biological parents with their kids and tapping the expertise of foster parents to assist the biological parents in a supportive coaching role regarding what worked with their kids parenting-wise and with parenting skill development. Additionally, Minuchin and his team collaborated with other involved larger systems professionals like: probation officers, social service agency case managers and therapists, child protective workers, drug counselors, school professionals, and so forth to build cooperative partnerships with them, both the biological and foster parents, and the children (Minuchin, Colapinto, & Minuchin, 1998). Some master couple and family therapists are using their approaches to transform healthcare, mental health, social service, substance abuse treatment delivery systems; change organizational dynamics and behaviors in corporate settings, and empowering people to have their voices heard and getting people working together in their communities

(Herzig & Chasin, 2006; Anderson & Goolishian, 1986; Imber-Black, 1986; Bloch, 1986; Cecchin & Fruggeri, 1986; Borwick, 1986; Friedman, 1986; Bokos & Schwartzman, 1985).

Mentoring and Supervising Advanced-Level Couple and Family Therapists

By mentoring and coaching advanced-level couple and family therapists, master-level couple and family therapists will find this work to be both intellectually stimulating and keep them on their toes in terms of ways they can and should improve upon their choice treatment approach. In fact, they will not only discover from their apprentices the gaps or limitations in their approaches but learn about new and creative therapeutic tools and strategies they have developed on their own before ever meeting their mentors. For master-level couple and family therapists, mentoring can be a professionally growth-producing experience and a reminder that knowledge is always on the way and that they can always learn something new from the next generation of advanced-level couple and family therapists (Goolishian & Anderson, 1988).

Serve on the Faculty of a Family Therapy Institute, a Marital and Family Therapy Program, or for Other Graduate School Programs

Often, master couple and family therapists get offers to join a family therapy institute training faculty or accept an appointment as part of a marital and family therapy graduate program faculty or serving as a faculty member in a graduate level psychology, counseling, or social work school. If this has not come their way, it can be quite rewarding to teach graduate level students and they should explore with area graduate school programs if there are any adjunct faculty positions available. Most students are highly enthusiastic, have a strong thirst for learning, and use their curiosity to pose intriguing questions. They can share stories about their early struggles and valuable lessons and practice wisdom they learned from pioneers in the field and other trainers and supervisors, which helped them to become competent couple and family therapists. Like supervising, mentoring, and coaching advance level couple and family therapists, both beginning and intermediate-level couple and family therapists will keep them on their toes with thought-provoking questions and share their constructive criticism about some of the therapeutic approaches and methods taught.

Expand the Possibilities with Your Signature Model by Applying it to an Existing but Unexplored Treatment Issue or Problem or a Newly Emerging Issue or Problem of Contemporary Couples and Families

Since master-level couple and family therapists are highly curious and looking to pioneer new directions in the couple and family therapy field, they can prospect for ways to apply their signature treatment approaches to certain treatment and emerging issues and types of presenting problems that contemporary couples and families are currently struggling with. Some examples are: developing systemically oriented family-based treatment programs for self-injuring and suicidal youth, domestic couple and family violence; developing new couple and family therapy approaches for opiate addiction, gambling, excessive video-gaming, and cyber-sex problems; new couple and family therapy approaches for veterans struggling with post-traumatic stress disorder; new couple and family therapy approaches to binge-eating, avoidant/restrictive food intake difficulties, obesity; and innovative couple and family resilience-enhancing treatment methods for the traumatic aftermath of COVID-19 and for mental and physical health maintenance for coping with future pandemics. Another important area that master-level couple and family therapists can get involved in as social activists and in helping families better cope with is the impact of global warming on them and the world. All of these couple and family difficulties are ripe for the expertise and leadership of master-level couple and family therapists to trailblaze innovative prevention and treatment programming for making a difference on a larger scale in our society.

Consider Doing Treatment Outcome Research

Stanton and Todd (1982) not only co-developed their structural-strategic family therapy approach after years of training with Minuchin and Haley but they were the first to research the efficacy of their treatment approach with one of the toughest populations to treat, adult heroin addicts. This was the first major family therapy treatment outcome study with substance abusers. The success of their research and demonstrating that close to 68–70% of the heroin addicts in their project either greatly reduced their use or achieved abstinence by changing their family systems, put them on the world map as the gold standard family treatment model of choice for both adolescent and adult substance abusers.

Master-level couple and family therapists should consider demonstrating through both qualitative and quantitative research methods that their models are effective. Once this can be proven, state and national certification boards will endorse them as empirically supported treatments that mental health and addiction professionals should get training in, which cannot only lead to helping their training businesses grow significantly but they will have a bigger impact on whole populations by training large numbers of professionals.

Keep Publishing on and Presenting Your Cutting-Edge Clinical Work

Master-level couple and family therapists often are passionate about their clinical work, training and educating therapists at all skill levels, and want to make their unique contribution to our field. They do this through regularly publishing articles, writing books, and presenting workshops on the local, national, and international levels. They also should consider joining an editorial board of a major couple and family therapy journal. Those that have become pioneers in the field are constantly expanding the possibilities with their approaches and coming up with increasingly more creative ways to use themselves as the catalysts for change with their clients and in the context of live consultations.

Serve as a Family Therapy Consultant for a Youth and Family Service Agency or Mental Health Clinic

Serving as a family therapy consultant for social service agencies and mental health programs is a great way to rapidly trouble-shoot with stuck and difficult cases. When doing consultations at agencies and mental health programs, master-level couple and family therapists should do a few live couple or family consultations, including the treating therapists and any other helping professionals involved. By using this consultation format, they can help the treating therapists get unstuck and they can demonstrate how to build cooperative relationships with the involved helping professionals. If the agency or clinic does not have one-way mirrors, a closed-circuit TV hook-up can be set up so that the larger group can observe the live consultations from a separate room. To help take the training to the next level, after the consultations are concluded, the participating couple or family clients can be asked to share what their experiences were like in their consultations and the consultant can share his or her therapeutic decision-making in the therapeutic process, that is why he or she chose to do what they did in different moments in the session. In my mind, there is no better way for master-level couple and family therapists to use to train therapists than this format. Additionally, having agency and clinic staff present videotape clips of their stuck or difficult couples is another great training method. When using this training format, I like to have consultees first show two places on the video where they thought they were brilliant and pleased with and then show two places in their sessions where they felt stuck.

Continue to Maintain a Small to Medium-Size Private Practice to Keep Up with Couples' and Families' Ever-Changing Problems and Struggles of the Day

There are some master-level couple and family therapists that have decided to stop seeing clients. Personally, I think this is a mistake because couples and families are constantly changing with the times and in order to stay up to date with these changes, it makes sense to maintain at least a small caseload of couples and families. Additionally, if master-level couple and family therapists are teaching and training beginning and intermediate-level couple and family therapists, they should know first-hand what are the contemporary struggles and challenges couples and families are dealing with, including particular problems that are more prevalent today.

Therapeutic Humility: Continue to Cultivate this Important Virtue

Master-level couple and family therapists over their long illustrious careers have come to discover that they are fallible just like their trainees and supervisees and have been at a loss for what to do with some difficult couples and families, have experienced clients dropping out of therapy, made big mistakes in sessions, and have had their share of treatment failures. They also have cultivated calm optimism that is, they have discovered by maintaining their presence and patience with their clients that even when feeling stuck and at a loss for what to do, they know through past similar experiences that together they will eventually come up with some useful ideas that could lead to the co-construction of solutions (Levitt & Piazza-Bonin, 2016; Roffman, 2014). Bradatan (2023) contends that humility is a life-enhancing virtue and greatly contributes to our personal growth. Master-level couple and family therapists need to drive home the message to all who they train, supervise, and teach that we are not, nor will never be God-like, all-knowing, always on top of our game, and to embrace that fact.

Training Exercises

In this last section of the chapter, I present ten training exercises that can be used by trainers and supervisors in any practice setting and in a workshop context to help further hone the conceptual, perceptual, and executive skills of couple and family therapists at any developmental stage in their use of themselves. I provide instructions for how to do each of the training exercises, the number of participants in a skill-building group, and what couple and family therapist skill level could benefit the most from each exercise.

"Let's Say Your Treatment Success was Completely Guaranteed with Your Toughest Couple or Family Clients. What daring and surprising things will you do in your next session with them?"

This exercise can be done in groups of twos or threes. Each participant takes turns sharing what they would try with the couple or family outside of their comfort zones. They also can share feedback with one another about the daring and surprising moves they will take and based on the clients' responses, where to go next with them. This exercise is useful for intermediate and advanced-level couple and family therapists.

Thriving in the Unknown: Creating Possibilities in a Session with Uncertainties, Doubts, and Embracing the Mysterious (Groups of Four: Intermediate- and Advanced-Level MFTs)

John Keats, the famous Irish poet, in describing in a letter to his two brothers George and Tom, introduced his concept of *negative capability* to them. What he meant by this concept was a man or woman's ability to thrive in uncertainty, when having doubts, and allow oneself to be intrigued by the mysterious (Keats, 2001). Keats also shared with his brothers in his letter that a wonderful example of thriving in negative capability was his highly admired literary hero William Shakespeare who had many great achievements and creative ideas. After I share Keats's negative capability concept with the supervisory or training group or workshop participants, they are to break up into groups of four. They are presented with the following client scenario:

> Suppose you had to conduct a session with a family where you have no information about them, not even anything about the nature of their presenting problems. All that you do know is that you are the tenth therapist they have been to.

They are to respond to the following questions:

- "Where would you begin with this family?"
- "What questions would you ask them?"
- "What therapeutic tools and strategies would you try based on their responses?"
- "What would you do next?"
- "After that?"

There are two options with this exercise. First, the groups can respond to the questions and decide together what would be the best way to proceed with this family. Second, you can do a simulation where the family is role-played and group members can take turns trying out what they think might work with this family as the therapist. This exercise can be used with intermediate, advanced, and master-level couple and family therapists.

Engaging Reluctant Adolescents

This exercise is done in groups of two with each partner sitting back-to-back. Each partner takes turns being the adolescent and the therapist. The therapist has to figure out a way outside of their comfort zone taking risks and/or using humor to turn the adolescent so that they can talk face-to-face. The adolescents will only turn if they hear something that really catches their attention, that is interesting, funny, or engaging about the therapist. The adolescents in the exercises can share with the larger group what specifically resonated with them that led to there being open to face their therapists and cooperating with them. The therapists can share both their frustrations, where they struggled, what seemed to work, and what the key takeaways for them from the exercise were. This exercise can be used with both beginning and intermediate-level couple and family therapists.

Thick Description

This exercise consists of having four team members, representing four different family therapy approaches, such as structural family therapy, narrative family therapy, solution-focused brief therapy, and collaborative language systems therapy (Goolishian and Anderson), observing live a colleague working with a family, viewing them through the lens of each of these different approaches, throughout the course of therapy. The team is to look for intersection points, what change would look like using these different approaches, where they could potentially be integrated, and how the different models can complement one another. The team will follow their colleague working with the same family until the therapy is completed trying out along the way major therapeutic tools and strategies from the different models in a purposeful way being sensitive to the family's unique needs, theories of change, and goals. This exercise is great to use with intermediate and advanced-level couple and family therapists. Three important takeaways with this exercise are:

1 There are many different ways to view and intervene with a family.
2 All family therapy approaches intersect at some point and are about changing the viewing and the doing with clients.
3 Trainees and supervisees learn about what models logically fit together and are worthwhile integrating to expand their therapeutic approach and range with the use of self.

Deliberate Practice with Couple and Family Simulations

This exercise can be used with training and supervision groups and in the context of in-house agency or clinic training contexts. Trainers and supervisors can have intermediate and advanced-level couple and family therapists practice their use of self-skills with a challenging couple or family presenting problem or scenario, such as: working with high-conflict couples deadlocked in an entrenched blame-counterblame destructive pattern of interaction; ways to ferret out what the clients are not talking about, such as a secret; rebalancing power and control in a couple relationship where one partner wields all of the power and is stonewalling, to name a few challenging clinical scenarios. A couple or family simulation (role-play) can be conducted and the therapists can take turns trying to create possibilities with the aforementioned challenging case situations. Using deliberate practice methods, the trainer or supervisor can offer them right on the spot support, recommendations to redirect them, and other feedback on their performances after they have taken their turns (Blow et al. 2023; Ericsson & Pool, 2017).

Question-Storming

This exercise can be used in the contexts of training or supervision groups, as a skill-building exercise in workshops or in-house training. They are to break-up into groups of 4-6 and craft intriguing and bold questions for the case presenter presenting his or her stuck case, to either ask the couple partners or family members directly and/or questions to ponder/reflect on for exploring alternative therapeutic directions or letting go of what is not working with their current way of viewing and intervening with the couple or family. They are first to respond to the following key question: "What are the essential questions that have not yet been asked about this couple or family's situation?" Next, they are to craft 5–6 questions beginning with qualifiers like: *What? What if? How? Why?* The questions co-constructed can either be designed to help the case presenter to think about new ways of viewing and intervening with his/her client's situation or questions to pose directly to the couple partners or family members that might be useful. The case presenter is to star those questions they found to be most useful. They are given thirty minutes as a group to do the exercise. The case presenters will share the starred questions with the larger group that they found most useful and what their future directions are with their cases. This exercise can be used with all couple and family therapist skill levels.

Famous Guest Consultants

This exercise can be done in group supervision, in the context of a workshop, or in-house training context. A supervisee or therapist presents a stuck couple or family case they are struggling with. Each supervisee or member of the workshop/in-house training break-out groups is to think of someone famous they have always admired and have been inspired by, such as: philosophers, historic figures, scientists, authors, artists, musicians, sports stars, well-known chefs, and so forth and put themselves in the minds of their selected people. They are to respond to the following question, "Based on what you know about what your famous people are known for, what ideas would they have for your colleague's stuck case?" The group is to co-generate two or more creative solutions for the stuck case. They will have thirty minutes to do the exercise. The case presenter will share with larger group the creative ideas their group came up with and what their future directions are with their cases. This exercise can be used with all couple and family therapist skill levels.

The Supervisor Shows a Videotape of their Worst All Time Couple or Family Session

This exercise can be used in group supervision or with a training group in a workshop or in-house training contexts with beginning and intermediate-level couple and family therapists. The group is shown a video of the trainer's or supervisor's worst all time couple or family session. As a group, they are to respond to the following question:

- "If you had a shot at this couple or family, what would you have done differently that you think might have made it a more productive session?"
- "What questions would you have asked?"
- "What in-session therapeutic tools and strategies would you have tried?"
- "In terms of your use of self, what daring things would you have said or tried?"

The Supervisory or Training Group Serves as the Supervisor's/Trainer's
Consultation Team with His or Her Difficult Couple or Family Case

This exercise can be done with either a supervisory or training group and gives them a great opportunity to team the supervisor or trainer and offer their creative input with therapeutic technique and strategy selection or using their own inventiveness to craft therapeutic experiments to offer the clients. With this exercise and the previous one, it normalizes for beginning and intermediate-level couple and family therapists that as supervisors and trainers we get stuck, make mistakes, and fail too with our clients.

Pretend a Miracle Happened Before Your Next Session
with Your Most Difficult Couple or Family Clients

This exercise can be done in groups of two. Each partner takes turn imagining that a miracle had happened with their most difficult couple or family client before their next sessions with them and all their problems are now solved. This exercise can be used with beginning and intermediate-level couple and family therapists. They are to share with one another their responses to the following questions:

- "How will you be able to tell that the miracle really happened?"
- "How will they look different in their interaction with themselves and with you?"
- "What else will be better with them?"
- "What will they be the most pleased with that you are doing differently with them?"
- "What else will they be pleased with that you are doing differently with them?"
- "How else will you be empowering them and consolidating their gains?"

In this chapter, I have presented a developmental framework for the use of self throughout one's professional career as a couple and family therapist. Recommended developmental tasks to attempt to achieve mastery with at the beginning, intermediate, advanced, and master levels are offered. Some of these developmental tasks may not be mastered until couple and family therapists accrue more practice experience and advance into the next developmental stage. The use of self-developmental framework can greatly benefit frontline couple and family therapists, trainees, supervisees, trainers, supervisors, and mentors in assessing where they are at developmentally with their use of self-skills and what tasks and sets of skills they need to pursue and master to move to the next developmental stage. Finally, I presented ten training exercises that are designed to further hone therapists' use of self, conceptual, perceptual, and executive skills that can be used in any practice and training setting.

9

The Therapist's Use of Self and Beyond

Major Themes and Implications for the Future

Major Themes of the Book

By now, my hope is that readers are feeling inspired to be more daring, playful, improvisational, and inventive outside of their comfort zones with the couples and families they work with. We began this reading journey with paying homage to ten true masters of the use of self: Milton H. Erickson, Michele Weiner-Davis, John H. Weakland, Harry Goolishian, Michael White, Virginia Satir, Peggy Papp, Salvador Minuchin, Harry Aponte, and Carl Whitaker. They regularly brought courage, passion, charisma, humor, absurdity, playfulness, metaphors, stories, and provocation to help liberate couples and families from their seemingly intractable difficulties and co-created workable realities with them. For those of you who missed the professional opportunity to train with some of these pioneers while they were still alive, I highly recommend that you read their seminal publications, and watch training DVDs, and YouTube videos of their masterful clinical work.

In Chapter 3, I discussed the advantages and disadvantages of relying solely on practice evidence-based wisdom and presented some important research on pattern recognition and wise therapists and individuals that can help inform our therapeutic decision-making. To help counter-balance the limitations of relying solely on practice evidence-based wisdom, I also discussed the importance of being mindful as a clinician of the eight mental traps and cognitive biases that could lead us to poor clinical decision-making and negative treatment outcomes.

Readers will find that the therapist's use of self-toolkit described in Chapter 4 offers them eleven different therapeutic tools and strategies they can use in a purposeful way to help open up space for therapeutic breakthroughs and preferred future realities for their clients. Case examples demonstrate each of these therapeutic tools and strategies in action.

Since we all have found ourselves getting stuck or lost in a client problem maze, particularly with highly complex and challenging couples and families, I offer in Chapter 5 several practical trouble-shooting guidelines for remedying what I call *therapeutic brick walls*. I discuss three major contributing factors to their occurrence, they are: therapist-generated, client-generated, and therapist-client-eco-systemic

DOI: 10.4324/9781003334460-9

generated factors. After discussing each of them, I offer effective ways to rapidly remedy them and unstick the treatment system.

The COVID-19 pandemic forced couple and family therapists and other helping professionals to turn to Zoom and other safe and confidential streaming systems to provide virtual tele-health therapy to their clients. For many therapists not used to doing virtual tele-health therapy, they found this counseling format to be stifling, unnatural, and to be a challenging constraint. However, what many couple and family therapists had discovered was that their clients were much more relaxed and opened up about issues and difficulties they may never had talked about in their offices before the pandemic. They lowered their drawbridges to us and gave us a real gift, by sharing their important pastimes, rituals, sharing their pets with us, showing us their highly cherished mementos and creations made by them, provided us with a live musical performance, and so forth. One of the major benefits of the constraints of the pandemic and working together in a virtual tele-health therapy context was that it sparked high levels of creativity and inventiveness from both the clients and us to co-produce high-quality solutions together.

As a way to help expand therapist's use of self-range and style, I made a case in Chapter 7 for outside of our brains and our couple and family therapy field, there is a goldmine of creative ideas and metaphors we can tap from such diverse fields as: art, architecture, film, theater, literature, philosophy, history, music, science and technology, and nature. I provided case examples to illustrate how we can use these ideas to craft bold and intriguing questions and use them to co-design therapeutic experiments with clients.

Finally, in the last chapter, I wanted to contribute a unique and practical use of self-developmental framework for frontline couple and family therapists, trainers, supervisors, and mentors that they can use in their own individual professional development and in training and supervisory contexts. Under each of the developmental stages, there are recommended tasks to strive to master that can advance yourself, trainees, supervisees, trainers, and supervisors to the next use of self-developmental stage. Even at the master's level, there is still much more to know and plenty of unchartered territory in the couple and family therapy field.

Implications for the Future

The therapist's use of self in couple and family therapy is a research area in need of more studies that attempt to isolate other important qualities and ingredients of what therapists do in the therapeutic process that clients report benefiting them, other than what we already know from their self-reports in treatment outcome studies about specific relationship and structuring skills that their therapists used with them. Finally, I hope to do future research on and allow my use of self-developmental framework to further evolve, particularly looking at the proposed tasks at each stage and how they contribute to the professional growth of couple and family therapists and what other tasks may be worthwhile adding to each of the stages of the use of self-skill-development. My hope is that readers will be enticed by this book to come up with their own novel and improvisational ways of using themselves with couples and families as the catalysts for change and do research in this area. So, what will your unique contribution be?

References

Ackerman, N.W. (1972). *The psychodynamics of family life: Diagnosis and treatment of family relationships*. New York: Basic.

Alexander, J.F., Waldron, H.B., Robbins, M.S., & Neeb, A.A. (2013). *Functional family therapy for adolescent behavior problems*. Washington, DC: American Psychological Association.

Allen, W. (1985). *The purple rose of Cairo*. [Film]. MGM Pictures.

Allen, W. (1983). *Zelig*. [Film]. Orion Pictures.

Alvord, L.A. & Chen-Van Pelt, E. (2000). *The scalpel and the silver bear: The first Navajo woman surgeon combines western medicine and traditional healing*. New York: Bantam.

Andersen, T. (1995). Reflecting processes; acts of informing and forming: You can borrow my eyes, but you must not take them away from me! In S. Friedman (Ed.), *The reflecting team in action: Collaborative practice in family therapy* (pp. 11–38). New York: Guilford.

Andersen, T. (1991). *The reflecting team: Dialogues and dialogues about the dialogues*. New York: Norton.

Anderson, H. (1997). *Conversation, language, and possibilities: A postmodern therapy approach to therapy*. York: Basic.

Anderson, H. & Gehart, D. (2007). *Collaborative therapy: Relationships and conversations that make a difference*. New York: Routledge.

Anderson, H. & Goolishian, H. (1988). Human systems as linguistic systems: Evolving ideas about the implications for theory and practice. *Family Process, 27*, 371–393.

Anderson, H. & Goolishian, H. (1986). Systems consultation with agencies dealing with domestic violence. In L.C. Wynne, S.H. McDaniel, & T.T. Weber (Eds.), *Systems consultation: A new perspective for family therapy* (pp. 284–300). New York: Guilford.

Anderson, H., Goolishian, H., & Winderman, L. (1986). Problem-determined systems: Towards transformation in family therapy. *Journal of Systemic and Strategic Therapies, 5*, 1–13.

Anderson, T., Crowley, M.J., Himawan, L., Holmberg, J.K., & Uhlim, B.D. (2016). Therapist facilitative interpersonal skills and training status: A randomized clinical trial on alliance and outcome. *Psychotherapy Research, 26*, 511–529.

Anderson, T. & Hill, C.E. (2017). The role of therapist skills in therapist effectiveness. In L.G. Gastonguay & C.E. Hill (Eds.), *How and why are some therapists better than others? Understanding therapist effects* (pp. 139–157). Washington, DC: American Psychological Association.

Andreas, S. (1991). *Virginia Satir: The patterns of her magic*. Palo Alto, CA: Science and Behavior Books.

Angelou, M. (2009). *I know why the cage bird sings*. New York: Ballantine.

Anker, M.G., Duncan, B.L., & Sparks, J. A. (2009). Using feedback to improve couple therapy outcomes: A randomized clinical trial in naturalistic settings. *Journal of Consulting and Clinical Psychology, 77* (4), 693–704.

Anker, M.G., Owen, J., Duncan, B.L., & Sparks, J.A. (2010). The alliance in couple therapy: Partner influence, early change, and alliance patterns in a naturalistic setting. *Journal of Consulting and Clinical Psychology, 78*, 635–645.

Aponte, H.J. (2016). The person-of-the-therapist model on the use of self in therapy. In H.J. Aponte & K. Kissel (Eds.), *The person of the therapist training model: Mastering the use of self.* (pp. 1–13). New York: Routledge.

Aponte, H.J. (1994). *Bread and spirit: Therapy with the new poor: Diversity of race, culture, and values.* New York: Norton.

Aponte, H.J., Powell, E.D., Brooks, S., Watson, M.F., Litzke, C., Lawless, J., & Johnson, E. (2009). Training the person of the therapist in an academic setting. *Journal of Marital and Family Therapy, 35* (4), 381–394.

Aponte, H.J. & Van Deusen, J.M. (1981). Structural family therapy. In A.S. Gurman & D.R. Kniskern (Eds.), *Handbook of family therapy* (pp. 310–361). New York: Brunner/Mazel.

Aponte, H.J. & Winter, J.E. (2013). The person and practice of the therapist: Treatment and training. In M. Baldwin (Ed). *The use of self in therapy*, 3rd ed. (pp. 141–166). New York: Routledge.

Aristotle. (1987). *Nicomachean ethics.* New York: Prometheus.

Aurelius, M. (2002). *Meditations.* New York: Modern Library.

Aviv, R. (2022). *Strangers to ourselves: Unsettled minds and the stories that make us.* New York: Farrer, Straus, & Giroux.

Bacon, S. (2018). *Practicing psychotherapy in constructed reality: Ritual, charisma, and enhanced client outcomes.* Lanham, MD: Lexington.

Bakewell, S. (2010). *How to live or a life of Montaigne in one question and twenty attempts at an answer.* New York: Other Press.

Bakker, N., Jansen, L., & Luijten, H. (2010). *The real Van Gogh: The artist and his letters.* London, UK: Royal Academy of Arts.

Baltes, P.B. & Staudinger, U.M. (2000). Wisdom: A meta-heuristic (pragmatic) to orchestrate mind and virtue toward excellence. *American Psychologist, 55* (1), 122–136.

Bandura, A. (2000). Cultivate self-efficacy for personal and organizational effectiveness. In E.A. Locke (Ed.), *Handbook of principles of organizational behavior* (pp. 120–136). Oxford, UK: Blackwell.

Bandura, A. (1997). *Self-efficacy: The exercise of control.* New York: Freeman.

Bar, M. (2022). *Mind wandering: How your constant mental drift can improve your mood and boost your creativity.* New York: Hachette.

Barkham, M., Lutz, W., Lambert, M.J., & Saxon, D. (2017). Therapist effects, effective therapists, and the law of variability. In L.G. Castonguay & C.E. Hill (Eds.), *How and why are some therapists are better than others? Understanding therapist effects* (pp. 13–36). Washington, DC: American Psychological Association.

Barlow, D. (2001). *Anxiety and its disorders: The nature and treatment of anxiety and panic.* New York: Guilford.

Barrie, J.M. (2017). *Peter and Wendy.* Scott's Valley, CA: CreateSpace Independent.

Battino, R. (2002). *Metaphoria: Metaphor and guided metaphor for psychotherapy and healing.* Williston, VT: Crown House Publishing.

Baumbach, N. (2005). *The squid and the whale.* [Film]. Sony Pictures.

Beck, J.S. (2011). *Cognitive therapy for challenging problems: What to do when the basics don't work.* New York: Guilford.

Bergman, J. (1985). *Fishing for barracuda: Pragmatics of brief systemic therapy.* New York: Norton.

Berns, G. (2022). *The self-delusion: The new neuroscience of how we invent and reinvent our identities.* New York: Basic.

Beutler, L., Harwood, T.M., Michelson, A., Song, X., & Holman, J. (2011). Reactance/reactance level. In J.C. Norcross (Ed.), *Psychotherapy relationships that work: Evidence-based responsiveness,* 2nd ed. (pp. 261–279). New York: Oxford University.

Beyebach, M. & Carranza, V.E. (1997). Therapeutic interaction and drop-out: Measuring relational communication in solution-focused therapy. *Journal of Family Therapy, 19* (3), 173–213.

Blight, D. (2018). *Frederick Douglas: Prophet of freedom.* New York: Simon & Schuster.

Bloch, D.A. (1986). The family therapist as consultant to health care organizations. In L.C. Wynne, S.H. McDaniel, & T.T. Weber (Eds.), *Systems consultation: A new perspective for family therapy* (pp. 139–150). New York: Guilford.

Blow, A.J., Seedall, R.B., Miller, D.L., Rousmaniere, T., & Vaz, A. (2023). *Deliberate practice in systemic family therapy.* Washington, DC: American Psychological Association.

Boag, Z. & C. Pury (2023). Worthwhile risks: An interview with Cynthia Pury. *New Philosopher, 38,* 64–72.

Bodin, A.M. (1981). The interactional view: Family therapy approaches of the Mental Research Institute. In A.S. Gurman & D.P. Kniskern (Eds.)., *Handbook of family therapy* (pp. 267–310). New York: Brunner/Mazel.

Bohart, A.C. & Tallman, K. (2022). Client expertise: The active client in psychotherapy. In J.N. Fuertes (Ed.), *The other side of psychotherapy: Understanding clients' experiences and contributions in treatment* (pp. 13–45). Washington, DC: American Psychological Association.

Bohart, A.C. & Tallman, K. (1999). *How clients make therapy work: The process of active self-healing.* Washington, DC: American Psychological Association.

Bohm, D. (1996). *On dialogue.* London, UK: Routledge.

Bokos, P.J. & Schwartzman, J. (1985). Family therapy and methadone treatment for opiate addiction. in J. Schwartzman (Ed.), *Families and other systems* (pp. 163–196). New York: Guilford.

Bordin, E. (1979). The generalizability of the psychoanalytic concept of the working alliance. *Psychotherapy: Theory, Research, and Practice, 16,* 252–260.

Borwick, I. (1986). The family therapist as business consultant. In L.C. Wynne, S.H. McDaniel, & T.T. Weber (Eds.), *Systems consultation: A new perspective for family therapy* (pp. 423–441). New York: Guilford.

Boscolo, L. & Bertrando, P. (1993). *The times of time: A new perspective in systemic therapy and consultation.* New York: Norton.

Boscolo, L., Cecchin, G., Hoffman, L., & Penn, P. (1987). *Milan systemic family therapy: Conversations in theory and practice.* New York: Basic Books.

Bowen, M. (1978). *Family therapy in clinical practice.* New York: Jason Aronson.

Brach, T. (2004). *Radical acceptance: Embracing your life with the heart of Buddha.* New York: Bantam.

Bradatan, C. (2023). *In praise of failure: Four lessons in humility.* Cambridge, MA: Harvard University.

Brassey, J., De Smet, A., & Kruyt, M. (2022). *Deliberate calm: How to learn and lead in a volatile world.* New York: Harper Business.

Brown, S. & Vaughn, C. (2016). *Play: How it shapes the brain, opens the imagination, and invigorates the soul.* New York: Avery.

Bryant, F.B., King, S., & Smart, C.M. (2005). Using the past to enhance the present: Boosting happiness through positive reminiscence. *Journal of Happiness Studies, 6,* 227–260.

Camillus, J. (2015, Winter). Feed-forward systems: Framing a future faced with wicked problems. *Rotman Management,* 52–60.

Campbell, J. (1973). *Hero with a thousand faces.* Princeton, NJ: Princeton University.

Camus, A. (2018). *The myth of Sisyphus.* New York: Knopf Doubleday.

Carr, D.W. (2006). *Velazquez.* London, UK: The National Gallery.

Carroll, L. (2018). *Alice in Wonderland.* Ware, UK: Wordsworth Editions.

Cassell, S. & Diamond, G. (2023). Therapist-adolescent therapeutic ruptures in attachment-based family therapy. In C.F. Eubanks, L.W. Samstag, & J.C. Muran (Eds,), *Rupture and repair in psychotherapy: A critical process for change,* (pp. 95–119). Washington, DC: American Psychological Association.

Catmull, E. (2014). *Creativity, Inc.: Overcoming the unseen forces that stand in the way of true inspiration.* New York: Random House.

Cecchin, G. & Fruggeri, L. (1986). Consultation with mental health systems teams in Italy. In L.C. Wynne, S.H. McDaniel, T.T. Weber (Eds.), *Systems consultation: A new perspective for family therapy* (pp. 103–115). New York: Guilford.

Cervantes, M. (2003). *Don Quixote.* New York: Penguin Classics.

Chodron, P. (2009). *Taking the leap: Freeing ourselves from old habits and fears.* Boston, MA: Shambhala.

Chow, D.L., Miller, S.D., Seidel, J.A., Kane, R.T., Thorton, J.A., & Andrews, W.P. (2015). The role of deliberate practice in the development of highly effective psychotherapists. *Psychotherapy, 52,* 337–343.

Clark, A. (2011). *Supersizing the mind: Embodied, situated, and distributed cognitive extension.* New York: Oxford University.

Clark, A. & Chalmers, D. (1998, January). Where does the mind stop? The extended mind. *Analysis,* 7–19.

Coelho, P. (1993). *The alchemist.* New York: Harper-Perennial.

Colapinto, J. (1991). Structural family therapy. In A.S. Gurman & D.R. Kniskern (Eds.), *Handbook of family Therapy, Vol. II* (pp. 417–444). New York: Brunner/Mazel.

Coleman, J.C. (1974). *Relationships in adolescence.* New York: Routledge & Kegan Paul.

Connell, G., Mitten, T., & Burberry, W. (1999). *Reshaping family relationships: The symbolic therapy of Carl Whitaker.* Philadelphia, PA: Taylor & Francis.

Constantino, M.J., Boswell, F., Coyne, A.E., Kraus, D.R., & Castonguay, L.G. (2017). Who works for whom and why? Integrating therapist effects analysis into psychotherapy outcome and process research. In L.G. Castonguay & C.E. Hill (Eds.), *How and why are some therapists better than others? Understanding therapist effects* (pp. 55–68). Washington, DC: American Psychological Association.

Coppock, T.E., Owen, J., Zagarskas, E., & Schmidt, M. (2010). The relationship between client hope and therapy outcomes. *Psychotherapy Research, 20* (6), 619–626.

Crits-Christoph, P., Connolly-Gibbons, M.B., & Mukherjee, D. (2013). Psychotherapy process research. In M.J. Lambert (Ed.), *Bergin and Garfield's handbook of psychotherapy and behavior change* (pp. 298–340). Hoboken, NJ: Wiley.

Csikszentmihalyi, M. (1997). *Finding flow.* New York: Basic.

Csikszentmihalyi, M. (1990). *Flow: The psychology of optimal experience.* New York: Harper and Row.

Cumming, R. (2020). *Art: A visual history,* 2nd ed. London, UK: DK.

DeFrain, J. (2007). *Family treasures: Creating strong families.* New York: iUniverse, Inc.

DeFrain, J. & Stinnett, N. (1992). Building on inherent strengths in families: A positive approach for psychologists and counselors. *Topics in Family Psychology and Counseling, 1* (1), 15–26.

De Shazer, S. (1999). John H. Weakland: Master of the fine art of "doing nothing." In W.A. Ray & S. De Shazer (Eds.), *Evolving brief therapies: In honor of John H. Weakland* (pp. 30–44). Galena, IL: Geist & Russell.

De Shazer, S. (1991). *Putting difference to work.* New York: Norton.

De Shazer, S. (1988). *Clues: Investigating solutions in brief therapy.* New York: Norton.

De Shazer, S. (1985) *Keys to solution in brief therapy.* New York: Norton.

De Shazer, S., Dolan, Y., Korman, H., Trepper, T., McCollum, E., & Berg, I.K. (2007). *More than Miracles: The state of the art of solution-focused brief therapy.* Binghamton, NY: Haworth.

De Shazer, S. & White, M. (1996, September). *Narrative solutions/Solution narratives.* Three-day conference sponsored by the Brief Family Therapy Center, Milwaukee, IL.

Dick, P.K. (2012). *The man in the high castle.* Boston, MA: Mariner.

Dick, P.K. (1996). *Do androids dream of electric sheep?* New York: Random House.

Diamond, G.S., Diamond, G.M., & Levy, S.A. (2014). *Attachment-based family therapy for depressed adolescents.* Washington, DC: American Psychological Association.

Doyle, A.C. (2016). *The memoirs of Sherlock Holmes: Silver Blaze.* Scotts Valley, CA: CreateSpace.

Duncan, B.L. (2019, November). *8 lessons learned from the Norway couple project.* Keynote presentation at the Harvard University's Treating Couples Conference, Cambridge, MA.

Duncan, B.L. (2010). *On becoming a better therapist.* Washington, DC: American Psychological Association.

Duncan, B.L. & Miller, S.D. (2000). *The heroic client: Doing client-directed, outcome-informed therapy.* San Francisco, CA: Jossey-Bass.

Durrant, M. & Coles, D. (1991). The Michael White approach. In T.C. Todd & M.D. Selekman (Eds.), *Family therapy approaches with adolescent substance abusers* (pp. 135–175). Needham Heights, MA: Allyn & Bacon.

Dweck, C.S. (2006). *Mindset: The new psychology of success.* New York: Ballantine.

Eastwood, M., Sweeney, D., & Piercy, F. (1987). The "no-problem problem:" A family approach for certain first-time adolescent substance abusers. *Family Relations, 36,* 125–128.

Eco, U. (1983). *The name of the rose.* New York: Harcourt.

Ellison, R. (1995). *Invisible man.* New York: Vintage.

Emmons, R.A. (2007). *Thanks! How the new science of gratitude can make you happier.* Boston, MA: Houghton-Mifflin.

Emmons, R.A. & McCullough, M.E. (2004). *The psychology of gratitude.* New York: Oxford University.

Epictetus. (1995). *The art of living: The classical manual on virtue, happiness, and effectiveness.* New York: Harper One.

Epstein, M. (2022). *The Zen of therapy: Uncovering a hidden kindness in life.* New York: Penguin.

Epstein, M. (2018). *Advice not given: A guide to getting over yourself.* New York: Penguin.

Epstein, M. (2013). *The trauma of everyday life.* New York: Penguin.

Epston, D. (2000, September). *Crafting questions in narrative practice with David* Epston. A three-day workshop sponsored by the Evanston Family Therapy Center, Evanston, IL.

Erickson, M.H. (1964). The confusion technique in hypnosis. *American Journal of Hypnosis, 6,* 183–207.

Erickson, M.H. (1954). Pseudo-orientation in time as a hypnotherapeutic procedure. *Journal of Clinical and Experimental Hypnosis, 2,* 261–283.

Ericsson, A. & Pool, R. (2017). *Peak: Secrets from the new science of expertise.* New York: HarperOne.

Erlich, E., Erlich, L.H., & Pepper, G.B. (Eds.). (1994). *Karl Jaspers: Basic philosophical writings.* Atlantic Highlands, NJ: Humanities Press.

Eubanks, C.F., Samstag, L.W., & Muran, J.C. (2023). Don't be afraid to get messy—points of convergence in rupture and repair. In *Rupture and repair in psychotherapy: A critical process of change,* In C.F. Eubanks, L.W. Samstag, & J.C. Muran (Eds.), (pp. 305–319). Washington, DC: American Psychological Association.

Farber, B.A. (2017). Gaining therapeutic wisdom and skills from creative others (writers, actors, musicians and dancers). In L.G. Castonguay & C.E. Hill (Eds.), *How and why are some therapists better than others? Understanding therapist effects* (pp. 215–231). Washington, DC: American Psychological Association.

Fisch, R. & Schlanger, K. (1999). *Brief therapy with intimidating cases: Changing the unchangeable.* San Francisco, CA: Jossey-Bass.

Fisch, R., Weakland, J.H., & Segal, L. (1982). *The tactics of change: Doing therapy briefly.* San Francisco, CA: Jossey-Bass.

Fishman, H.C. (2022). *Performance-based family therapy: A therapist's guide to measurable change.* New York: Routledge.

Fletcher, A. (2021). *Wonderworks: Literary invention and the science of stories.* New York: Simon & Schuster.

Fluckiger, C., Del Re, A.C., Wampold, B.E., Symonds, D., & Horvath, A.O. (2012). How central is the alliance in psychotherapy? A multi-level longitudinal meta-analysis. *Journal of Counseling Psychology, 59,* 10–17.

Fogarty, T. (1976a). System concepts and the dimensions of self. In P.J. Guerin (Ed.)., *Family therapy: Theory and practice* (pp. 144–154). New York: Gardner.

Fogarty, T. (1976b). Marital crisis. In P.J. Guerin (Ed.)., *Family therapy: Theory and practice* (pp. 325–335). New York: Gardner.

Foster, C. (2020). *My Octopus Teacher.* [Film]. Netflix.

Frankl, V.E. (1992). *Man's search for meaning.* Boston, MA: Beacon.

Fredrickson, B.L. (2009). *Positivity: Groundbreaking research reveals how to embrace the hidden strength of positive emotions, overcome negativity, and thrive.* New York: Crown.

Friedlander, M.L. & Escudero, V. (2023). A close look at the complex rupture and repair process in family therapy. In C.F. Eubanks, L.W. Samstag, & J.C. Muran (Eds), *Rupture and repair in psychotherapy: A critical process for change*, (pp. 73–95). Washington, DC: American Psychological Association.

Friedlander, M.L., Escudero, V., Heatherington, L., & Diamond, G. (2011). Alliance in couple and family therapy. In J.C. Norcross (Ed.), *Psychotherapy relationships that work: Evidence-based responsiveness*, 2nd ed. (pp. 92–110). New York: Oxford University.

Friedman, E. (1986). Emotional process in the marketplace: The family therapist as consultant in work systems. In L.C. Wynne, S.H. McDaniel, & T.T. Weber (Eds.), *Systems consultation: A new perspective for family therapy* (pp. 398–423). New York: Guilford.

Fuller, B.R. & Tanaka, H. (1982). *The critical path*, 2nd ed. New York: St. Martin's Griffin.

Furr, N. & Furr, S.H. (2022). *The upside of uncertainty: A guide to finding possibility in the unknown*. Boston, MA: Harvard Business Review Press.

Gabriel, P. (1994). *Secret world live*. [CD]. Geffen Records, B000000OTY.

Gardner, H. (2008). *5 minds for the future*. Boston, MA: Harvard Business.

Garfield, J.L. (2022). *Losing ourselves: Learning to live without a self*. Princeton, NJ: Princeton University.

Garofalo, R., Wolf, R.C., Wissow, L., Woods, E.R., & Goodman, E. (1999). Sexual orientation and risk of suicide attempts among a representative sample of youth. *Archives of Pediatrics and Adolescent Medicine, 153*, 487–493.

Geller, S.M. & Greenberg, L.S. (2012). *Therapeutic presence: A mindful approach to effective therapy*. Washington, DC: American Psychological Association.

Gelso, C.J. & Perez-Rojas, A.E. (2017). Inner experience and the good therapist. In L.G. Gastonguay & C.E. Hill (Eds.), *How and why are some therapists better than others? Understanding therapist effects* (pp. 101–115). Washington, DC: American Psychological Association.

Gilbert, P. (2007). *Stumbling on happiness*. New York: Viking.

Gingerich, W.J, de Shazer, S., & Weiner-Davis, M. (1988). Constructing change: A research view of interviewing. In E. Lipchik (Ed.), *Interviewing* (pp. 21–33). Rockville, MD: Aspen Publications.

Gino, F. & Pisano, G.P. (2022, Summer). Why leaders don't learn from success. *Harvard Business Review*, 10–18.

Gluck, J. (2019). The development of wisdom during adulthood. In R.J. Sternberg & J. Gluck (Eds.), *The Cambridge handbook of wisdom* (pp. 323–346). Cambridge, UK: Cambridge University Press.

Gluck, J. & Weststrate, N. M. (2022). The wisdom researchers and the elephant: An integrative model of wise behavior. *Personality and Social Psychology Review*, https://doi.org/10.1177/10888683221094650.

Goldenberg, S. (2022). *Radical curiosity: Questioning commonly held beliefs to imagine flourishing futures*. New York: Crown.

Goleman, D. (2013). *Focus: The hidden driver of excellence*. New York: Harper.

Goodwin, D.K. (2005). *Team of rivals: The political genius of Abraham Lincoln*. New York: Simon & Schuster.

Goolishian, H. (1991, October). *The dis-diseasing of mental health*. Plenary address at the Annual Houston-Galveston Family Institute Conference, San Antonio, TX.

Goolishian, H. & Anderson, H. (1988, November). *The therapeutic conversation*. Three-day workshop, Institute of Systemic Therapy, Chicago, IL.

Gottman, J.M. & Silver, N. (2015). *The seven principles for making marriage work*. New York: Harmony.

Grayling, A.J. (2019). *The history of philosophy*. New York: Penguin.

Greaves, A. (2022). Clients' agentic and self-healing activities in psychotherapy. In J.N. Fuertes (Ed.), *The other side of psychotherapy: Understanding clients' experiences and contributions in treatment* (pp. 159–203). Washington, DC: American Psychological Association.

Green, R.J. (2019). Same-sex couples: Successful coping with minority stress. In M. McGoldrick & K.V. Hardy (Eds.), *Re-visioning family therapy: Addressing diversity in clinical practice* (pp. 388–403). New York: Guilford.

Greene, R. (2012). *Mastery*. New York: Penguin.

Greene-Morton, E. & Minkler, M. (2020). Cultural competence or cultural humility? Moving beyond the debate. *Health Promotion Practice, 21* (1), 142–145.

Grossmann, I. (2017). Wisdom in context. *Perspectives on Psychological Science,* 12 (2), 233–257.

Grossman, I. & Kross, E. (2014). Exploring Solomon's paradox: Self-distancing eliminates the self-other asymmetry in wise reasoning about close relationships in younger and older adults. *Psychological Science, 25* (8), 1571–1580.

Guerin, P.J., Fay, L.F., Burden, S.L., & Kautto, J.G. (1987). *The evaluation and treatment of marital conflict: A four stage approach*. New York: Basic.

Guzman, M. (2022a). *I never thought of it that way: How to have furiously curious conversations in dangerously divided times*. Dallas, TX: Ben Bella Books, Inc.

Guzman, M. (2022b, April). *An interview and book presentation with Monica Guzman*. Sponsored by the Family Area Network, Winnetka, IL.

Haley, J. (1985a). *Conversations with Milton H. Erickson, MD, Volume II: Changing couples*. Williston, VT: Crown House Classics.

Haley, J. (1985b). *Conversations with Milton H. Erickson, MD, Volume III: Changing children and families*. Williston, VT: Crown House Classics.

Haley, J. & Madanes, C. (1986, November). *Four-day live supervision training in strategic family therapy with Jay Haley and Chloe Madanes*. Gestalt Integrated Family Institute, Chicago, IL.

Halifax, J. (2018). *Standing at the edge: Finding freedom where fear and courage meet*. New York: Flatiron.

Hancock, H. & Dickey, L. (2014). *Possibilities*. New York: Viking.

Haneke, M. (2005). *Caché*. [Film]. Canal +.

Hanh, T.N. (2019). *How to see*. Berkeley, CA: Parallax.

Hanh, T.N. (2011, Fall). After the honeymoon. *Buddhadharma: The Practitioner's Quarterly*, 26–33.

Hanh, T.N. (2001). *Anger: Wisdom for cooling the flames*. New York: Riverhead.

Hanh, T.N. (1998). *The heart of Buddha's teaching: Transforming suffering into peace, joy, and liberation*. New York: Broadway.

Hanh, T.N. (1991). *Peace is every step: The path of mindfulness in everyday life*. New York: Bantam.

Hannah, S.T., Sweeney, P.J., & Lester, P.B. (2010). The courageous mind-set: A dynamic personality system approach to courage. In C.L.S. Pury & S.J. Lopez (Eds.), *The psychology of courage: Modern research on an ancient virtue* (pp. 125–149). Washington, DC: American Psychological Association.

Hansen, B.P., Lambert, M.J., & Vlass, E.N. (2015). Sudden gains and sudden losses in the clients of a "super-shrink": 10 case studies. *Journal of Pragmatic Case Studies in Psychotherapy, 11*, 154–201.

Hanson, R. (2013). *Hardwiring happiness: The new brain science of commitment, calm, and confidence.* New York: Harmony.

Hanson, R. & Mendius, R. (2009). *Buddha's brain: The practical neuroscience of happiness.* Oakland, CA: New Harbinger.

Hardy, K.V. (2019). Toward a psychology of the oppressed: Understanding the invisible wounds of trauma. In M. McGoldrick & K.V. Hardy (Eds.), *Re-visioning family therapy: Addressing diversity in clinical practice,* 3rd Ed., (pp.133–151). New York: Guilford.

Hardy, K.V. & Laszloffy, T.A. (2005). *Teens who hurt: Clinical interventions to break the cycle of adolescent violence.* New York: Guilford.

Havens, R.A. (1996). *The wisdom of Milton H. Erickson: The complete volume.* Williston, VT: Crown House.

Hayes, J.A. & Vinca, M. (2017). Therapist presence, absence, and extraordinary presence. In L.G. Castonguay & C.E. Hill (Eds.), *How and why are some therapists better than others? Understanding therapist effects* (pp. 85–99). Washington, DC: American Psychological Association.

Heinlein, R.A. (2018). *Stranger in a strange land.* New York: ACE.

Henggeler, S.W. & Sheidow, A.J. (2011). Empirically supported family-based treatments for conduct disorder and delinquency in adolescents. *Journal of Marital and Family Therapy, 38* (1), 30–58.

Herzig, M. & Chasin, L. (2006). *Fostering dialogue across divides: A nuts and bolts guide from Essential Partners.* Cambridge, MA: Essential Partners.

Hibbert, C. (1999). *The house of Medici: Its rise and fall.* New York: William Morrow.

Hoffman, L. (1988). A constructivist position for family therapy. *Irish Journal of Psychology, 9,* 110–129.

Horvath, A.O., Del Re, A.C., Fluckiger, C., & Symonds, D. (2011). Alliance in individual psychotherapy. *Psychotherapy, 48,* 9–16.

Ibsen, H. (1992). *A doll's house.* New York: Dover.

Imber-Black, E. (1988). *Families and larger systems: A family therapist's guide through the labyrinth.* New York: Guilford.

Imber-Black, E. (1986). The systemic consultant and human-service provider systems. In L.C. Wynne, S.H. McDaniel, & T.T. Weber (Eds.), *Systems consultation: A new perspective for family therapy* (pp. 357–375). New York: Guilford.

Isaacson, W. (2003). *Benjamin Franklin: An American life.* New York: Simon & Schuster.

Itzchakov, G., DeMarree, K.G., Kluger, A.N., & Turjeman-Levi, Y. (2018). The listener sets the tone: High-quality listening increases attitude clarity and behavior-intention consequences. *Personality and Social Psychology Bulletin, 44*(5), 762–778.

Jackson, M. & Shorter, W. (2023, May). Wayne Shorter: A final interview. *Downbeat Magazine, 90* (5), 22–30.

Jennings, L., d'Rozario, V., Goh, M., Soveriegn, A., Brogger, M., & Skovholt, T.M. (2008). Psychotherapy expertise: A qualitative investigation. *Psychotherapy Research, 18* (5), 508–522.

Jennings, L. & Skovholt, T.M. (1999). The cognitive, emotional, and relational characteristics of master therapists. *Journal of Counseling Psychology, 46* (1), 3–11.

Jones, S.D. When I breathe in peace. [CD].

Kahneman, D. (2011). *Thinking, fast and slow.* New York: Farrar, Straus, and Giroux.

Kahneman, D., Lovallo, D., & Sibony, O. (2015, Winter). Before you make that big decision. In *Leadership: The art of decision-making. Harvard Business Review Onpoint,* 31–41.

Kahneman, D., Sibony, O., & Sunstein, C.R. (2021). *Noise: A flaw in human judgment*. New York: Little, Brown Spark.

Kanter, R.M. (2023, Spring). Zoom in, zoom out. *Harvard Business Review*, Special Issue: How to think more strategically, 29–35.

Kantor, D. & Lehr, W. (1975). *Inside the family*. San Francisco, CA: Jossey-Bass.

Keats, J. (2001). *Complete poems and selected letters*. New York: The Modern Library.

Kegan, R. & Lahey, L.L. (2001). *How the way we talk can change the way we work: Seven languages for transformation*. San Francisco, CA: Jossey-Bass.

Keith, D.V. (2015). *Continuing the experiential approach of Carl Whitaker: Process, practice, and magic*. Phoenix, AZ: Zeig, Tucker, & Theisen.

Keith, D.V., Connell, G.M., & Connell, L.C. (2001). *Defiance in the family: Finding hope in therapy*. Philadelphia, PA: Taylor & Francis.

Kelley, R.D.G. (2009). *Thelonious Monk: The life and times of an American original*. New York: Free Press.

Keltner, D. (2023). *Awe: The new science of everyday wonder and how it can transform your life*. New York: Penguin.

Kendall, P.C. (2011). *Child and adolescent therapy: Cognitive-behavioral procedures*, 4th ed. New York: Guilford.

Kim, Y., Nusbaum, H.C., & Yang, F. (2022). Going beyond ourselves: The role of transcendent experiences in wisdom. *Cognition and Emotion*, 1–19.

Klein, G. (2013). *Seeing what others don't: The remarkable ways we gain insights*. New York: Public Affairs.

Klein, G. (2002). *Intuition at work*. New York: Currency Doubleday.

Klein, G. (1998). *Sources of power: How people make decisions*. Cambridge, MA: MIT.

Knobloch-Fedders, L.M., Pinsof, W.M., & Mann, B.J. (2007). Therapeutic alliance and treatment progress in couple psychotherapy. *Journal of Marital and Family Therapy*, *33*, 245–257.

Knox, S., Butler, M.C., Kaiser, D.J., Knowlton, G., & Hill, C.E. (2017). Something to laugh about: Humor as a characteristic of effective therapists. In L.G. Castonguay & C.E. Hill (Eds.), *How and why are some therapists better than others? Understanding therapist effects* (pp. 285–307). Washington, DC: American Psychological Association.

Kort, J. (2008). *Gay affirmative therapy for the straight clinician: An essential guide*. New York: Norton.

Kulhan, B. & Crisafulli, C. (2017). *Getting to "yes and": The art of business improv*. Stanford, CA: Stanford University.

Kunzmann, U. & Gluck, J. (2019). Wisdom and emotion. In R.J. Sternberg & J. Gluck (Eds.), *The Cambridge handbook of wisdom* (pp. 575–601). Cambridge, UK: Cambridge University Press.

Kurosawa, A. (1950). *Rashomon*. [Film]. Criterion.

Labalme, V. (2021). *Risk forward: Embrace the unknown and unlock your hidden genius*. Carlsbad, CA: Hay House.

Lambert, M.J. (2010). *Prevention of treatment failure: The use of measuring, monitoring, and feedback in clinical practice*. Washington, DC: American Psychological Association.

Lax, W. (1995). Offering reflections: Some theoretical and practical considerations. In S. Friedman (Ed.), *The reflecting team in action: Collaborative practice in family therapy* (pp. 145–167). New York: Guilford.

Lebow, J. (2004). Separation and divorce issues in couple therapy. In A.S. Gurman (Ed.), *Clinical handbook of couple therapy*, (pp. 459–477). New York: Guilford.

Led Zeppelin (2014). *Led Zeppelin II, Remastered*. [CD]. Atlantic Catalog Group, BOOIXHBQUK.

Lester, P.B., Vogelgesang, G.R., Hannah, S.T., & Kimmey, Jr., T. (2010). Developing courage in followers: Theoretical and applied perspectives. In C.L.S. Pury & S.J. Lopez (Eds.), *The psychology of courage: modern research on ancient wisdom* (pp. 187–209). Washington, DC: American Psychological Association.

Levitt, H.M. & Grabowski, L.M. (2019). Professional wisdom: Functions and processes of psychotherapeutic and judicial wisdom. In R.J. Sternberg & J. Gluck (Eds.), *The Cambridge handbook of wisdom* (pp. 676–698). Cambridge, UK: Cambridge University Press.

Levitt, H.M. & Piazza-Bonin, E. (2016). Wisdom and psychotherapy: Studying expert therapists' clinical wisdom to explicate common processes. *Psychotherapy Research, 26* (1), 31–47.

Levitt, H.M. & Williams, D.C. (2010). Facilitating client change: Principles based upon the experience of eminent psychotherapists. *Psychotherapy Research, 20*, 337–352.

Levy, A. (2022). *Saxophone colossus: The life and music of Sonny Rollins*. New York: Hachette.

Levy, S.A. (2023, March). *Engaging the family in suicide care: An attachment-based family therapy approach*. Webinar presented at the Second Annual Suicide Safer Care in Clinical Practice Conference, New York, IL.

Linehan, M.M. (1993). *Cognitive-behavioral treatment in borderline personality disorder*. New York: Guilford.

Lipchik, E. (2002). *Beyond technique in solution-focused therapy*. New York: Guilford.

Losey, J. (1973). *A doll's house*. [Film]. British Lion.

Lum, W. (2002, March). The use of self of the therapist. *Contemporary Family Therapy, 24*(1), 181–197.

Maeschalck, C.L. & Barfnecht, L.R. (2017). Using client feedback to inform treatment. In D.S. Prescott, C.L. Maeschalck, & S.D. Miller (Eds.). *Feedback-informed treatment in clinical practice: Reaching for excellence* (pp. 53–79). Washington, DC: American Psychological Association.

Maisel, R., Epston, D., & Borden, A. (2004). *Biting the hand that starves you: Inspiring resistance to anorexia/bulimia*. New York: Norton.

Marinoff, L. (2003). *The big questions: Therapy for the sane or how philosophy can change your life*. London, UK: Bloomsbury.

Marlatt, G.A., Bowen, S., Chawla, N., & Witkiewitz, K. (2008). Mindfulness-based relapse prevention for substance abusers: Therapist training and therapeutic relationships. In S.F. Hick & T. Bien (Eds.), *Mindfulness and the therapeutic relationship* (pp. 107–122). New York: Guilford.

Martin, R. (2007). *The opposable mind: How successful leaders win through integrative thinking*. Boston, MA: Harvard Business School.

Mauboussin, M.J. (2009). *Think twice: Harnessing the power of counter-intuition*. Boston, MA: Harvard Business.

McGoldrick, M. & Gerson, R. (1986). *Genograms in family assessment*. New York: Norton.

McGoldrick, M., Giordano, J., & Garcia-Preto, N. (Eds.). (2005a). Overview: Ethnicity and family therapy. In M. McGoldrick, J. Giordano, & N. Garcia-Preto (Eds.), *Ethnicity and family therapy*, 3rd edition (pp. 1–40). New York: Guilford.

McGoldrick, M., Giordano, J., & Garcia-Preto, N. (Eds.). (2005b). *Ethnicity in family therapy, 3rd Ed.* New York: Guilford.

McGoldrick, M. & Hardy, K.V. (Eds.). (2019). *Re-visioning family therapy: Addressing diversity in clinical practice*, 3rd edition New York: Guilford.

McKeel, J. (2012). What works in solution-focused brief therapy: A review of change process research. In C. Franklin, T.S. Trepper, W.J. Gingerich, & E.E. McCollum (Eds.), *Solution-focused brief therapy: A handbook of evidence-based practice* (pp. 130–144). New York: Oxford University.

McLeod, J. (1997). *Narrative and psychotherapy.* London, UK: Sage.

Miller, G. (1997). *Becoming miracle workers: Language and meaning in brief therapy.* New York: Aldine De Gruyter.

Miller, S.D., Mee-Lee, D., Plum, W., & Hubble, M.A. (2005). Making treatment count: Client-directed, outcome-informed clinical work with problem drinkers. In J.L. Lebow (Ed.), *Handbook of clinical family therapy* (pp.281–309). Hoboken, NJ: Wiley.

Miller, A.L., Rathus, J.H., & Linehan, M.M. (2007). *Dialectical behavior therapy with suicidal adolescents.* New York: Guilford.

Minuchin, P., Colapinto, J., & Minuchin, S. (1998). *Working with families of the poor.* New York: Guilford.

Minuchin, S. (1986, September). *Four-day live supervision training in structural family therapy.* Gestalt Integrated Family Institute, Chicago, IL.

Minuchin, S. (1974). *Families and family therapy.* Cambridge, MA: Harvard University.

Minuchin, S. & Fishman, H.C. (1981). *Family therapy techniques.* Cambridge, MA: Harvard University.

Minuchin, S., Montalvo, B., Guerney, B.G., Rosman, B.L., & Schumer, F. (1967). *Families of the slums: An exploration of their structure and treatment.* New York: Basic.

Minuchin, S., Reiter, M.D., & Borda, C. (2021). *The craft of family therapy: Challenging certainties*, 2nd ed. New York: Routledge.

Minuchin, S., Rosman, B.L., & Baker, L. (1978). *Psychosomatic families: Anorexia nervosa in Context.* Cambridge, MA: Harvard University.

Moffit, P. (2012). *Emotional chaos to clarity: Move from the chaos of the reactive mind to the clarity of the responsive mind.* New York: Plume.

Montgomery, A., Barber, C., & McKee, P. (2002). A phenomenological study of wisdom later in life. *International Journal of Aging and Human Development, 54* (2), 139–157.

Mudd, P. (2015). *The head game: High-efficiency analytic decision-making and the art of solving complex problems quickly.* New York: Liveright.

Muñiz de la Pena, C., Friedlander, M.L., Escudero, V., & Heatherington, L. (2012). How do therapists ally with adolescents in family therapy? An examination of relational communication in early sessions. *Journal of Counseling Psychology, 59* (3), 339–351.

Muran, J.C. & Eubanks, C.F. (2020). *Therapist performance under pressure: Negotiating emotion, difference, and rupture.* Washington, DC: American Psychological Association.

Muran, J.C., Eubanks, C.F., & Samstag, L.W. (2023). Rupture in a wicked and wonderful world. In C.F. Eubanks, L.W. Samstag, & J.C. Muran (Eds.), *Rupture and repair in psychotherapy: A critical process for change*, (pp. 3–21). Washington, DC: American Psychological Association.

Murphy-Paul, A. (2021). *The extended mind: The power of thinking outside the brain.* Boston, MA: Houghton Mifflin.

Napier, A.Y. & Whitaker, C.A. (1978). *The family crucible: The intense experience of family therapy*. New York: HarperCollins.

Nealy, E.C. (2019). Working with LGBTQ families. In M. McGoldrick & K.V. Hardy (Eds.), *Re-visioning family therapy: Addressing diversity in clinical practice* (pp. 363–388). New York: Guilford.

Neff, K. (2015). *Self-compassion: The proven power of being kind to yourself*. New York: William Morrow.

Neret, G. (2022). *Dali: The paintings*. Bonn, Germany: Taschen.

Neruda, P. (2001). *The book of questions*. Port Townsend, WA: Copper Canyon.

Niebauer, C. (2019). *No self no problem: How neuropsychology is catching up to Buddhism*. San Antonio, TX: Hierophant Publishing.

Nisbett, R.E. (2015). *Mindware: Tools for smart thinking*. New York: Farrar, Straus, & Giroux.

Nisker, W. (1990). *Crazy wisdom: A provocative romp through the philosophies of east and west*. Berkeley, CA: Ten Speed.

Nissen-Lie, H.A., Monsen, J.T., Ulleberg, P., & Ronnestad, M.H. (2013). Psychotherapists self-reports of their interpersonal functioning and difficulties in practice as predictors of patient outcome. *Psychotherapy Research, 23*, 86–104.

Norcross, J.C., Krebs, P.M., & Prochaska, J.O. (2011). Stages of change. In J.C. Norcross (Eds.), *Psychotherapy relationships that work: Evidence-based responsiveness, 2nd Ed* (pp. 279–301). New York: Oxford University.

Norcross, J.C. & Lambert, M.J. (2013). Compendium of evidence-based relationships. *Psychotherapy In Australia, 19* (3), 34–37.

Norcross, J.C. & Lambert, M.J. (2011). Evidence-based relationships. In J.C. Norcross (Ed.), *Psychotherapy relationships that work: Evidence-based responsiveness, 2nd Ed* (pp. 3–25). New York: Oxford University.

Nylund, D. & Corsiglia, V. (1994). Becoming solution-focused forced in brief therapy: Remembering something important we already know. *Journal of Systemic Therapies, 13*, 5–13.

Oettingen, G. (2014). *Rethinking positive thinking: Inside the new science of motivation*. New York: Current.

O'Farrell, T.J. & Fals-Stewart, W. (2006). *Behavioral couples therapy for alcoholism and drug abuse*. New York: Guilford.

O'Hanlon, W.H. (1987). *Taproots: Underlying principles of Milton H. Erickson's therapy and hypnosis*. New York: Norton.

O'Hanlon, W.H. & Hexum, A.L. (1990). *An uncommon casebook: The complete clinical work of Milton H. Erickson*. New York: Norton.

O'Hanlon, W.H. & Weiner-Davis, M. (1989). *In search of solutions: A new direction in psychotherapy*. New York: Norton.

Orwell, G. (1961). *1984*. New York: Signet Classic.

Osgarby, S.M. & Halford, W.K. (2013, December). Couple relationship distress and observed expression of intimacy during reminiscence about positive relationship events. *Behavior Therapy, 44* (4), 686–700.

Ott, T.E. & Eisenhardt, K.M. (2020). Decision-weaving: Forming novel, complex strategy in entrepreneurial settings. *Strategic Management Journal, 41* (12), 2275–2314.

Owen, J., Duncan, B., Anker, M., & Sparks, J. (2012). Initial relationship goal and couple therapy outcomes at post and six-month. *Journal of Family Psychology, 26* (2), 179–186.

Owen, J., Duncan, B., Reese, R.J., Anker, M., & Sparks, J. (2014). Accounting for therapist variability in couple therapy outcomes: What really matters? *Journal of Sex and Marital Therapy, 40* (6), 488–502.

Palazzoli, M.S., Boscolo, L., Cecchin, G., & Prata, G. (1980). The problem with the referring person. *Journal of Marital and Family Therapy, 6* (1), 3–9.

Palazzoli, M.S., Cecchin, G., Prata, G., & Boscolo, L. (1978). *Paradox and counter-paradox: A new model in the therapy of the family in schizophrenic transaction.* New York: Jason Aronson.

Papp, P. (2000a). New directions for therapists. In P. Papp (Ed.), *Couples on the fault line: New directions for therapists,* (pp. 1–29). New York: Guilford.

Papp, P. (2000b). Gender differences in depression: His or her depression. In P. Papp (Ed.)., *Couples on the fault line: New directions for therapists* (pp. 130–152). New York: Guilford.

Papp, P. (1983). *The process of change.* New York: Guilford.

Parker, C. (2006). *Charlie Parker: Complete Jazz at Massey Hall.* [CD]. The Jazz Factory, 22856.

Pereira, J.A. & Barkham, M. (2015). An exceptional, efficient, and resilient therapist: A case study in practice-based evidence. *Journal of Pragmatic Case Studies in Psychotherapy, 11,* 216–223.

Pittampalli, A. (2016). *Persuadable: How great leaders change their minds to change the world.* New York: Harper Business.

Planas, C.R. (2001). *Picasso's las meninas.* Barcelona, Spain: Editorial Meteora.

Pollak, S.M., Pedulla, T., & Siegel, R.D. (Eds.). (2014). *Sitting together: Essential skills for mindfulness- based psychotherapy.* New York: Guilford.

Popper, K.A. (1965). *Conjectures and refutations: The growth of scientific method.* New York: Harper & Row.

Post, S. & Niemark, J. (2007). *Why good things happen to good people: The exciting new research that proves the link between doing good and living a longer, healthier, and happier life.* New York: Broadway.

Prochaska, J.O., Norcross, J.C., & DiClemente, C.C. (1994). *Changing for good: A revolutionary six-stage program for overcoming bad habits and moving your life positively forward.* New York: William Morrow.

Prochaska, J.O. & Prochaska, J.M. (2016). *Changing to thrive: Using the stages of change to overcome the top threats to your health and happiness.* Center City, MN: Hazelden.

Puett, M. & Gross-Loh, C. (2016). *The path: A new way to think about everything.* New York: Simon & Schuster.

Pury, C.L.S., Lopez, S.J., & Key-Roberts, M. (2010). The future of courage research. In C.L.S. Pury & S.J. Lopez (Eds.), *The psychology of courage: Modern research on ancient virtue* (pp. 229–237). Washington, DC: American Psychological Association.

Pury, C.L.S. & Starkey, C.B. (2010). Is courage an accolade or a process? A fundamental question for courage research. In C.L.S. Pury & S.J. Lopez (Eds.), *The psychology of courage: Modern research on an ancient virtue* (pp. 67–89). Washington, DC: American Psychological Association.

Rabu, M. & McLeod, J. (2018). Wisdom in professional knowledge: Why it can be valuable to listen to the voices of senior psychotherapists. *Psychotherapy Research, 28* (5), 776–792.

Rathus, J.H. & Miller, A.L. (2015). *DBT skills manual for adolescents.* New York: Guilford.

Rennie, D.L. (1994). Storytelling in psychotherapy: The client's subjective experience. *Psychotherapy: Theory, Research, & Practice, 31* (2), 234–243.

Rennie, D.L. (1992). Qualitative analysis of the client's experience of psychotherapy: The unfolding of reflexivity. In S.G. Toukamanian & D.L. Rennie (Eds.), *Psychotherapy process research: Paradigmatic and narrative approaches* (pp. 211–233). London, UK: Sage.

Richtel, M. (2022). *Inspired: A journey through art, science, and the soul.* Boston, MA: Mariner.

Rinpoche, L.Z. (1993). *Transforming problems into happiness.* Boston, MA: Wisdom.

Rittel, H.W. & Webber, M.M. (1973). Dilemmas in a general theory of planning. *Policy Sciences, 4* (2), 155–169.

Robbins, M.S., Turner, C.W., Dakof, G.A. & Alexander, J.F. (2006). Adolescent and parent therapeutic alliances as predictors of dropout in multidimensional family therapy. *Journal of Family Psychology, 20*, 108–116.

Roberto, L.G. (1991). Symbolic-interactional family therapy. In A.S. Gurman & D.R. Kniskern (Eds.), *Handbook of family therapy, Vol. II* (pp. 444–479). New York: Brunner/Mazel.

Roffman, A.E. (2014). Rigor, imagination, humility, and love: Systemic wisdom in psychotherapy practice. *Journal of Systemic Therapies, 33* (2), 1–15.

Rogers, S. & Ogas, O. (2022). *This is what it sounds like: What the music you love says about you.* New York: Norton.

Rolling, J.K. (2000). *Harry Potter and the goblet of fire.* New York: Scholastic.

Sander, L.W. (2002). Thinking differently principles in process in living systems and the specificity of being known. *Psychoanalytic Dialogues, 12* (1), 11–42.

Satir, V. (2013). The therapist story. In M. Baldwin (Ed.)., *The use of self in therapy, 3rd ed,* (pp. 19–28). New York: Routledge.

Satir, V. (1988). *The new peoplemaking.* Mountain View, CA: Science and Behavior Books.

Satir, V. (1983). *Conjoint family therapy*, 3rd ed. Mountain View, CA: Science and behavior Books.

Satir, V. (1972). *Peoplemaking.* Palo Alto, CA: Science and Behavior Books.

Satir, V. (1967). *Conjoint family therapy: A guide to theory and technique.* Palo Alto, CA: Science and Behavior Books.

Satir, V. & Baldwin, M. (1984). *Satir step by step: A guide to creating change in families.* Mountain View: Science and Behavior Books.

Satir, V., Banmen, J., Gerber, J., & Gomori, M. (2006). *The Satir model: Family therapy and beyond.* Mountain View, CA: Science and Behavior Books.

Schon, D.A. (1983). *The reflective practitioner: How professionals think in action.* New York: Basic.

Schucklard, E., Miller, S.D., & Hubble, M.A. (2017). Feedback-informed treatment: Historical and empirical foundations. In D. S. Prescoitt, C.L., Maeschalck, S.D. Miller (Eds.), *Feedback-informed treatment in clinical practice: Reaching for excellence,* (pp. 13–37). Washington, DC: American Psychological Association.

Schwartz, J.M. & Gladding, R. (2011). *You are not your brain: The 4-step solution for changing bad habits, ending unhealthy thinking, and taking control of your life.* New York: Avery.

Segal, L. (1991). Brief therapy: The MRI approach. In A.S. Gurman & D.R. Kniskern (Eds.), *Handbook of family therapy: Volume II,* (pp. 171–200). New York: Brunner/Mazel.

Selekman, M.D. (2023). Breaking free from a gang lifestyle: The use of a solution-determined collaborative team to help transform a challenging and complex adolescent case situation. *Journal of Clinical Psychology: Case Reports, 79* (6), 1537–1550.

Selekman, M.D. (2021, March). COVID–19 as a transformative opportunity for families and therapists: Harnessing the possibilities that constraints offer us. *Australian & New Zealand Journal of Family Therapy, 42* (1), 70–84.

Selekman, M.D. (2018, Winter). Question-storming: Co-Creating compelling future realities with couples and families. *Psychotherapy Section Review, 62,* 7–16.

Selekman, M.D. (2017). *Working with high-risk adolescents: A collaborative strengths-based approach.* New York: Guilford.

Selekman, M.D. (2010). *Collaborative brief therapy with children.* New York: Guilford.

Selekman, M.D. (2009). *The adolescent and young adult self-harming treatment manual: A collaborative strengths-based brief therapy approach.* New York: Norton.

Selekman, M.D. (2006). *Working with self-harming adolescents: A collaborative strengths-based therapy approach.* New York: Norton.

Selekman, M.D. (2005). *Pathways to change: Brief therapy with difficult adolescents, 2nd Ed.* New York: Guilford.

Selekman, M.D. (1996). Turning out the light on a seasonal affective disorder. *Journal of Systemic Therapies, 15* (3), 40–52.

Selekman, M.D. (1995). Rap music with wisdom: Peer reflecting teams. In S. Friedman (Ed.), *The reflecting team in action: Collaborative practice in family therapy* (pp. 205–223). New York: Guilford.

Selekman, M.D. (1991). "With a little help from my friends": The use of peers in the family therapy of adolescent substance abusers. *Family Dynamics of Addiction Quarterly,* 1 (*1*), 69–77.

Selekman, M.D. & Beyebach, M. (2013). *Changing self-destructive habits: Pathways to solutions with couples and families.* New York: Routledge.

Seneca, L.A. (2007). *Dialogues and essays.* Oxford, UK: Oxford University Press.

Sheinberg, M. (1985). The debate: A strategic technique. *Family Process,* 24 (2), 259–271.

Shetty, J. (2020). *Think like a monk: Train your mind for peace and purpose every day.* New York: Simon & Schuster.

Short, D. (2020). *From William James to Milton Erickson: The care of human consciousness.* Bloomington, IN: Archway.

Small, A. & Schmutte, K. (2022). *Navigating ambiguity: Creating opportunity in a world of unknowns.* New York: Ten Speed Press.

Smith, J.E. & Meyers, R.J. (2023). *The CRAFT treatment manual for substance abuse problems: Working With family members.* New York: Guilford.

Soll, J.B., Milkman, K.L., & Payne, J.W. (2015, Winter). Outsmart your own biases. In *Leadership: The art of decision-making. Harvard Business Review OnPoint,* 2–48.

Sparks, J.A. & Duncan, B.L. (2010). Common factors in couple and family therapy: Must all have prizes? In B.L. Duncan, S.D. Miller, B.E. Wampold, & M.A. Hubble (Eds.)., *The heart and soul of change: Delivering what works in therapy,* 2nd ed. (pp. 357–393). Washington, DC: American Psychological Association.

Spetzler, C., Winter, H., & Meyer, J. (2016). *Decision quality: Value creation from better business decisions.* Hoboken, NJ: Wiley.

Sprenkle, D.H., Davis, S.D., & Lebow, J. L. (2009). *Common factors in couple and family therapy: The overlooked foundation of effective practice.* New York: Guilford.

Stanton, M.D. & Todd, T.C. (1982). *The family therapy of drug abuse and addiction.* New York: Guilford.

Stearns, M. (2004). *Conscious courage: Turning everyday challenges into opportunities.* Seminole, FL: Enrichment.

Sternberg, R.J. (2019). Why people prefer wise guys to guys who are wise: An augmented balance theory of the production and reception of wisdom. In R.J. Sternberg & J. Gluck (Eds.), *The Cambridge handbook of wisdom* (pp. 162–181). Cambridge, UK: Cambridge University Press.

Stierlin, H., Rucker-Embden, I., Wetzel, N., & Wirsching, M. (1980). *The first interview with the family*. New York: Brunner/Mazel.

Stiles, W.B. & Horvath, A.O. (2017). Appropriate responsiveness as a contribution to therapist effects. In L.G. Castonguay & C.E. Hill (Eds.), *How and why some therapists are better than others? Understanding therapist effects* (pp. 71–84). Washington, DC: American Psychological Association.

Stinnett, N. & O'Donnell, M. (1996). *Good kids: How you and your kids can successfully navigate the teen years*. New York: Doubleday.

Stylistics (2013). *The very best of the Stylistics*. [CD]. Spectrum Audio UK, B00B1OWGXS.

Suddendorf, T. & Redshaw, J., & Bulley, A. (2023). *The invention of the tomorrow: A natural history of foresight*. New York: Basic.

Summers, R.F. & Barber, J.P. (2010). *Psychodynamic therapy: A guide to evidence-based practice*. New York: Guilford.

Swift, J.K. & Greenberg, R.P. (2015). *Premature termination in psychotherapy: Strategies for engaging clients and improving outcomes*. Washington, DC: American Psychological Association.

Symonds, B.D. & Horvath, A.O. (2004). Optimizing the alliance in couple therapy. *Family Process, 43*, 443–455.

Szapocznik, J. & Hervis, O.E. (2020). *Brief strategic family therapy*. Washington, DC: American Psychological Association.

Taffel, R. & Blau, M. (2001). *The second family: How adolescent power is challenging the American family*. New York: St. Martin's.

Taschen, B. (1994). *Dali*. Bonn, Germany: Taschen.

Tervalon, M. & Murray-Garcia, J. (1998). Cultural humility versus cultural competence: A critical distinction in defining physician training outcomes in multicultural education. *Journal of Health Care for the Poor and Underserved, 9* (2), 117–125.

Tetlock, P. & Gardner, D. (2015). *Super-forecasting: The art and science of prediction*. New York: Crown.

Thoreau, H.D. & Cramer, J.S. (2004). *Walden: A fully annotated edition*. New York: Harper Perennial.

Todd, T.C. & Selekman, M.D. (1991a). Beyond structural-strategic family therapy: Integrating brief systemic therapies. In T.C. Todd & M.D. Selekman (Eds.), *Family therapy approaches with adolescent substance abusers* (pp. 241–271). Needham Heights, MA: Allyn & Bacon.

Todd, T.C. & Selekman, M.D. (Eds.). (1991b). *Family therapy approaches with adolescent substance abusers*. Needham Heights, MA: Allyn & Bacon.

Tomm, K. (1988). Interventive interviewing: Part III. Intending to ask lineal, circular, strategic, and reflexive questions. *Family Process, 27*, 1–15.

Tomm, K. (1987). Interventive interviewing: Part II: Reflexive questioning as a means to enable Self-healing. *Family Process, 26* (1), 167–183.

Tomm, K. & White, M. (1987, October). Externalizing problems and internalizing directional choices. Workshop presented at the Annual American Association for Marriage and Family Therapy Conference, Chicago, IL.

Tremblay, N., Wright, J., Mamodhouseen, S., McDuff, P., & Sabourin, S. (2008). Refining therapeutic mandates in couple therapy outcome research: A feasibility study. *American Journal of Family Therapy, 36*, 137–148.

Tryon, G. S. & Winograd, G. (2011). Goal consensus and collaboration. In J.C. Norcross (Ed.), *Psychotherapy relationships that work: Evidence-based responsiveness*, 2nd ed. (pp. 153–168). New York: Oxford University.

Turkle, S. (2011). *Alone together: Why we expect more from technology and less from each other.* New York: Basic.

Tzu, C. & Watson, B. (1968). *The complete works of Chuang Tzu.* New York: Columbia University.

Von Foerster, H. (1981). *Observing systems.* Cambridge, MA: Intersystems.

Vonnegut, K. (1973). *Slaughter-house five.* New York: Dell.

Wampold, B.E. (2010). The research evidence for common factors model: A historically situated perspective. In B.L. Duncan, S.D. Miller, B.E. Wampold, & M.A. Hubble (Eds.), *The heart and soul of change: Delivering what works in therapy*, 2nd Ed, (pp. 49–83). Washington, DC: American Psychological Association.

Wampold, B.E., Baldwin, S.A., Holtforth, M.G., & Imel, Z.E. (2017). What characterizes effective therapists? In L.G. Castonguay & C.E. Hill (Eds.), *How and why are some therapists are better than others? Understanding therapist effects* (pp. 37–53). Washington, DC: American Psychological Association.

Watzlawick, P., Weakland, J.H., & Fisch, R. (1974). *Change: Principles of problem formation and problem resolution.* New York: Norton.

Weiner-Davis, M. (1992). *Divorce-busting: A revolutionary and rapid program for staying together.* New York: Summit.

Weiner-Davis, M., de Shazer, S., & Gingerich, W.J. (1987). Building on pretreatment change to construct the therapeutic solution: An exploratory study. *Journal of Marital and Family Therapy, 13* (4), 359–363.

Wells, H.G. (2005). *The time-machine.* New York: Penguin Classics.

Westerhof, G.J., Bohlmeijer, E., & Webster, J.D. (2010). Reminiscence and mental health: A review of recent progress in theory, research, and interventions. *Ageing & Society, 30*, 697–721.

Weststrate, N.M. (2019). The mirror of wisdom: Self-reflection as a developmental precursor and core competency of wise people. In R.J. Sternberg & J. Gluck (Eds.), *The Cambridge handbook of wisdom* (pp. 500–519). Cambridge, UK: Cambridge University Press.

Whitaker, C.A. (1975). Psychotherapy of the absurd: With a special emphasis on the psychotherapy of aggression. *Family Process, 14* (1), 1–16.

Whitaker, C.A. & Keith, D.V. (1981a). Symbolic-experiential family therapy. In A.S. Gurman & D.P. Kniskern (Eds.), *Handbook of family therapy* (pp. 187–226). New York: Brunner/Mazel.

Whitaker, C.A. & Keith, D.V. (1981b, July). Play therapy: A paradigm for work with families. *Journal of Marital Therapy, 7* (3), 243–255.

Whitaker, C.A. & Malone, T.P. (1981). *The roots of psychotherapy.* New York: Brunner/Mazel.

Whitaker, C.A. & Napier, A.Y. (1978). *The family crucible.* New York: Harper & Row.

Whitaker, C.A. & Napier, A.Y. (1977). Process techniques of family therapy. *Interaction, 1* (1), 4–19.

Whitaker, C.A. & Ryan, M.O. (1989). *Midnight musings of a family therapist.* New York: Norton.

White, M. (2007). *Maps of narrative practice.* New York: Norton.

White, M. (1995). *Re-authoring lives: Interviews and essays.* Adelaide: Dulwich Centre.

White, M. (1988a, Summer). Externalizing the problem and the re-authoring of lives and relationships. *Dulwich Centre Newsletter, 5*–28.

White, M. (1988b). Two-day workshop in narrative therapy with Michael White. Gestalt Integrated Family Institute, Chicago, IL.

White, M. (1987). Anorexia nervosa: A cybernetic approach. In J.E. Harkaway (Ed.), *Eating-disorders* (pp. 117–131). Rockville, MD: Aspen.

White, M. (1986, Spring). The conjoint therapy of men who are violent and the women with whom they live. *Dulwich Centre Newsletter,* 101–105.

White, M. (1985). Fear busting and monster taming: An approach to the fears of young children. *Dulwich Review,* 107–113.

White, M. & Epston, D. (1990a). Consulting your consultants: The documentation of alternative knowledges. *Dulwich Centre Newsletter, 4,* 25–35.

White, M. & Epston, D. (1990b). *Narrative means to literary ends.* New York: Norton.

Whitfield, S. (1992). *Magritte.* London, UK: South Bank Centre.

Whitlock, J., Muehlenkamp, J., & Eckenrode, J. (2008). Variation in non-suicidal self-injury: Identification and features of latent classes in a college population of emerging adults. *Journal of Clinical Child and Adolescent Psychology, 37* (4), 725–735.

Wucker, M. (2021). *You are what you risk: The new art and science of navigating an uncertain world.* New York: Pegasus.

Zeavin, H. (2021). *The distance cure: A history of telehealth therapy.* Cambridge, MA: MIT Press.

Zeytinoglu, S. (2016). The POTT program: Step-by-step. In H.J. Aponte & K. Kissil (Eds.), *The person of the therapist training model: Mastering the use of self* (pp. 14–26). New York: Routledge.

Index

Mirroring the text, therapeutic strategies are written in *italics*. Locators in *italics* refer to figures.